Animal Abuse

Helping Animals and People

FSC
www.fsc.org
MIX
Paper from responsible sources
FSC® C013604

Think occasionally of the suffering of which you spare yourself the sight.

Albert Schweitzer

No act of kindness, no matter how small, is ever wasted.

Aesop

Animal Abuse

Helping Animals and People

Catherine Tiplady

Centre for Animal Welfare and Ethics
University of Queensland
Australia

www.cabi.org

CABI is a trading name of CAB International

CABI
Nosworthy Way
Wallingford
Oxfordshire OX10 8DE
UK

Tel: +44 (0)1491 832111
Fax: +44 (0)1491 833508
E-mail: info@cabi.org
Website: www.cabi.org

CABI
38 Chauncey Street
Suite 1002
Boston, MA 02111
USA

Tel: +1 800 552 3083 (toll free)
Tel: +1 (0)617 395 4051
E-mail: cabi-nao@cabi.org

A catalogue record for this book is available from the British Library, London, UK.

Library of Congress Cataloging-in-Publication Data

Tiplady, Catherine.
Animal abuse: helping animals and people / by Catherine Tiplady.
p. ; cm.
Includes bibliographical references and index.
ISBN 978-1-84593-983-0 (alk. paper)
I. C.A.B. International. II. Title.
[DNLM: 1. Animal Welfare. 2. Animal Assisted Therapy. 3. Forensic Medicine--methods. 4. Veterinary Medicine--methods. HV 4708]
636.0832--dc23

2012042151

ISBN: 978 1 84593 983 0

Commissioning editor: Sarah Hulbert
Editorial assistant: Alexandra Lainsbury
Production editor: Tracy Head

Typeset by SPi, Pondicherry, India.
Printed and bound in the UK by CPI Group (UK) Ltd, Croydon, CR0 4YY.

Contents

Contributors

Mr Phil Arkow is coordinator of the National Link Coalition (http://www.nationallinkcoalition.org), Chair of the Latham Foundation's Animal Abuse and Family Violence Prevention Project and consultant to both the American Society for the Prevention of Cruelty to Animals and the Animals & Society Institute. Mr Arkow trains internationally on a variety of topics for veterinarians, animal shelters, child protection agencies, domestic violence programmes, adult protective services, judges and law enforcement and has authored numerous articles, chapters and reference books. E-mail: arkowpets@snip.net

Dr David Bailey is a veterinarian and a qualified forensics scientist. He runs a private company offering research and consultancy advice services to industry, academia, government, legal, veterinary and training organizations. Website: www.forensicvet.com

Moo Baulch runs the Lesbian, Gay, Bisexual, Transgender and Intersex Domestic and Family Violence Project as part of the work of ACON's Anti-Violence Project (formerly the AIDS Council of New South Wales, Australia). She is a member of the NSW LGBTIQ Domestic and Family Violence Interagency and helped coordinate the first Australian conference on LGBTIQ domestic and family violence in late 2011. The Interagency is responsible for Another Closet, a world first online and hardcopy resource designed specifically for LGBTIQ people affected by violence in intimate partnerships and their families and to assist domestic and family violence service providers to support people of diverse sex, sexuality and gender. She loves her job! Websites: www.anothercloset.com.au; www.acon.org.au. E-mail: mbaulch@acon.org.au

Michael Byrne QC, Barrister-at-Law, Queensland Bar was first called to the Bar in 1977 and took silk in 1993. Michael specializes in criminal law and has appeared in a number of the seminal High Court cases emanating from Queensland, Australia. He was, formerly, an Acting Judge of the District Court and the Queensland Deputy Director of Public Prosecutions. He presently has chambers in Brisbane. Michael was the Vice President of the Queensland Bar Association for the years of 2008 and 2009. E-mail: byrneqc@qldbar.asn.au

Dr David Chamberlain BVetMed, GPCert(FelP), MRCVS qualified from the Royal Veterinary College in 1987 and worked in mixed practice for 22 years. He invented the world's first microchip cat flap and worked as a consultant to a global pet accessory manufacturer. Currently he is the State's Veterinary Officer for the Island of Guernsey, where he is responsible for animal health and welfare, public health with regard to the slaughterhouse and zoonotic disease, and the artificial insemination centre.

Dr Cam Day BVSc, BSc, MACVS (Animal Behaviour) is a veterinarian, media presenter and full-time veterinary behaviour consultant (www.pethealth.com.au). Cam is committed to animal welfare and he is the inaugural and current Chair of the Queensland State Government Animal Welfare Advisory Committee, a role he has maintained since 2004. He is also an Adjunct Associate Professor (animal behaviour) with the University of Queensland Veterinary School. Cam has previously worked for the RSPCA in the positions of Animal Welfare Policy Officer, Operations Manager and Community Liaison Manager.

Cassandra Day is an animal therapy trainer who works alongside Cam Day and uses positive reinforcement-based training with gentle, reward-based techniques. Cassandra regularly works to rehabilitate animals from abusive and neglectful pasts.

Dr Stephen J. Drew BVM&S, MRCVS graduated from the Royal (Dick) School of Veterinary Studies, Edinburgh in 1999 obtaining the degree of Bachelor of Veterinary Medicine and Surgery with Credit, as well as the Norman Dobson Memorial Prize in Veterinary Pathology and the Highland and Agricultural Society of Scotland Medal in Large Animal Surgery. Working in clinical veterinary practice ever since, except for a period as a Defra Veterinary Inspector during the 2001 Foot and Mouth Disease outbreak, Stephen currently works as a companion animal veterinary practitioner in the East Neuk of Fife, Scotland. He is nearing completion of the European School of Veterinary Postgraduate Studies General Practitioner Certificate in Forensics and Law and is also studying for the Royal College of Veterinarians Certificate in Advanced Veterinary Practice.

Jenny Edwards works as a Special Animal Crimes Investigator and has been instrumental in the arrest and conviction of animal sex offenders in Washington, Tennessee, Ohio and Florida, USA. She is a certified Private Investigator and has taught Law Enforcement officers as well as Animal Control Officers all over the USA. Jenny is a contributor to the University of Missouri Law Enforcement Training Institute, National Animal Cruelty Investigator Schools, and has authored multiple print and online publications. In 2006 Jenny worked on and appeared in the documentary film *Zoo*. Jenny may be reached at jenny.edwards@ChandlerEdwards.org. Currently, Jenny works in the Pacific Northwest region of the USA.

Tracy-Lynne Geysen, Partner – Couper Geysen – Family and Animal Law (www.coupergeysen.com.au), is a lawyer who practises both family law and animal law – her firm is the first law firm practising in this area in Australia. Tracy-Lynne is one of the founding members of BLEATS (Brisbane Lawyers Educating and Advocating for Tougher Sentences; www.bleats.com.au), a group set up in 2007 and currently consisting of some 300 lawyers, including six Senior Counsel and three Queens Counsel, and about 150 support staff, including psychiatrists and a psychologist, prosecuting matters on a pro bono basis for the RSPCA. The group have saved the RSPCA more than approximately AU$1,900,000 in legal fees (their annual budget is AU$50,000). E-mail: tracy-lynne.geysen@coupergeysen.com.au

Zoe Hinds B Ed (Grad), B Comn, CertIV TAA is the Education Director at Animal Welfare League, Queensland, Australia. Website: awlqld.com.au. E-mail: education@awlqld.com.au

Dr Natasha Lee is a Veterinary Programmes Manager at the World Society for the Protection of Animals (www.wspa-international.org), in charge of the tertiary education programme in Asia. She can be reached at NatashaLee@wspa-asiapacific.org.

Jenna Ooi is a Domestic Violence Child Support Worker at the Macleod Accommodation Support Service, Inc., Queensland, Australia. E-mail: childsupport@macleod.org.au

Allie Phillips is an author, attorney and advocate for protecting vulnerable victims and promoting human–animal interactions. She is the founder of Sheltering Animals & Families Together (SAF-T)™ (http://www.animalsandfamilies.org). She is a former prosecuting attorney from Michigan (USA), who works for the National District Attorneys Association specializing in the linkage of animal abuse to violence against people. At NDAA, she launched the National Center for Prosecution of Animal Abuse where she is the Director, and is the Deputy Director of the National Center for Prosecution of Child Abuse. She was the Vice President of Public Policy and Vice President of Human-Animal Strategic Initiatives for the American Humane Association. She has been working with crime victims since 1993, training criminal justice professionals since 1997, and since 2000 has been helping abused and abandoned animals. Ms Phillips is licensed to practice law in Michigan and Maryland. She has conducted over 200 trainings nationally and has authored over 50 publications on these topics, including *Defending the Defenseless: A Guide to Protecting and Advocating for Pets* (2011) and *How Shelter Pets are Brokered for Experimentation: Understanding Pound Seizure* (2010). She is on the steering committee of the National Link Coalition, Vice President of No Paws Left Behind (an organization to help foreclosure animals), a council board member of the State Bar of Michigan's Animal Law Section, co-founder of Michiganders for Shelter Pets and Friends of Ingham County Animal Shelter, and volunteer with King Street Cats in Alexandria, Virginia. Allie is also a certified Usui Reiki Master-Teacher and Integrated Energy Therapy® Master-Instructor, who provides energy healing to abused, neglected and homeless shelter pets. To read more about Allie's work, please visit http://www.alliephillips.com and http://www.manifestedharmony.com.

Professor Clive Phillips MA, PhD, BSc (Hons) has approximately 30 years of experience researching the welfare of farm, companion and captive wild animals. Clive is the Foundation Chair of Animal Welfare at the University of Queensland's Centre for Animal Welfare and Ethics (www.uq.edu.au/vetschool/cawe).

Dr Howard Ralph BVSc (Hons1), MBBS (Hons), MVS (Wildlife Medicine), JCCA Accred. (Anaesth), Dip TESL, A/Dip Fine Arts, Cert Ed NSW is an experienced wildlife veterinarian, who works to rescue and rehabilitate waterbirds injured during the legal waterbird shooting season. Website: www.southerncrosswildlifecare.org.au

Dr Pippa Swan BVSc CertWEL MRCVS has worked as a small animal clinician for 16 years, acted for the RSPCA, and carried out inspection and management of standards for KFC, McDonald's and Assured Food Standards. She has also acted as an examiner in Welfare, Ethics and Law for the Royal College of Veterinarians. Currently, Pippa works in Northern Ireland.

Catherine Tiplady BVSc, BAppSci (Hons 1), is a veterinarian who has worked in both private clinical practice and shelter environments. Prior to graduation, Catherine had worked as animal attendant and veterinary nurse and she has also undertaken voluntary work in a range of settings – such as processing animal cruelty complaints at an RSPCA call centre, visiting schools to speak to children about animal welfare with the Australian Veterinary Association PetPEP programme, visiting an Australian Indigenous community to undertake dog desexing with the Animal Management in Rural and Remote Indigenous Communities group and providing veterinary care to animals in emergency evacuation centres after a natural disaster. Currently, Catherine is researching animal abuse and human interpersonal violence at the Centre for Animal Welfare and Ethics, University of Queensland.

Dr Deborah Walsh BSW, MSW, PhD, GCHEd, MAASW is a social work practitioner, trauma counsellor, lecturer and clinical supervisor in the area of domestic and family violence and is currently employed by the University of Queensland.

Preface and Acknowledgments

I have always been upset by animal cruelty and, although I knew it existed, I was unprepared for the cases of animal abuse (often linked with child abuse, elder abuse or domestic violence) that I encountered after graduating as a veterinarian. While most owners provide adequate care for their animals, being confronted with those who deliberately hurt, neglected and exploited animals affected me quite badly and I found emotional support hard to find. People I worked with had their own problems and others outside work weren't keen to hear upsetting stories about my day. When I volunteered to visit schools to talk about animal welfare I was shocked to hear children speak of abuse – one young boy proudly told me how he had assaulted his puppy, punching his fist into her mouth and pushing her off the trampoline. The cycle of violence was clearly evident when the teacher told me how the boy's mother had lost teeth from being punched in the mouth by her partner.

On my days off I volunteered in the RSPCA call centre and learned more about the extent of abuse and neglect occurring in our society every day. I wondered why animal abuse had been barely mentioned at university, let alone the connection to human interpersonal violence and how veterinarians could assist. The issue of mental health in veterinarians was similarly not given adequate attention despite vets being a high-risk group for suicide. After graduation, I worked in an animal welfare organization, which allowed owners options of paying off treatment, or rehoming unwanted animals at their shelter rather than euthanizing healthy, sociable animals. I thought this would place me in the best position to save lives and although I have certainly helped, it was heartbreaking to see animals that you knew or suspected had been abused. At no fault of their own, these cringing, fearful, poorly socialized animals clearly had less chance of successful rehoming unless lengthy and committed rehabilitation could be undertaken. During my time as a vet, I have seen horrific cases of animal abuse (such as a mutilated kitten, which was wrapped in a towel and dumped at the vet clinic with his legs cut off). Not surprisingly, I have also met extremely violent people. Sometimes, owners seemed totally callous or indifferent to animal suffering. One such owner had left her small terrier dog with a severe leg injury for weeks, resulting in the leg needing amputation. Extensive dental work (multiple tooth extractions) was needed as well as clipping of very matted hair. The owner was unwilling or unable to pay for any treatment so I suggested the dog be surrendered for treatment and rehoming, at no cost to the owner. The owner's response was merely to shrug and say scornfully 'Who'd want the dog anyway, it's just so ugly'. After reporting this owner to the RSPCA for neglect it was found that the dog's mother was living in a similar state of neglect in the same home. The owner was required to bring the mother dog in for treatment and the dog's offspring was treated and rehomed.

Euthanasia is one way in which animal victims of abuse can be helped, but many owners demand 'convenience euthanasia' of pets that are completely healthy, and this can be an added source of stress for veterinary and shelter staff.

One night, after an owner demanded a 'convenience' euthanasia of her beautiful, affectionate and heavily pregnant tabby cat (which I refused to do but another vet was pressured into doing), I felt totally despondent. It seemed being a vet was doing more harm than good and no matter what I did, the endless supply of unwanted animals, cases of neglect, hoarding, puppy farmers, disinterest and outright animal abuse continued. Animals are viewed by some people as disposable items – one man laughed when I outlined treatment options for his injured kitten with thoracic trauma, informing me 'It's not worth treating! I'll just get another one – kittens like that are a dime a dozen.' Looking back, I realize I had developed all the signs of compassion fatigue but couldn't recognize it as I didn't know what it was.

That's when I wished there was a book about working with animal abuse, if only to know that I wasn't alone in my emotional turmoil and disillusionment with being a veterinarian. Luckily, at this point I contacted CAB International commissioning editor Sarah Hulbert, who put my book idea forward to CAB International staff and persevered, alongside editorial assistant Alex Lainsbury and other staff until the book was completed. I am very grateful for their support and patience.

Many others have also assisted in this project, with much-needed advice, encouragement and information. These include Professor Frank Ascione, John and Margaret Cooper, Ian Robertson (vet and lawyer), Jan Allen, Julia Hardaker and Sophie Constable of AMRRIC (Animal Management in Rural and Remote Indigenous Communities), Sy Woon, Francesca Riccomini, Annabel Buchanan (chief inspector (prosecutions) for RSPCA Queensland) for advice on reporting cruelty cases and Ricky Hunter for bravely sharing her experiences as a survivor of domestic violence. My PhD supervisors at the University of Queensland, Professor Clive Phillips and Dr Deborah Walsh, have been a constant source of encouragement.

Grateful thanks are also due to the following contributors: Allie Phillips, Phil Arkow, Deborah Walsh, Clive Phillips, Howard Ralph, Michael Byrne QC, Tracy-Lynne Geysen, David Bailey, Pippa Swan, David Chamberlain, Stephen Drewe, Marc Cooper, Moo Baulch, Zoe Hinds, Jenna Ooi, Cassandra Day, Cam Day, Jenny Edwards, Natasha Lee and Lucia de Vries and to the many other people mentioned in the text who provided me with quotes and information.

Thank you also to these inspiring people who gave up their time to be interviewed about their work with animal abuse: Carol J. Adams, Andrew Knight, Jan Creamer, Jade Norris, Diane Balkin, Jed Goodfellow, Sarah Ferguson and Laurie Levy.

A range of people and organizations have kindly allowed me to use their excellent photographs and/or case studies, including Animal Defenders International, Animals Australia, Animal Welfare League Community Veterinary Clinic at Ipswich, Adam Turnbull, Robert Reisman at ASPCA, Marc Cooper at RSPCA England and Wales, David Bailey and colleagues, SHAC, WSPA, IFAW, PETA, Howard Ralph, Allie Phillips, Jacqueline Reid, Lucia de Vries, Natasha Lee, Jutamart Jattuchai and David Bomgardner for his image of the Magerius Mosaic. Thank you to my brother Stephen for creating the graphs.

Finally, thank you to my family, friends and colleagues for supporting me throughout this project, to my parents for welcoming homeless animals into the home and especially to my mother for always encouraging my compassion for animals and believing in me.

I sincerely hope this book will help us better understand and support the animals and people who experience the trauma of abuse and will be of assistance to those who care for them.

Catherine Tiplady
Brisbane
July 2012

This book includes interviews and contributions from a diverse range of people who work in the field of animal care/advocacy and includes their personal opinions, which may not necessarily be the views of the author or the publishers. No offence is intended by the language used and the ideas expressed by others. As well as frank discussion of sensitive topics such as religion, child abuse, domestic violence, animal sexual abuse and other matters of a sexual nature, this book includes graphic images and descriptions of animal abuse.

Introduction

Clive Phillips

Catherine Tiplady has been involved in research on animal abuse for several years and as a veterinarian has also first-hand experience of abuse cases. She initially studied the role of pets in domestic violence situations in her Veterinary Honours programme, and she continued this theme in her postgraduate degree. Under the guidance of supervisor Deborah Walsh, a specialist in domestic violence, and myself, Catherine has developed a keen understanding of this topic in a short space of time. In her initial studies she demonstrated the particular vulnerability of dogs in domestic violence situations, but it is clear that all animals are at risk of both verbal and physical abuse.

In this book she brings together several years of research on animal abuse, as well as including contributions from key workers in this field, such as Allie Phillips, the celebrated lawyer who specialises in cases involving animal abuse, David Bailey, forensic veterinarian, Howard Ralph, wildlife veterinarian and volunteers from aid agencies. Case studies provide the detail to keep the reader closely in touch with the real world, and interviews with key people provide an intensely personal experience of abuse. Phil Arkow describes how veterinarians can make a difference by having a critical eye to detect and report animal abuse, giving them a central role and responsibility in managing abuse cases. The vital function that animal cruelty organizations fulfil is recognized; with their protective role and that of veterinarians it may be unclear to readers how widespread abuse is allowed to happen. The fallibility of human nature and inadequate resources are regrettably too often the reason.

With many terms in this area being emotive, Catherine has used her scientific background to first define and then confine her discussions to her clear understanding of these terms. Abuse is described in relation to the uses of animals by humans that are most commonly found in the Western world. This is entirely logical because as the many instances of abuse in provision of food and fibre for humans are presented, it becomes only too clear that humans are selfish individuals, tolerating cruelty far more readily when we have something to gain from it. These are widespread instances of abuse, but Catherine also successfully charts many less common forms of abuse, from bear baiting to bestiality.

Pet abuse is a field that receives little publicity, unlike farm animal abuse, yet it is apparent from Catherine's major focus on this topic that may be very common. Pet ownership is more popular than ever, yet the pressures of modern living can reduce the animals' welfare, with busy working hours for both partners, high-density living and many possibilities for alternative uses of leisure time. However, pets' important role in many households inevitably brings them into close proximity with domestic violence, rendering them vulnerable to abuse.

Catherine outlines some of the best known historical examples of animal cruelty, by the Romans for example, which leaves the reader wondering whether abuse has always been part of human society, rather than just a modern scar on society. As I stood on the steps of the colosseum in Rome earlier this year I wondered what sort of society would applaud such evil deeds. Yet when we witness the slaughter of livestock today, it is clear that nothing has changed except perhaps that we have distanced ourselves from many of the most confronting issues. Other evidence that animal abuse is a continuous problem in human society, a pernicious thorn in our side, comes from the large number of complaints about cruelty being made directly to the animal advocacy groups. As human society grows in intensity and complexity, there is greater temptation to prosper through the use, and abuse, of animals.

In discussions of the topic, which are sometimes provocative and at times even challenging to read, Catherine leaves the reader with a clear sense that something has to be done about abuse to animals. Throughout the book she searches for the reasons why animals are abused. Perversely, the animals involved are often the ones that we have bred to be docile, so that they best fulfil their function, some companion dogs, for example, or cows used for meat and milk production. Regrettably, in a pressured society humans are all too ready to pass on aggression to animals, but there are some common elements in the abuse cycle that Catherine explores, such as the role of women. Women often are the interlocutors in abuse situations, the ones who inform the veterinarian, who intervene in violent households to protect the children or the animals. The prevalence rates of domestic violence are sobering, with some regions reporting abuse in one in four households. Reasons for the abuse are varied, but point to a breakdown in societal relationships, which is all too common today. Catherine highlights the fact that animals are particularly vulnerable to abuse in such situations and much of it is remains undetected. The vital role of education and training are emphasized, with a focus on prevention strategies that instruct children to be empathetic to animals. She does not shy away from the issue that nearly all abusers are male, and that we need to instil a sense of responsibility in our males at a young age to avert the societal perversion that is animal abuse.

It takes a special type of person to be able to address the issues discussed here without becoming disillusioned with humans' ability to manage animals. Often Catherine wisely resorts to using scientific methods to evaluate the importance of abuse cases, but throughout she has shown herself to be that kind of person, who can present the book dispassionately and with meticulous detail. She has produced a much-needed book that focuses on the worst instances of humans' interactions with animals, which will both enthral and inform. If it reduces the amount of abuse by just one animal, it will have served its purpose.

Clive Phillips
Centre for Animal Welfare and Ethics
University of Queensland

Part I

Animal Abuse: Defining the Problem

Animal abuse is an international problem, which has been part of human civilization for millennia. Despite this, consensus has not been reached on a single definition for animal abuse. This section includes a discussion of the various definitions proposed by experts, a historical perspective of animal abuse and, importantly, examines reasons why some people may be cruel to animals whereas others are caring. To enhance our understanding of the motivations to abuse animals, theories and hypotheses for violent behaviour are explained, as well as an insight into animal rights activists and their campaigns. The incidence of animal abuse among certain members of society, such as children, serial killers and perpetrators of domestic violence is described, along with case study analysis and quotes from animal abusers.

1 What is Animal Abuse?

Catherine Tiplady

Definitions

Animal abuse is the *deliberate* harm, neglect or misuse of animals by humans resulting in the animals suffering physically and/or emotionally. Not only animals but entire communities can be affected by the impact of animal abuse (Fig. 1.1).

Can the terms animal abuse and animal cruelty be used interchangeably and what do they mean? The word 'cruelty' is derived from the Latin 'crudelem' or 'morally rough' (Nell, 2006, p. 211) and 'abuse' from the Latin 'abusus' meaning to 'misuse' or 'take a bad advantage of' (Britannica, 1962).

Abuse has been defined as misuse or maltreatment and cruelty as indifference or pleasure in another's pain (*The Concise Oxford Dictionary*, 1974). From this it appears that 'abuse' can be more widely applied in the context of human–animal relationships whereas 'cruelty' focuses on the abuser's perceptions of the act. It has also been argued that abuse is caused through ignorance but cruelty implies intent by the perpetrator (Rowan, 1993).

There have been a number of attempts to define animal abuse/cruelty and one which is widely adopted is by Professor Frank Ascione. He has defined cruelty as 'an emotional response of indifference or taking pleasure in the suffering and pain of others, or as actions that unnecessarily inflict such suffering and pain' (Ascione, 1993, p. 226) and cruelty specifically to animals as 'socially unacceptable behaviour that intentionally causes unnecessary pain, suffering, or distress to and/or the death of an animal' encompassing physical, sexual, emotional/psychological abuse and neglect (p. 228). Others have defined cruelty as 'the wilful infliction of harm, injury and intended pain on a non-human animal' (Kellert and Felthous, 1985, p. 1114). It has been stated that a feature of abuse is that perpetrators take delight in the harm they cause (Nell, 2006), although some may argue that the perpetrator's frame of mind is of little consequence to the animals that suffer.

Animal abuse can be physical and/or mental. Physical abuse can be active (including mutilation and assault) or passive (such as failure to provide food and water); mental abuse can similarly be classified as active maltreatment (e.g. instilling fear in the animal) or passive neglect (such as depriving the animal of affection) (Vermeulen and Odendaal, 1993). Merck (2009, p. 65) takes a broad and pragmatic approach, considering that animal cruelty is 'basically any action or lack of action that results in illness, injury or death of an animal'. Even continuing to use malfunctioning or broken stunning equipment in an abattoir can be considered an act of abuse (Grandin, 2010). Others may consider habitat

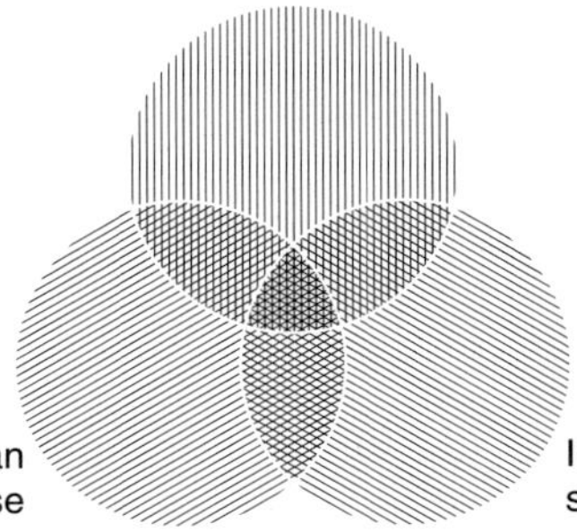

Fig. 1.1. Venn diagram showing overlap between animals, abusers of animals and the rest of society. Abuse of animals is often linked to abuse of people and has impacts on wider society.

destruction and extinction of species to constitute animal abuse.

Many people consider animal abuse and cruelty to have the same meaning and use the terms interchangeably. One author defines abuse and cruelty as significant harm to animals when a person actively and intentionally harms or fails to act appropriately towards an animal for which he or she is responsible (Olsson, 2010). Most legal definitions require intentionality on the part of the abuser, but this does not affect the impact on the animal. Edwards (2010) defines animal abuse as a deliberate act that inflicts obvious, unnecessary harm and suffering such as starvation, beating, torture, poking out eyes and depriving of water. The National Society for the Prevention of Cruelty to Children (NSPCC, n.d.) also describes animal abuse as the intentional harm of an animal. This raises interesting questions about whether *unintentional* harm of animals could be considered abuse – the dog accidentally run over as he runs out to greet you, the kitten hiding under a cushion, which is sat on and killed, the chick squeezed to death by a small child. If all of these occur unknowingly and unintentionally, then they are not strictly abuse but rather accidents that have resulted in animal harm.

Children may lack a clear definition of animal abuse. Pagani *et al.* (2010) asked children for their thoughts on animal cruelty, and they raised a range of valid points such as whether cruelty included killing flies, going fishing, not cleaning your fish tank and keeping birds in a cage. The issue of children and animal abuse will be discussed further in Chapter 3.

For the purposes of this book, abuse and cruelty will be used interchangeably and unless otherwise specified, deliberate neglect will be included as part of abuse or cruelty. 'Animals' will be the term used rather than the correct but more cumbersome 'non-human animals' and although 'he' or 'she' will be used to refer to animals where possible, if an animal's gender is not known the pronoun 'it' will be used.

Types of Animal Abuse

Animal abuse can occur through omission (neglect of the animal's needs) or commission (knowing abuse) (Phillips, 2005), and determining which it is can be difficult. Beating a dog to death obviously involves commission but some examples of omission (such as failing to supply adequate food and water to an animal) can be undertaken knowingly. This may have the aim of preventing later animal suffering. Intentional overstocking in sheep, as a method to prevent over-fatness and subsequent dystocia, is an example of this (Joyce *et al.*, 1976).

Where Can Animal Abuse Occur?

Animal abuse may occur:

- in the home;
- in wild animals living free;
- in hunted and fished animals;
- in zoos, tourist attractions or animal sanctuaries;
- where animals are used in sport, work or leisure;
- in farmed animals;
- in guard, guide, draught and work animals;
- in research animals;
- in animals in veterinary clinics, shelters or pounds; and
- in animals you have met.

Abuse can occur anywhere that humans and animals interact.

Issues Impacting on our Acceptance of Animal Abuse

Cultural aspects of animal abuse

People's attitudes toward and acceptance of animal abuse may vary depending on their culture, the species of animal and the animal's intended use.

Cock fighting and bear baiting, for example are generally considered cruel in Western culture yet considered sport in others. Slaughter methods and husbandry techniques may also be considered cruel by some cultures but acceptable by others. In most legal texts, 'harm to animals is not considered cruelty or abuse if it takes place within accepted agricultural, management or research practice and if the harm is not greater than considered necessary to obtain the purpose' (Olsson, 2010, p. 16). This means that those animals in agricultural or research systems are potentially vulnerable to legally sanctioned abuse.

Many people accept some types of animal abuse, dependent on the species of animal. When developing an interview to assess childhood cruelty to animals, Ascione *et al.* (1997) differentiated between invertebrates (e.g. worms, insects), cold-blooded vertebrates (e.g. reptiles, fish) and warm-blooded vertebrates (e.g. mammals and birds), with abuse of the latter being considered the most severe. 'Speciesism' such as this was refuted by Singer (1995), whose book *Animal Liberation* compared speciesism to racism and sexism and inspired the Animal Liberation movement when it was first published in 1975. People's perceptions towards animals may be affected by other factors. Arluke and Sanders (1996) describe a sociozoological scale where people rate animals as morally more or less important according to a number of factors such as the animal's perceived 'cuteness' and usefulness to humans.

Even within the same species, some animals are abused in the name of sport or food production and others seen as valuable. An example of this is cattle – valuable draught animals in developing nations, considered sacred in India, tortured in bullfighting, pushed to their physical limits as dairy and meat animals and occasionally subjected to terrible abuse during husbandry procedures and slaughter (see Figs 1.2–1.4).

People who work with abused animals will rely on legal definitions of animal abuse or cruelty in order to prosecute offenders, but it is still important that you develop your own perspective on what animal abuse is in your own mind and how it affects you and those around you. Just as every case of abuse affects individual animals in different ways, individual people will be affected differently by seeing and working with the effects of animal abuse.

The aims in writing this book are:

- to help the animal victims;
- to help you understand where there may be connection between human and animal abuse;
- to help you understand why and how abuse happens;
- to help you identify possible cases of abuse; and
- to support those who see, treat or work with abused animals and their carers.

While it is acknowledged that animals may harm or kill other animals (for example,

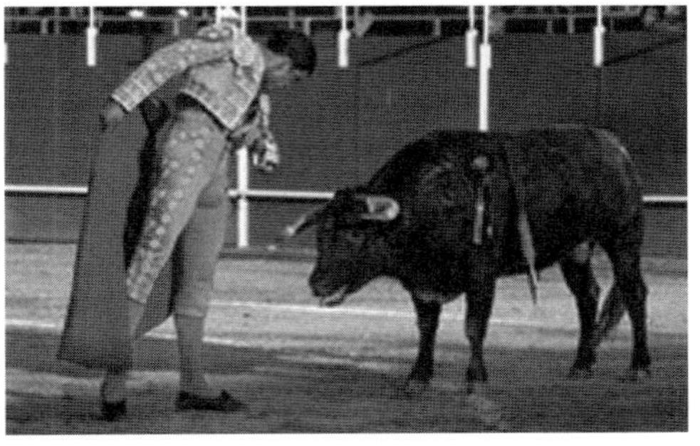

Fig. 1.2. A bullfight in Juriquilla, Querétaro, México. Bullfighting is a strong part of the national identity in several countries and until the actual fight, the welfare of the animal is very good. Can a generally well cared for life ever outweigh the suffering inflicted during death? (Photograph courtesy of WSPA.)

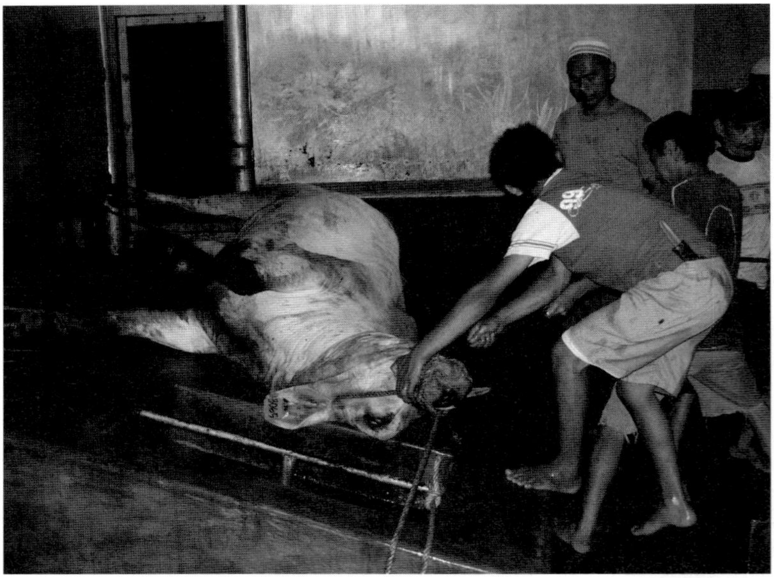

Fig. 1.3. Distressed, roped Australian steer exported to Indonesia for slaughter, vocalizing prior to slaughter on Meat and Livestock Australia-installed equipment. (Photograph courtesy of Animals Australia.)

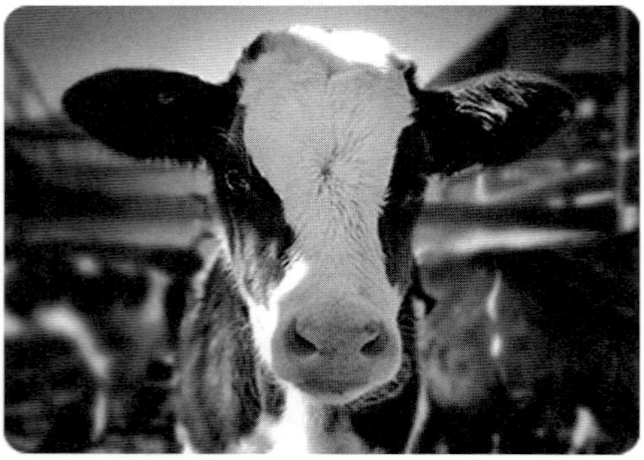

Fig. 1.4. A pen of dairy calves. Around the world millions of dairy calves are removed from their mothers every year and sold for slaughter at less than a week of age. Calves of this age would naturally suckle from their mothers 5–10 times a day (Broom and Fraser, 2007). Standards have been proposed to deny transported calves food for up to 30 h, stating this will 'improve the welfare of calves' (Dairy Australia, 2011). (Photograph courtesy of Animals Australia.)

animals fighting with each other or killing other animals to eat), that is not the focus of this book. An exception to this is where human interference is directly responsible for the animal's harm (for example, using trained terriers to hunt badgers). It is recognized that all animals can potentially have a negative impact on other species and the environment, yet human mismanagement (for example, overgrazing land, habitat destruction, dumping of unwanted domestic animals or allowing them to stray) is often the reason behind this.

Before we discuss how to help animals and people affected by abuse, it is first necessary to examine the issue of animal abuse from a global and historical perspective. Knowledge of the way animals were treated in the past will assist our understanding of current and future motivations to protect or abuse animals.

References

Arluke, A. and Sanders, C.R. (1996) *Regarding Animals.* Temple University Press, Philadelphia, Pennsylvania.

Ascione, F.R. (1993) Children who are cruel to animals: a review of research and implications for developmental psychopathology. *Anthrozoös* 6(4), 226–247.

Ascione, F.R., Thompson, T.M. and Black, T. (1997) Childhood cruelty to animals: assessing cruelty dimension and motivation. *Anthrozoös* 10(4), 170–173.
Britannica (1962) *Britannica World Language Edition of the Oxford Dictionary*. Oxford University Press, London, UK.
Broom, D.M. and Fraser, A.F. (2007) *Domestic Animal Behaviour and Welfare*, 4th edn. CAB International, Wallingford, UK.
Dairy Australia (2011) Handling bobby calves during transport. Available at: http://www.dairyaustralia.com.au/Animals-feed-and-environment/Animal-welfare/Calf-welfare/Managing-bobby-calf-welfare/Handling-bobby-calves-during-transport.aspx (accessed 19 September 2011).
Edwards, L.N. (2010) Animal well-being and behavioural needs on the farm. In: Grandin, T. (ed.) *Improving Animal Welfare: a Practical Approach.* CAB International, Wallingford, UK, pp. 139–159.
Grandin, T. (2010) Improving livestock, poultry and fish welfare in slaughter plants with auditing programmes. In: Grandin, T. (ed.) *Improving Animal Welfare: a Practical Approach.* CAB International, Wallingford, UK, pp. 160–185.
Joyce, J.P., Clarke, J.N., MacLean, K.S., Lynch, R.J. and Cox, E.H. (1976) The effect of level of nutrition on the productivity of sheep of different genetic origin. *Proceedings of the New Zealand Society of Animal Production* 36, 170–178.
Kellert, S.R. and Felthous, A.R. (1985) Childhood cruelty toward animals among criminals and noncriminals. *Human Relations* 38(12), 1113–1129.
Merck, M. (2009) Animal cruelty: recognition, reporting and testifying. In: *Australian Small Animal Veterinary Association Proceedings Australian Veterinary Association Annual Conference 2009*, Darwin Convention Centre 17–22 May, pp. 65–68.
Nell, V. (2006) Cruelty's rewards: the gratifications of perpetrators and spectators. *Behavioral and Brain Sciences* 29, 211–257.
NSPCC (n.d.) Understanding the Links. The National Society for the Prevention of Cruelty to Children, London. Available at: http://www.nspcc.org.uk/Inform/publications/downloads/understandingthelinks_wdf48177.pdf (accessed 18 May 2012).
Olsson, A. (2010) Animal abuse. In: Mills, D.S., Marchant-Forde, J.N., McGreevy, P.D., Morton, D.B. and Nicol, C.J. (eds) *The Encyclopedia of Applied Animal Behaviour and Welfare.* CAB International, Wallingford, UK, p. 16.
Pagani, C., Robustelli, F. and Ascione, F.R. (2010) Investigating animal abuse: some theoretical and methodological issues. *Anthrozoös* 23(3), 259–276.
Phillips, C. (2005) How animal welfare science assists in defining cruelty to animals. In: *RSPCA Australia Proceedings of the 2005 RSPCA Australia Scientific Seminar* held at the Telstra Theatre, Australian War Memorial, Canberra, Australia, 22 February, pp. 29–37.
Rowan, A.N. (1993) Cruelty to animals. *Anthrozoös* 6, 218–220.
Singer, P. (1995) *Animal Liberation.* Pimlico, London.
The Concise Oxford Dictionary (1974) 5th edn. Oxford University Press, Oxford, UK.
Vermeulen, H. and Odendaal, J.S.J. (1993) Proposed typology of companion animal abuse. *Anthrozoös* 6(4) 248–257.

2 History of Animal Abuse

Catherine Tiplady

Animal abuse has long been part of human society and features in philosophy, religion, science, art and literature dating back centuries. Legal protection of animals against cruelty dates back to the 18th century BC and is mentioned in the *Codex Hammurabi* of ancient Babylon and the Hindu *Atharva Veda* (Olsson, 2010).

Animal Abuse in Ancient Civilizations

The juxtaposition of caring for some animals and abusing others has been a feature of ancient and modern societies and it is likely that animal abuse co-evolved along with compassion towards animals.

Scenes of animals being hunted and killed have been depicted in artworks since prehistoric times; however, it can be difficult to differentiate cruelty from predatory behaviour in these images of primeval hunting practices (Phillips, 2009). Ancient cultures appear to have regarded animals in a similar way as modern society, with some animals protected from harm and others abused, even within the same species. Treatment of cats in Ancient Egypt is an interesting example. Felines were deified by the Ancient Egyptians and harsh penalties enacted for anybody who harmed or killed one, yet radiographs of mummified cats and kittens show displaced cervical vertebrae, suggesting that their necks had been broken (Clutton-Brock, 1993). It is proposed that Ancient Egyptian priests deliberately bred cats to be sacrificed as votive offerings (Clutton-Brock, 1993). Cervical dislocation, when performed by trained operators, can be a humane method of euthanasia for rats, mice and poultry (AVMA, 2007) but it is more difficult in animals over 1 kg in weight (Keller, 1982). In ancient civilizations cervical dislocation may well have been the most humane option available for cat euthanasia; however, there is the ethical concern that animals may have been bred and killed purely for religious sacrifice.

Ancient Rome

The slaughter of animals by the Ancient Romans has been described as an 'extravagant carnage' possibly unsurpassed in human history (Lindstrøm, 2010, p. 312), yet in modern times, the carnage certainly continues on an enormous scale. (An estimated 70 billion wild fish are caught and killed per year worldwide (Phillips, 2009), but this is for food production rather than entertainment.) It is interesting to consider why such large-scale animal cruelty ever became a popular form of entertainment for the masses in Ancient Rome, particularly as the people had a lot of admiration for the beauty of animals. One author comments on this:

> One of the most outstanding paradoxes of the Roman mind – that a people that was so much alive to the interest and beauty of the animal kingdom, that admired the intelligence and skill to be found in so many of its representatives, that never seemed to tire of the sight of rare and unfamiliar specimens, that displayed such devotion to pets, should yet have taken pleasure in the often hideous sufferings and agonizing deaths of quantities of magnificent and noble creatures.
>
> (Toynbee, 1973, p. 21)

In Rome and throughout the Roman Empire, entertainment known as 'Ludi' was made freely available to the public in circuses, arenas and amphitheatres. Ludi consisted of a variety of events: chariot races, theatrical plays, musical processions, gladiator contests, animal exhibits, animal fights and staged hunts (venationes) with a climax of mass animal killing (Lindstrøm, 2010). Ludi served to strengthen the popularity and position of the person who gave them (Harries, 2003) and were an influential method of gaining votes for rising politicians (Fig. 2.1). Ludi increased in frequency and magnitude until nearly half the year was devoted to them by the end of the 4th century CE (Lindstrøm, 2010). The scale of animal killing was massive – 8000 animals were killed in 2 days to celebrate the opening of the Colosseum in Rome and 11,000 were killed following Emperor Trajan's military victory in Dacia (Preece and Chamberlain, 1993).

There is a range of reasons proposed as to why animal killing became such popular entertainment among the Ancient Romans. Repeated

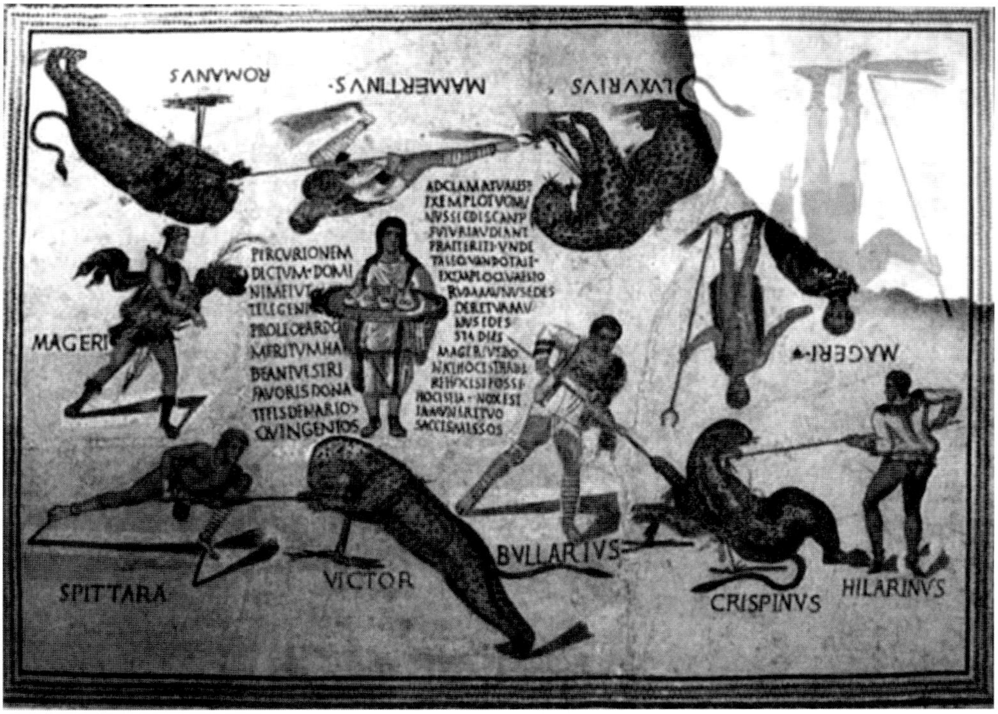

Fig. 2.1. The *Magerius Mosaic.* The mosaic shows the sponsor of the event (the politician, Magerius) in the centre with a tray of money. He is surrounded by leopards, which are being stabbed by hunters. The fact that the leopards are named and wearing garlands suggests the animals were actually tame and kept and trained for the deliberate purpose of killing (*Current Archaeology*, 2011), much like the bulls killed by matadors today. The blood seen spurting out of the leopards may have represented a blood sacrifice to ensure fertility for the following season (*Current Archaeology*, 2011). (Photograph courtesy of David Bomgardner.)

exposure to horrifying stimuli can desensitize the viewer (Schwartz, 1989) and so, to continue to elicit feelings of excitement, surprise and horror desired by the audience, the cruelty had to escalate (Lindstrøm, 2010). Another reason for the escalation of violence was politically motivated. Every new Ludus had to be bigger and better than those given by the opponents or predecessors, becoming increasingly expensive and with no concerns for the animals' welfare (Lindstrøm, 2010).

The choice of killing exotic and ferocious animals (such as bears, lions, leopards and elephants) demonstrated to the audience the strength of the Roman Empire, simultaneously reassuring and warning them of the Empire's power (Lindstrøm, 2010). Peer pressure may also have coerced people into attending the events and 'bystander apathy' decreased the likelihood of anyone protesting at the cruelty (Latane and Darley, 1969), even if there were some who objected.

The large-scale animal cruelty ended around the 5th century CE – not because the Romans realized their treatment of animals was cruel but because the Roman Empire collapsed and could no longer afford the expense of mass animal slaughter for entertainment (Preece and Chamberlain, 1993). Despite the popularity of animal killing, the Romans were not alone in enjoying the sight of animals (and people) being tormented and killed (Fagan, 2011). Such cruelty continues today with 'snuff' or 'crush' videos, in which people and animals are abused until they die, and public animal baiting and fighting events.

Animal abuse in the Medieval and Renaissance era

In the years 1000–1400 CE, animals continued to be abused as part of entertainment, mostly in sports such as cockfighting, bull-baiting and bear-baiting, in which dogs were let loose to attack a blinded bear, which was tethered to a stake (Kiser, 2007). Performing animals, trained to perform human-like behaviours, such as dancing, travelled across medieval Europe with their trainers to entertain royalty and the wealthy (Kiser, 2007). Hunting was important to the medieval people – hounds, horses and falcons were used in social hunting parties by the aristocracy who could afford to keep and train such animals (Smets and Van Den Abeele, 2007). Vivisection became a popular form of scientific research and even as public entertainment.

History of Animal Abuse in Experimentation/Research

Vivisection, 'the partial dissection of, or surgical intervention on, living animals for the purpose of research' (Maehle and Trohler, 1987, p. 14), has been widely practised since ancient times, acquiring a degree of popularity before becoming a controversial issue in the late 1800s (Rupke, 1987). Much of the public debate appeared to have been from a moral standpoint against animal cruelty, but some scientists had been having doubts about the validity of animal experimentation for some time. Early vivisection was intrinsically linked with pain and suffering as effective anaesthesia was not widely available until the mid-19th century CE (Kandela, 1998).

Public displays of vivisection in the 16th century CE were extremely cruel. A vivisectionist called Colombo (1515–59) performed vivisection on a pregnant bitch, removing and torturing her puppy to provoke the mother's furious barking and then allowing her to lick it tenderly (Colombo 1559 in Rupke, 1987). High-ranking clergymen attended these public vivisections and took great pleasure observing evidence of the maternal love between the bitch and her puppy (Colombo, 1559 in Rupke, 1987).

In recent times, animal experiments commonly cause public outrage when images are revealed. This monkey, known as Elisa (Fig. 2.2), had electrodes inserted into her head as part of brain experiments at the Institute of Neurology, London.

In Renaissance Europe of the 15th and 16th centuries CE, pet ownership increased in popularity although medieval practices of bear- and bull-baiting and performing animals continued (Boehrer, 2007). During this time, fear of witchcraft was growing, causing widespread panic and changing people's attitudes towards animals.

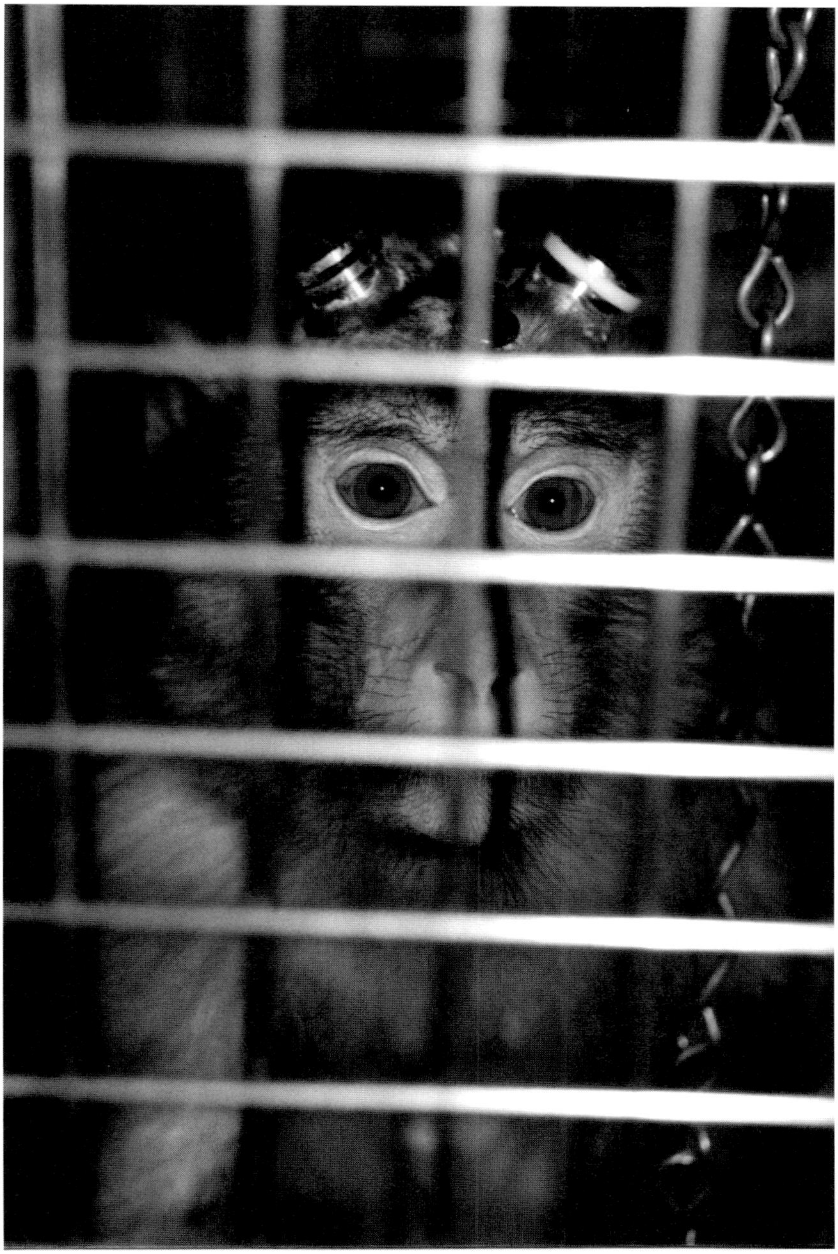

Fig. 2.2. Photograph of Elisa. (Photograph copyright Animal Defenders International.)

Witchcraft and Animal Abuse

The word 'witch' is derived from the Anglo-Saxon word 'wicce' (feminine form) or 'wicca' (masculine form), meaning 'wise one' (Illes, 2010). Witches were usually women (but could also take the form of men or animals) and were believed to communicate with the devil to perform supernatural acts of witchcraft (Britannica, 1962). Animals were frequently implicated in witch-hunts due to their role as companions or 'familiars' of witches. Familiars included cats, dogs, foxes, pigs, bats, corvid (crow-like) birds, owls, rabbits, raccoons and wolves (Illes, 2010).

Cats were the main targets during the witch-hunts as medieval Christianity distrusted these 'unruly' and 'lascivious' animals (di Simplicio, 2006, p. 174). In the 15th century CE, Pope Innocent VIII issued a decree denouncing cats and their owners – cats (familiars) and their owners (witches) were to be captured and killed by burning en masse, even those cats without an owner (Illes, 2010). Black cats were regarded as demons incarnate and were slaughtered by peasants all over Europe to destroy the witches who bewitched them (Tuczay, 2006). Other species were also vulnerable in the witch-hunt hysteria but to a lesser extent. In Salem, Massachusetts, dogs accused of being witches' accomplices were hanged to death (Illes, 2010). 'Proof' that an animal was actually a witch was obtained by harming the animal and seeing if the same injuries appeared on its human counterpart (Tuczay, 2006).

Witchcraft and spells could also involve animal sacrifice, such as live geese boiled alive (Hanafi, 2006) and snakes and roosters thrown into a cauldron to summon up a storm (Zika, 2006).

Witchcraft is not confined to the past. In current times, ritualistic animal mutilation and sacrifice may be practised by followers of Satanism, Vampirism, Voodoo, Santeria and Palo Mayombe (Merck, 2007). Followers of animist religions (including Voodoo) believe in spiritual powers of gods, demons, witches and forces of nature and use magic, rituals, sacrifice and trance (Plan, 2010). Fear of witches continues in some communities today and is taken very seriously (Fig. 2.3). In 2011 in Kagiso, near Johannesburg, a vervet monkey was beaten, pelted with stones, shot at, doused with petrol and burned to death due to fears the monkey was a talking witch that would bring bad luck to the community (Globalpost, 2011).

Nazism and Animal Abuse

> In many respects, the Nazis were more like the rest of us than we care to acknowledge
>
> (Sax, 2000, p. 165)

The Holocaust was orchestrated by Nazi Germany and resulted in the deaths of over 6 million Jewish people between 1939 and 1945. The atrocities of the Nazi regime and World War II resulted in countless people losing their lives and loved ones. What did the Nazis think about animals? The Law on Animal Protection (passed by then Chancellor Adolf Hitler in 1933) reveals what appears to be a surprisingly humane approach to animal welfare. For example, from Section 1, Cruelty to Animals, 'It is forbidden to unnecessarily torment or roughly mishandle an animal'; Section 2, Measures for the Protection of Animals states 'It is forbidden to so neglect an animal in one's ownership, care or accommodation that it thereby experiences appreciable pain or appreciable damage', as well as forbidding painful procedures on animals performed in an 'unprofessional' manner or without anaesthesia. People violating the laws could be permanently banned from keeping certain animals and punishment for animal cruelty was up to 2 years in prison, a fine, or both (Law on Animal Protection, 1933). Despite these animal protection laws, there were reports of horrific animal abuse perpetrated by the Nazis. It is alleged that SS soldiers would spend months working closely with German shepherd dogs only to be instructed by an officer to break the dog's neck in order to demonstrate teamwork, discipline and obedience to the Führer (Radde, 1991). It is suggested by Sax (2000) that the Nazis were 'like us', as they showed an extreme manifestation of a mentality present in Western society since at least the start of the modern era – namely, the ability to be kind to (certain) animals and cruel to (certain) people. Such selective compassion and cruelty to certain groups of people and animals continues today.

Animal Abuse in War

Regardless of which side people are fighting on, animals have become innocent victims of war, forced to work in carrying messages, for guarding, protection, bomb detection, draught animals and for experimentation. Some of the harm to animals during war includes the following (Fowler, 2010):

- Carrier pigeons being shot at while flying through occupied countries in World War I.

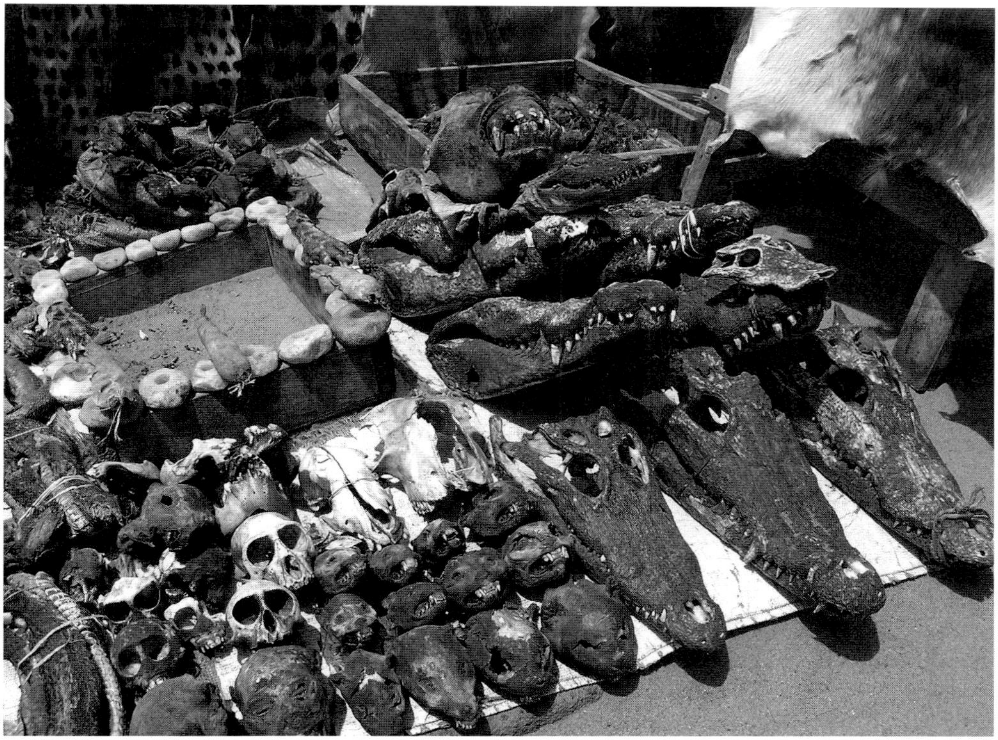

Fig. 2.3. Poached pieces of African wildlife at an animist market. Items on display in Lomé, Togo at a 'Marché fétiche' – a market for animist practices and Africans preferring traditional medicine. At the open market many parts of protected species are offered for sale including big-cat skins, big-cat heads, shark jaws, turtles, birds, gorillas, porcupine quills, horns, chimps, monkeys, antelope skins and heads, lion blubber, crocodile as well as live monkeys and live turtles in cages. Despite many protected species available at the market, authorities take no action to close it down because animist practices are feared by many including the agents (IFAW). (Photograph courtesy of IFAW.)

- Military dogs and horses abandoned to fend for themselves when troops move on.
- Mules used as draught animals in the jungles of Burma had their vocal cords severed to silence them during the campaign against the Japanese.
- Animals destroyed inhumanely rather than enter enemy hands, for example 2500 messenger pigeons were burnt alive in 1914 in Belgium.
- A donkey was loaded with explosives, sent into crowds and deliberately blown up in 2003 in Jerusalem.

Animal experimentation to determine the impact of biological, physical and chemical agents of warfare continues. A major centre for warfare research is Porton Down in Wiltshire, UK, where animals are used for a range of military experiments. One experiment involves detonating bombs near pigs to investigate the possible effects of bomb blasts on humans injured in terrorist attacks. Pigs are anaesthetized and a bomb is detonated near them, a third of their blood then deliberately removed to replicate haemorrhaging (Garner *et al.*, 2009). If the pigs are unable to feel the bomb blast, does that mean this is acceptable research?

The Animals in War memorial sculpture in London (by sculptor David Backhouse) is dedicated to the animals that served and died alongside British and allied troops – the monument depicts two mules, a horse and a dog and lists the numbers of animals lost during wars. The inscription reads:

> This monument is dedicated to all the animals that served and died alongside British and Allied forces in wars and campaigns throughout time. They had no choice.

Animal Abuse Today – Is Animal Abuse Increasing?

The number of animal cruelty complaints investigated by services such as the UK RSPCA is steadily increasing (Fig. 2.4). Does this mean that we as a society are becoming increasingly cruel? That is possible but it is likely there are many more factors involved, such as welfare groups increasing the funding of investigation and prosecution of cruelty or increased public awareness and expectations thanks to the media promotions of groups such as the RSPCA.

Similarly, interest in animal abuse research has been growing since the late 1990s, particularly in investigating the connection between abuse of humans and animals. An online literature search using ISI web found that the number of publications with 'animal cruelty' or 'animal abuse' in the title or abstract increased from 16 in the 5 years between 1995 and 1999, to 33 (2000–2004) and 54 (2005–2009). Much of the research has taken a human, rather than veterinary focus – cross-disciplinary research combining human health and veterinary expertise is essential for advancing our understanding of animal abuse.

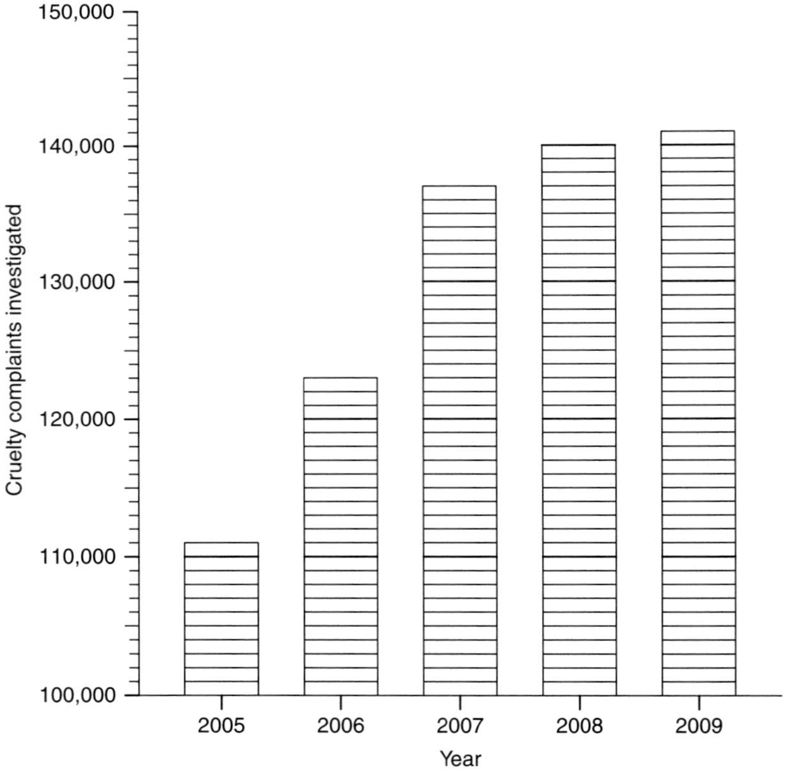

Fig. 2.4. The number of cruelty complaints investigated by the RSPCA in the UK between 2005 and 2009. Numbers have steadily increased since 2005 (RSPCA, 2011). In Malaysia, the number of cruelty cases attended by the ASPCA has also increased from 657 in 2009 to 762 in 2011 (Kelvin Cheah, personal communication, 11 January 2012).

The influence of animal advocacy groups continues to grow, largely due to undercover investigations of animal cruelty, which are then revealed to the public via the media.

Why would anybody want to abuse animals? Why would anybody want to protect animals? Reasons for people's motivations to abuse or protect animals will be discussed in the next chapter.

References

AVMA (2007) American Veterinary Medical Association guidelines on euthanasia. Available at: http://www.avma.org/issues/animal_welfare/euthanasia.pdf (accessed 16 March 2012).

Boehrer, B. (2007) Introduction. In: Boehrer, B. (ed.) *A Cultural History of Animals in the Renaissance*. Berg, Oxford, UK, pp. 1–26.

Britannica (1962) *Britannica World Language Edition of the Oxford Dictionary*. Oxford University Press, London.

Clutton-Brock, J. (1993) *Cats, Ancient and Modern*. Harvard University Press, Cambridge, Massachusetts.

Colombo, R. (1559) *De re anatomica libri XV* (Ex Typographia Nicolai Beuilacquae, Venetiis, 1559, Reprint Culture et Civilisation, Bruxelles, 1983). Cited in: Maehle, A.H. and Trohler, U. (1987) Animal experimentation from antiquity to the end of the eighteenth century: attitudes and arguments. In: Rupke, N.A. (ed.) *Vivisection in Historical Perspective*. Croom Helm, Beckenham, UK, p. 18.

Current Archaeology (2011) *The Magerius Mosaic*. Available at: http://www.archaeology.co.uk/cwa-2/world-news/the-magirius-mosaic.htm (accessed 17 September 2011).

di Simplicio, O. (2006) Cats. In: Golden, R.M. (ed.) *Encyclopedia of Witchcraft: The Western Tradition*. ABC-CLIO, Abingdon, UK, pp. 174–175.

Fagan, G.G. (2011) *The Lure of the Arena – Social Psychology and the Crowd at the Roman Games*. Cambridge University Press, Cambridge.

Fowler, K. (2010) *Animals – the Hidden Victims of War*. Animal Aid, Tonbridge, UK.

Garner, J.P., Watts, S., Parry, C., Bird, J. and Kirkman, E. (2009) Development of a large animal model for investigating resuscitation after blast and hemorrhage. *World Journal of Surgery* 33(10), 2194–2202.

Globalpost (2011) Monkey 'witch' burned by South African township mob. Available at: http://www.globalpost.com/dispatch/news/regions/africa/south-africa/110601/south-africa-wildlife-animal-welfare-monkey-witch-burned June 1 (accessed 18 September 2011).

Hanafi, Z. (2006) Natural magic. In: Golden, R.M. (ed.) *Encyclopedia of Witchcraft: The Western Tradition*. ABC-CLIO, Abingdon, UK, p. 705.

Harries, J. (2003) Favor populi: pagans, Christians and public entertainment in late Antique Italy. In: Lomas, K. and Cornell, T. (eds) *Bread and Circuses: Euergetism and Municipal Patronage in Roman Italy*. Routledge, London, pp. 125–141.

Illes, J. (2010) *The Weiser Field Guide to Witches*. Weiser Books, San Francisco, California.

Kandela, P. (1998) Sketches from *The Lancet* – which anaesthetic? *The Lancet* 352(9136), 1321.

Keller, G.L. (1982) Physical euthanasia methods. *Laboratory Animals* 11, 20–26.

Kiser, L.J. (2007) Animals in Medieval sports, entertainment and menageries. In: Resl. B. (ed.) *A Cultural History of Animals in the Medieval Age*. Berg, Oxford, UK, pp. 103–126.

Latane, B. and Darley, J.M. (1969) Bystander apathy. *American Scientist* 57, 224–268.

Law on Animal Protection (1933) signed by A. Hitler, Frick and Gürntner, cited in Sax, B. (2000) *Animals in the Third Reich – Pets, Scapegoats, and the Holocaust*. Continuum International Publishing Group, New York, pp. 175–179.

Lindstrøm, T.C. (2010) The animals of the arena: how and why could their destruction and death be endured and enjoyed? *World Archaeology* 42(2), 310–323.

Maehle, A.H. and Trohler, U. (1987) Animal experimentation from antiquity to the end of the eighteenth century: attitudes and arguments. In: Rupke, N.A. (ed.) *Vivisection in Historical Perspective*. Croom Helm, Beckenham, UK, p. 14.

Merck, M. (2007) *Veterinary Forensics: Animal Cruelty Investigations*. Blackwell Publishing, Ames, Iowa.

Olsson, A. (2010) Animal cruelty. In: Mills, D.S., Marchant-Forde, J.N., McGreevy, P.D., Morton, D.B. and Nicol, C.J. (eds) *The Encyclopedia of Applied Animal Behaviour and Welfare*. CAB International, Wallingford, UK, p. 18.

Phillips, C. (2009) *The Welfare of Animals – the Silent Majority*. Springer, Dordrecht, the Netherlands.

Plan (2010) What is Animism? Available at: http://www.plan.org.au/myplan/faq/childsponsorship/religions/2807 (accessed 15 September 2011).
Preece, R. and Chamberlain, L. (1993) *Animal Welfare and Human Values.* Wilfrid Laurier University Press, Waterloo, Ontario.
Radde, G. (1991) cited in Arluke, A. and Sax, B. (1992) Understanding Nazi Animal Protection and the Holocaust. *Anthrozoös* 5(1), 6–31.
RSPCA (2011) The Welfare State: Five years measuring animal welfare in the UK. Available at: http://www.rspca.org.uk/in-action/whatwedo/animalwelfareindicators (accessed 18 February 2011).
Rupke, N.A. (1987) Introduction. In: Rupke, N.A. (ed.) *Vivisection in Historical Perspective.* Croom Helm, Beckenham, UK, pp. 1–13.
Sax, B. (2000) *Animals in the Third Reich – Pets, Scapegoats, and the Holocaust.* Continuum International Publishing Group, New York.
Schwartz, B. (1989) *Psychology of Learning and Behaviour.* Norton, London.
Smets, A. and Van Den Abeele, B. (2007) Medieval hunting. In: Resl, B. (ed.) *A Cultural History of Animals in the Medieval Age.* Berg, Oxford, UK, pp. 59–79.
Toynbee, J.M.C. (1973) *Animals in Roman Life and Art.* Johns Hopkins University Press, Baltimore, Maryland.
Tuczay, C. (2006) Animals. In: Golden, R.M. (ed.) *Encyclopedia of Witchcraft: The Western Tradition.* ABC-CLIO, Abingdon, UK, pp. 41–42.
Zika, C. (2006) Cauldron. In: Golden, R.M. (ed.) *Encyclopedia of Witchcraft: The Western Tradition.* ABC-CLIO, Abingdon, UK, pp. 176–177.

3 Why Some People are Cruel to Animals

Catherine Tiplady

Why Do Some People Start to Abuse Animals?

To end tyranny we must first understand it.
Singer (1995, p. 185)

To understand why some people start to abuse animals it is first necessary to define human aggression and develop an understanding of the psychology involved in human behaviour and motivations. This chapter combines case studies and research from around the world to examine people's motivations to abuse animals.

Human aggression has been defined as 'behaviour performed by a person (the aggressor) with the deliberate intention of harming another person (the victim) who is believed by the aggressor to be motivated to avoid that harm' (Gullone, 2009, p. 38). Harm in this context includes physical harm (such as punching someone), psychological harm (such as verbal abuse) and indirect harm, such as damaging someone's property (Gullone, 2009). As an animal can be both victim as well as someone's 'property' they are at increased risk of abuse.

Why Do People Abuse or Care for Animals?

Before we examine more deeply why people may abuse animals it is worthwhile to consider the various attitudes people may hold towards animals.

A typology of ten basic attitudes humans hold toward animals has been listed (Kellert, 1980):

1. Naturalistic – interest in and affection for wildlife and the outdoors.
2. Ecologistic – concern for the environment and the interrelationships between wildlife species and natural habitats.
3. Moralistic – concern for the right and wrong treatment of animals, with strong opposition to cruelty toward and exploitation of animals.
4. Scientistic – interest in the physical attributes and biological functioning of animals.
5. Aesthetic – interest in the symbolic and artistic characteristics of animals.
6. Humanistic – interest in and strong affection for individual animals, primarily pets.
7. Utilitarian – concern for the practical and material value of animals.
8. Dominionistic – satisfactions from mastery and control over animals, typically in sporting situations.
9. Negativistic – primary orientation an active avoidance of animals due to fear or dislike.
10. Neutralistic – primary orientation a passive avoidance of animals due to indifference and lack of interest.

Rather than attempt to neatly slot ourselves or others into one of these ten categories, it is more likely that people have a mixture of these attitudes, and these may change over time and depending on personal experiences with the type of animal involved. For example, many view 'pest' animals differently to companion animals. There is no single category that is pathognomonic for an abuser. Animal hoarders, for example may initially be motivated by moralistic and humanistic attitudes to rescue and house unwanted animals that would otherwise be euthanized. Soon, however, these people may be overwhelmed and neglect and suffering of animals is the result. Does this mean that the cat hoarder is actually negativistic? Or even dominionistic by forcing animals to live confined in filthy cages and rooms? How to identify and help the people and animals involved in hoarding situations will be discussed further in Chapter 8.

There are various theories and hypotheses to help us understand why some people perform abusive acts. A few of these which will be briefly discussed include:

- social learning theory;
- progression or graduation hypothesis; and
- deviance generalization theory.

Social learning theory

The theory of social learning is that every individual is socialized to seek approval and affection from those they love (Dollard and Millar, 1950). When this is successful, both parties feel satisfied; however, when this does not occur the resulting frustration and anger may be transferred toward 'weaker creatures' (such as animals) that cannot retaliate (Wright and Hensley, 2003). According to the theory of social learning, violent behaviours are learned from early childhood (Bandura, 1973; Reitzel-Jaffe and Wolfe, 2001). A study involving over 1000 children and adolescents in Italy found that those who had witnessed their friends and mothers abusing animals were more likely to abuse animals themselves (Baldry, 2003). Similarly, a study involving 281 adolescents in Australia found that animal abuse was more common among those who had observed animal abuse by a parent, sibling, relative or friend (Thompson and Gullone, 2006). Figure 3.1 shows a group of young men smiling as their companion strangles a puppy.

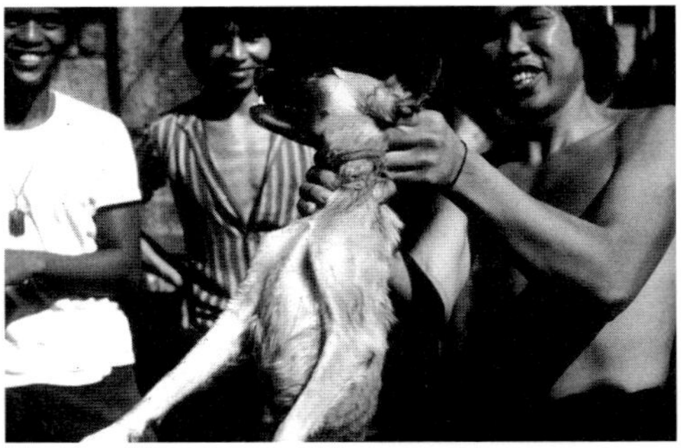

Fig. 3.1. Young male strangling a puppy while others watch. (Photograph courtesy of IFAW.)

Progression or graduation hypothesis

This hypothesis proposes that those who abuse animals during childhood will 'progress' or 'graduate' to harming humans as adults. This theory forms part of what is commonly referred to as 'the link/s', which is widely promoted among animal advocacy groups around the world (e.g. The Links Group UK, The Linkage Project USA and First Strike campaigns by the Scotland SPCA and the Humane Society of the United States). Although many people believe there is a connection between animal and human abuse, among them veterinarians (Green and Gullone, 2005) and members of the public (Taylor and Signal, 2006), some researchers criticize a perceived lack of rigorous research to provide evidence of such a link (Beirne, 2004; Patterson-Kane and Piper, 2009). Other researchers argue that the 'graduation' of abuse may not necessarily start with animals and progress to people, but move from 'distant' to 'intimate' victims (Arluke *et al.*, 1999). Following this idea, people could start by abusing people and later harm animals. A (human) stranger for example, may be considered 'distant' yet the abuser's own puppy be considered 'intimate'.

Deviance generalization theory

The deviance generalization theory rejects the hypothesis that there is an inevitable progression of animal abuse leading to human abuse. Animal abuse is instead viewed as a form of antisocial behaviour that may occur before, after or concurrently with other antisocial behaviour directed toward humans (Arluke *et al.*, 1999).

A study of criminals and members of the public found that animal abusers were more likely to perform a range of other antisocial behaviours (e.g. drug, property, interpersonal violence and public disorder offences) but animal abuse did not precede violence toward humans (Arluke *et al.*, 1999). In another study, owners of so-called high-risk or 'vicious' dogs had significantly more criminal convictions than owners of low-risk dogs (Barnes *et al.*, 2006).

Motivations for Animal Abuse

Researchers interviewed over 150 criminals and found that 25% of aggressive criminals reported five or more acts of animal cruelty, compared to 6% among moderate and non-aggressive criminals and none in the non-criminal group (Kellert and Felthous, 1985). From the stories of the respondents, Kellert and Felthous (1985) developed a classification scheme of nine animal cruelty motivations:

1. To control an animal (e.g. using abuse as discipline).
2. To retaliate against an animal.
3. To satisfy prejudice against a breed or species (e.g. hatred of cats).
4. To express aggression through an animal (e.g. organized dog fighting).
5. To enhance one's own aggressiveness (e.g. using animals as target practice).
6. To shock people for amusement.
7. To retaliate against another person (e.g. hurting an animal to upset the owner).
8. To displace hostility from a person to an animal (e.g. a person physically abused as a child displacing the violence on to an animal).
9. To act out non-specific sadism.

A study of 112 prison inmates who had abused animals were asked about their motivations for animal cruelty (Hensley and Tallichet, 2005). Respondents could indicate more than one motivation (Table 3.1). Anger was the most common motivation, followed by fun, dislike for the animal and wishing to control the animal (Hensley and Tallichet, 2005).

The article in Box 3.1 is a case study of animal abuse that highlights motivations. This report originally appeared in the *Daily Mercury* newspaper and is provided courtesy of the journalist, Bruce McKean (2009).

Table 3.1. Frequencies and percentages of inmates who had committed childhood and/or adolescent animal cruelty and their motivations for engaging in these acts ($n = 112$) (From Hensley and Tallichet, 2005).

Motivation	Number (n)	Percentage
Anger	54	48.2
For fun	43	38.4
Dislike for the animal	25	22.3
To control the animal	25	22.3
Fear of the animal	24	21.4
Imitation	17	15.2
Sexual purposes	16	14.3
Revenge against someone	16	14.3
To impress someone	11	9.8
To shock people	5	4.5

From the case study, it is evident that the perpetrators of the abuse had planned the animal cruelty as an act of revenge on the dog's owner. Key parts from this newspaper article are as follows:

1. The animal cruelty was not a random attack. The animal was deliberately abused as an act of revenge toward the woman owner.
2. The cruelty was filmed.
3. The perpetrators thought their actions were amusing.
4. The perpetrator had a history of violent crime.
5. People who heard details of the cruelty were emotionally upset.

Can you think of any other points that stand out in this case?

Animal Abuse and the Internet

Animal abusers may use the Internet to search for scenes of animal abuse, to learn animal abuse techniques or to post footage and images of themselves abusing animals. This has led to arrests of the abusers in a number of cases. A 22-year-old Chicago man and a 13-year-old boy were arrested and charged with several

Box 3.1. Case study: Maximum term for torture of dog

Bruce McKean, 4 September 2009

Several people wept in the public gallery as details of the cruel and callous torture and death of seven-month-old puppy Peanut were read in the District Court in Mackay yesterday.

Peanut's horrifying mutilation and death, which his killers videotaped on a mobile phone, beggars belief and the case has been described as the worst case of animal cruelty in Australian history.

After kidnapping Peanut in the middle of the night, Jonathon Blake and another man took him to a park behind the Moranbah rodeo grounds.

They mutilated and decapitated the small dog.

Parts of his body were found around the area by residents.

Prosecutor David Morters said that, by looking at the video: 'It is quite clear that both Blake and his co-accused are enthusiastic about their actions. They are laughing and making comments.

Their purpose in cutting off his legs was to severely disable the dog. It is also clear in the video that the dog is in excruciating pain.

The torture of the dog obviously resulted in great suffering, Mr Morters said.

Blake, now aged 25, pleaded guilty to seven charges, including burglary and killing an animal.

Blake was jailed for sex offences in 2006 and served 21 months; when he was released he was given employment by the Neilsen family in Moranbah. He was allowed to sleep in their home when he had nowhere else to sleep. The Neilsen family even lent him a car.

He had a falling out (with) Peanut's owner, Danielle Neilsen, and kidnapped and killed the dog for revenge.

After killing Peanut, Blake drove off and crashed his borrowed car through a council fence. He was arrested for drink-driving and it was then that police checked his mobile phone and found the horrific images of the killing of Peanut.

Judge Michael Shanahan said it was one of the worst cases he'd ever heard and said the details 'beggar belief'.

He was invited to watch the three videos but refused to see them, saying the details read out were enough for him to impose the maximum sentence of three years in jail.

However, Judge Shanahan followed usual legal practice and ordered parole release after one-third of the sentence (was served).

He ordered the videotapes be destroyed.

counts of animal cruelty and torture after videos on YouTube allegedly showed them suspending a dog from a leash and violently spinning it around, throwing dogs into the air and letting them drop and hiding a mother dog's young puppies from her as a form of psychological abuse (Mirabelli, 2012). The abusers identified themselves by name in the videos and had distinctive tattoos, which aided authorities in matching them to the posts (Mirabelli, 2012).

It is disturbing that people are filming animal cruelty as a form of entertainment, but particularly so when a child is involved in the animal abuse.

Animal Abuse as Part of Other Crime

According to the ASPCA (2012), intentional animal abuse can be one of the most visible parts of a history of antisocial and aggressive behaviour and is often seen with other crime, such as weapons violations, drug offences, domestic violence, sexual assault and gang activity.

There are many incidents of animals being threatened and injured during burglary, particularly dogs being threatened, stabbed or shot by intruders and of rapists threatening or harming their victim's animals. Service animals such as police dogs and horses are at risk of abuse from members of the public during their work. In one such case, violence broke out after a football game in London, resulting in 47 police officers and 26 police horses being injured when crowds threw bricks and paving stones at them and used 'thunder flash' devices and incendiary flares (Steele, 2002).

Sometimes, animals are abused as a rehearsal for violent crimes against humans. The most extreme example of this is the case of mass and serial murderers.

Animal Abuse, Mass Murderers and Serial Murderers

> I will never forget the howl she made. It sounded almost human. We laughed and hit her more.

This is an excerpt from the diary of Luke Woodham, a 16-year-old boy who is describing how he killed his dog, Sparkles. Later, Woodham stabbed his mother to death and shot nine schoolmates, two of them fatally (Hewitt *et al.*, 1997).

A serial murderer is somebody who murders four or more people over a period of days, weeks, months or years (Levin, 2008) and a mass murderer is someone who kills several people within moments or hours (Hickey, 2006). Although murder may be preceded by known or alleged abuse of animals and humans this is not always the case. In his manifesto published on the Internet, Anders Behring Breivik (quoted by McLaughlin, 2011) stated:

> As all my friends can attest to I wouldn't be willing to hurt a fly and I have never used violence against others.

Later, Breivik went on to shoot 69 people and kill eight others in a bomb attack, causing injuries to over 200 more people (BBC News Europe, 2012).

While some serial murderers have apparently enjoyed abusing living animals, more appear to prefer the dissection and exploration of deceased animals – it is even proposed that this curiosity of cutting into dead animals may facilitate the development of deviant sexual fantasies (Hickey, 2006).

An examination of 354 cases of serial murderers found that 75 (over 21%) were *known* to have abused animals (Wright and Hensley, 2003). While not wishing to minimize the importance of animal cruelty as a possible predictor of violent crime, another way of expressing this could be 'Over three-quarters of a sample of 354 serial murderers were not known to have committed cruelty toward animals'. Should we be bothered? Yes, because any harm of animals or humans is something we need to be concerned about.

In a case study analysis of five adult male serial murderers in the USA (Wright and Hensley, 2003), common features in the history of each murderer were as follows:

- verbal/physical abuse in the home;
- feelings of humiliation, frustration and anger toward one or more parent; and
- release of this frustration, first by abusing and killing animals, then later, humans, often using the same style of killing.

In a study of school shootings, Verlinden (2000) reported that of nine school shootings in the USA (from 1996 to 1999) five of the 11 perpetrators (45%) had histories of alleged animal abuse.

Learning more about violent criminals and their experiences with animals is an important way to uncover possible predictors of violence but focuses on a small group of people, and gathering data can be particularly difficult in the case of murderers, some of whom are now deceased. Ideally, further research in human/animal abuse would involve longitudinal studies of a large sample of children from various backgrounds, following them at regular intervals as they progress through life, working with their parents or guardians. Regular surveying of this group would provide valuable data to uncover the nature of any exposure to and perpetration of abuse against animals or humans.

Fortunately, there appear to be relatively few violent criminals living among us. So, what about animal abuse among the 'nice' people in the general community? Could our neighbours, our friends or even the local veterinarian be animal abusers? This will now be examined as we attempt to uncover the prevalence of animal abuse.

Animal Abuse in the Community

What is the prevalence and incidence of animal abuse in the general community?

> To the question, 'how much animal abuse is there?' one is tempted to answer, 'as much as you are willing to find'.
>
> (Beirne, 2004, p. 43)

As there is a lack of large-scale self-report studies on animal abuse (Beirne, 2004) and a lack of a clear definition of animal abuse (Munro, 1999) that is widely accepted, it is currently difficult to know the true extent of animal abuse in the wider community.

Several researchers have, however, attempted to uncover the prevalence of animal abuse within certain subsections of the community, with 'prevalence' defined as the number of cases in a population at any one time (Munro, 1999). A survey of children aged 7–17 years in Italy found that over 50% admitted being involved with at least one form of animal cruelty (Baldry, 2003), while 20.5% of a sample of university students in America reported that they had engaged in animal cruelty (Miller and Knutson, 1997).

Major problems when comparing studies of prevalence are that the definition of animal abuse or cruelty used by the researchers or participants may vary between studies, researchers are reliant on the accuracy of people's memory and people may not tell the truth for reasons such as social desirability. Some previous studies, while very informative, have also focused on animal abuse among groups that cannot be generalized to the wider community, for example, jailed criminals (Tingle *et al.*, 1986) or people in violent homes.

In homes where there is domestic violence, the prevalence of animal abuse has been found to be higher than in the general community. A case-control study in Victoria surveyed 104 women who had experienced domestic violence and 102 women who had not experienced violence (Gullone *et al.*, 2004). Among violent households, 53% of women reported pets had been abused by their partner compared to no reported pet abuse by partners in the non-violent control households. Domestic violence, child abuse and animal abuse are discussed further in Chapter 11.

Who Are the Abusers of Animals?

Anybody can be an abuser of animals and, just as in cases of human interpersonal abuse (see section on Working with Perpetrators by Deborah Walsh, Chapter 14), animal abusers can be experts at presenting a caring public persona. Animal abuse may be performed privately or publicly, perpetrated by a lone abuser or with a group of others. In group abuse, the cruelty may be part of initiation or an activity encouraged by the peer group. Human violence research has found there are greater levels of violence and injury to a victim of gang rape (or 'multiple perpetrator rape') compared to rape by a lone perpetrator (Horvath, 2011). It is possible that abuse of animals by multiple perpetrators involves similarly increased levels of violence and injury.

Are males more likely to abuse animals than females?

Males outnumber females in aggressive tendencies by a ratio of approximately ten to one (Gullone, 2009), with most aggressive incidents occurring between the ages of 15 and 24 years (Anderson and Huesmann, 2003).

According to a US pet abuse monitoring website (pet-abuse.com, 2012), the following data of abusers were collated:

- Of 13,916 reported animal abuse cases in the USA, the most common age group for male animal abusers was the 31–40-year age range (2169 men) and for women the 41–50-year age range (831 women).
- Of over 8000 cases, 64% involved the owner or caregiver of the animal as the abuser.
- The neighbour was the reporter of the animal abuse in 37% of cases.

Despite this, men and boys should not automatically be viewed with suspicion as there are women and girls who also abuse animals. Although there are more males who physically abuse animals and more females who are hoarders (see Figs 3.2 and 3.3), for the sake of the animals we all need to be open minded about who an abuser could be.

Animal abuse may be perpetrated by people we would not expect to be cruel.

Munro and Munro (2008) state that we should not assume owners with a disability will not abuse their support dogs or that pets with a disability (for example deaf dogs) will not be abused if the owner becomes frustrated with the animal.

A group of people who would never be expected to be animal abusers are veterinarians and, although the abusers are likely to form a small minority of the profession, this issue needs to be discussed.

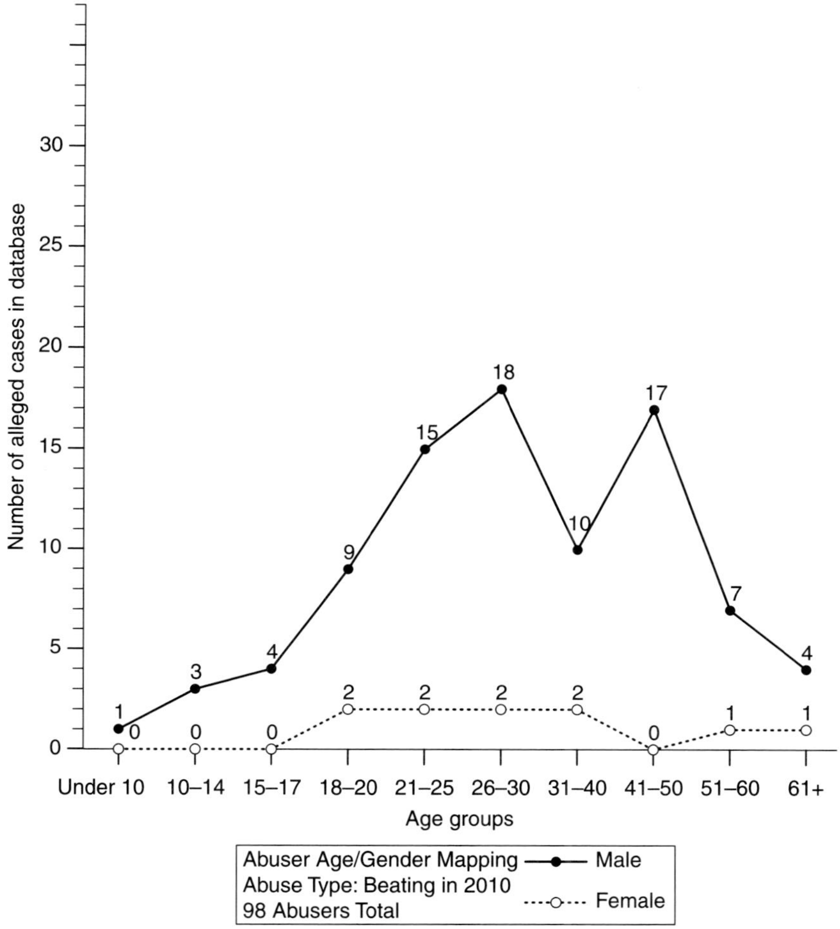

Fig. 3.2. Graph of alleged animal abuse (beating) cases with gender and age groups of abusers. (Source: pet-abuse.com and the AARDAS Project (accessed 2 April 2012)).

When the animal abuser is a veterinarian

> The veterinarian was making the young farm hand continually use the electric goad on the faces of the cattle moving down the race. The boy didn't want to do this but the vet was demanding he do this. The cattle became increasingly distressed.
>
> (Visitor to a large cattle property)

Veterinarians and veterinary staff can be animal abusers just as can anybody else. Overly forceful methods of restraint, extreme use of force as discipline or punishment, shouting and swearing at animals may be seen by colleagues or (less likely) customers of veterinarians. This is distressing to see, particularly when this violent approach is copied by other staff and used for all animals, even the quiet, frightened or affectionate. Patronek (2004) states that although there may be times when use of force in animal handling is unavoidable in order to protect the safety of animals, staff and the public, this should be limited to the extent needed and never used as a form of punishment. Managers of clinics and shelters must promote staff training in the correct use of equipment (such as bite-proof gloves, squeeze cages and nets), non-abusive handling techniques and use of tranquillizers and sedative drugs so staff can safely and humanely handle a variety of

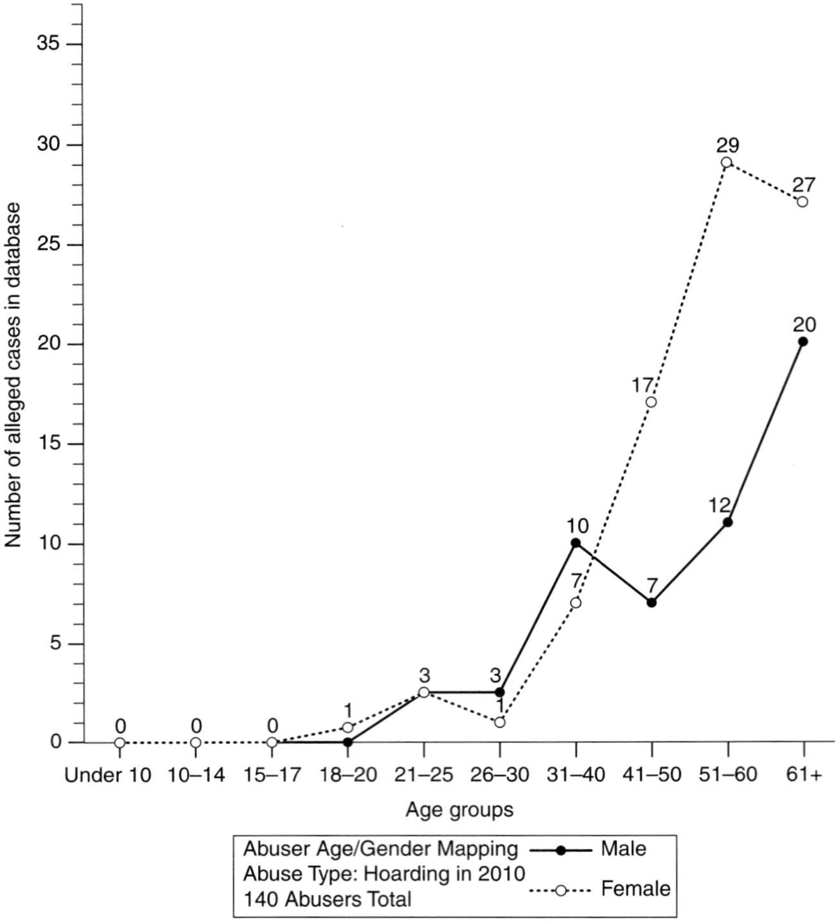

Fig. 3.3. Graph of alleged animal abuse (hoarding) cases with gender and age groups of abusers. (Source: pet-abuse.com and the AARDAS Project (accessed 2 April 2012)).

animals. Other areas of concern in some clinics include poorly performed surgery, inadequate analgesia (e.g. 'Why would I bother giving post-operative pain relief after spaying a feral cat? If they're feral and they're in pain, they'll be sitting still and that's good.') and a preference to euthanize animals rather than perform diagnostic work-ups and treatment. In cases of actual or suspected abuse the concerned customer or staff member could initially approach the manager of the veterinary clinic to complain. If this is not preferable or feasible (for example if the manager is the perpetrator of the abuse) then contact the Veterinarians Board, SPCA, humane society or other governing body for advice on how to lodge a complaint. Animal abuse can become commonplace within certain clinics and shelters, with more outspoken, aggressive personalities over-riding quieter, compassionate staff who are also often the target of offensive jokes. Unfortunately, those who care deeply for animal welfare often choose to leave an abusive workplace and, so, the culture of cruelty continues and the abusers have won.

Clinical veterinary staff who are cruel to animals have no place in animal welfare but unfortunately they are found, as seen in the following quote of a veterinarian talking about his first boss:

> He wouldn't use drugs to sedate the cats which came in for surgery. Instead, he would make his

> hand into a fist and then knock it down, hard, on top of each cat's head. That would make the cat unconscious.

Veterinarians and animal scientists undertaking research can also be cruel. One PhD student undertaking behavioural research in animal emotions wanted to research whether animals grieved. She spoke with enthusiasm how she intended to undertake this research – by slowly killing one rat whilst its pair-bonded companion watched on, helplessly. With so many animals and people pining for deceased or absent animal companions, research of this nature could easily be undertaken without killing. It is unnecessary, unethical and callous to cause animals to suffer in order to obtain a PhD in 'animal welfare'. Fortunately, other ways were found for that student to undertake her research.

The farmer as abuser

> I injected a sick old ewe with weed killer and left her out in the paddock to die. The next morning there were wild pigs laying dead around the paddock, they'd eaten her and got poisoned (laughs).
>
> (Farmer speaking to a veterinarian and veterinary student on farm animal placement with him)

Cruelty and neglect perpetrated by some farmers can be extreme. Regardless of situations where farmers are themselves suffering due to economic or personal problems, they have responsibility to care for the animals on their farm. If they are unable or unwilling to provide this care then they need to consider another career.

Some farm workers appear to view animals as mere money-making objects rather than living, sentient beings. Some of this may be due, again, to the culture of violence prevalent within some workplaces. In other cases, lack of training, lack of access to veterinary care, no money (or unwillingness) to pay for treatment and no equipment to humanely euthanize animals may be involved.

In the example given above, the farmer involved did have access to a gun and could have chosen to shoot the sick ewe rather than take the bizarre and cruel decision to inject her with weed killer and leave her to die. I know this because while at the farm I treated the farmer's dog for a bullet wound. The farmer told me he had shot his dog in the shoulder as punishment for not coming when he was called.

Issues with Accuracy in Assessing the Extent of Animal Abuse

There is always going to be a potential risk of inaccuracy when trying to determine the extent of animal abuse within a population.

In the prison inmate community, potential issues of inaccuracy when using retrospective data of childhood animal abuse include difficulty recollecting what happened, exaggeration to appear more aggressive, withholding information to appear less aggressive and inaccurate information being given because the question was not understood (Kellert and Felthous, 1985). Another issue is that there is often a poor response rate in studies involving the inmate community – typically over 50% decline to participate (Arluke *et al.*, 1999). Parental reporting of their child's treatment of animals also carries the risk of inaccuracy – abuse may be performed secretly or parents may choose to minimize known incidents of animal cruelty to present their child in a positive light.

Self-reporting by members of the general community also carries risks of inaccuracy. People often want to present the best possible side of themselves and are less likely to disclose violent behaviour. This can vary however, depending on their mood or peer group at the time. For example, an adolescent may behave in totally different ways toward animals (and in general) when among peers compared to when with a parent or teacher. An area where this is particularly notable is 'status' dogs owned by young people in gangs.

Status Dogs, Youth and Crime

The term 'status dogs' is defined by the Department for Environment, Food and Rural Affairs (Defra, 2010) as:

> the ownership of certain types of dogs which are used by individuals to intimidate and harass

> members of the public. These dogs are traditionally, but not exclusively, associated with young people on inner city estates and those involved in criminal activity.

These dogs may be used as weapons in fighting or as 'tough-looking' status symbols, and even though the owners can form very strong bonds and attachments with their status dog, they may not provide the safe environment and care that dogs require (SCAS, 2010).

Status dogs are at risk of abuse and neglect in the following ways (Metropolitan Police Service, n.d.):

- Their owners mistreat them.
- Sometimes the dogs will be kicked, beaten or even stabbed.
- Some status dogs end up being abandoned or left for dead.
- Sometimes the dogs are made to endure cruel training methods, such as hanging from branches by their teeth to strengthen their jaws.

More about the treatment and rehabilitation of fighting dogs is seen in Chapter 18.

In recent years, incidents, attacks and fighting of status dogs have increased with some incidents resulting in the deaths of children (Defra, 2010). It is believed that the increasing numbers of aggressive dogs owned by young people is linked to the rise in gang culture (SCAS, 2010).

Governments and animal welfare groups realize that status dogs pose a risk to human and animal well-being and in some areas have joined forces to try to manage this problem. The Metropolitan Police Authority in London has formed a Status Dog Unit and is working alongside animal welfare groups such as the RSPCA, Dogs Trust and The Blue Cross. In the USA, the Humane Society's 'End Dogfighting' programme offers owners of street-fighting dogs in Chicago the support, education and dog training skills to better care for their dogs and strengthen the human–animal bond. The Humane Society (HSUS, 2012) explains why they decided to offer a range of services to help these dogs and their owners:

> As we got to know people in these communities, we developed a keener understanding of how under-served they've been by animal care and welfare organizations. So we started offering a wider range of support: vaccinations, pet care information, veterinary wellness services (such as spay/neuter), health care and advice, etc.

Any attempt to help with the issue of status dogs needs to consider why young people feel the need to own these animals in the first place. A veterinarian who encounters status dogs and animal abuse in his work as director of the RSPCA Harmsworth Hospital in London is Dr David Grant. He describes owners of status dogs as 'the finished product of a conveyor belt of social deprivation that begins at birth' and advises that 'Focus should be on the social deprivation conveyor belt at its beginning, not at its end' (Grant, 2010).

Discussion needs to involve all relevant parties (such as the dog owners, police, veterinarians, social workers) to examine the social problems that are making gang life and status dogs so attractive to some.

Although owners of status dogs are typically young adults and adolescents, learning to abuse animals starts even earlier – during childhood.

Children who Abuse Animals

What motivates children to be cruel to animals?

> Ride your bike into (dog's name) as hard as you can and make her fall over! Don't worry, you won't kill her...
>
> (Four-year-old boy speaking to his younger brother)

Ascione *et al.* (1997) found that children's motivations for animal cruelty included the following:

- peer pressure;
- mood enhancement;
- exploration or curiosity;
- forced abuse;
- sexual gratification;
- attachment to an animal;
- animal phobias;
- identification with the child's abuser;
- post-traumatic play;

- imitation;
- as a vehicle for emotional abuse;
- self injury; and
- rehearsal for interpersonal violence.

Children may abuse animals because their parent or another person encourages or demands that they do so, for example as part of a domestic violence/child abuse situation.

Some parents threaten to harm, kill or give away pets to intimidate, punish and control the child, or to frighten the child from revealing their own abuse – repetition of this pattern can diminish the child's compassion towards animals (Loar and Colman, 2004).

One family therapist believes some abused children mimic their own mistreatment by abusing pets and suggests this could indicate a preoccupation with death or even serve as a rehearsal for the child's own suicide (Gill, 1994).

Children in violent homes are in a very stressful position as far as their relationship with animals is concerned. While animals are often the only source of comfort and safety these children have, they are regularly faced with the harm, death and disappearance of pets (Loar and Colman, 2004). The loss of this emotional support can have a profound effect on the children.

One child wrote of her pet loss (Raphael *et al.*, 1999, p. 25):

> I had too many pets that died.
> I really don't want to write about it.
> I can't tell you about them either.
> I just don't want to.
> It makes me too sad.
> Don't ask me any more.
> I will cry into the ocean.

It is essential that children's relationships with animals are taken seriously by their parents, teachers, medical staff and veterinarians. Children and animals can suffer physically and emotionally in violent homes and may constantly live with the fear of abuse. Not only are these children more likely to abuse animals, there are long-term detrimental effects on having healthy relationships as adults. It has been found that adults who abused animals as children were more likely to accept corporal punishment and hitting wives as part of family life (Flynn, 1999).

To stop this cycle of violence continuing, we need to consider where the abused and abusive children of today may be heading tomorrow without our intervention. A combined effort by veterinary and human health professionals will be most effective in identifying and helping humans and animals at risk.

References

Anderson, C.A. and Huesmann, L.R. (2003) Human aggression: a social-cognitive view. In: Hogg, M.A. and Cooper, J. (eds) *The Sage Handbook of Social Psychology.* Sage Publications, Thousand Oaks, California, pp. 296–323.

Arluke, A., Levin, J., Luke, C. and Ascione, F. (1999) The relationship of animal abuse to violence and other forms of antisocial behaviour. *Journal of Interpersonal Violence* 14, 963–975.

Ascione, F.R., Thompson, T.M. and Black, T. (1997) Childhood cruelty to animals: assessing cruelty dimensions and motivations. *Anthrozoös* 10(4), 170–197.

ASPCA (2012) The connection between domestic violence and animal cruelty. American Society for the Prevention of Cruelty to Animals. Available at: http://www.aspca.org/fight-animal-cruelty/domestic-violence-and-animal-cruelty.aspx (accessed 11 April 2012).

Baldry, A.C. (2003) Animal abuse and exposure to interparental violence in Italian youth. *Journal of Interpersonal Violence* 18(3), 258–281.

Bandura, A. (1973) *Aggression: A Social Learning Analysis.* Prentice Hall, Englewood Cliffs, New Jersey.

Barnes, J.E., Boat, B.W., Putnam, F.W., Dates, H.F. and Mahlman, A.R. (2006) Ownership of high-risk ('vicious') dogs as a marker for deviant behaviors: implications for risk assessment. *Journal of Interpersonal Violence* 21(12), 1616–1634.

BBC News Europe (2012) Anders Behring Breivik: Oslo bomb survivor testifies. 26 April. Available at: http://www.bbc.co.uk/news/world-europe-17852176 (accessed 26 April 2012).

Beirne, P. (2004) From animal abuse to interhuman violence? A critical review of the progression thesis. *Society and Animals* 12(1), 39–65.

Defra (2010) Public consultation on dangerous dogs. Department for Environment, Food and Rural Affairs, 9 March. Available at: http://webarchive.nationalarchives.gov.uk/20110202125928/http://www.defra.gov.uk/corporate/consult/dangerous-dogs/100309-dangerous-dogs-condoc.pdf (accessed 21 April 2012).

Dollard, J. and Miller, N. (1950) *Personality and Psychotherapy*. McGraw-Hill, New York.

Flynn, C. (1999) Animal abuse in childhood and later support for interpersonal violence in families. *Society and Animals* 7(2), 161–172.

Gill, E. (1994) Children and animals: a clinician's view. *The Animal's Agenda*, March/April, pp. 20–21.

Grant, D. (2010) cited in Morris, A. 'Status dogs: A reflection of a wider problem in society'. *Veterinary Record* 167(14), 508–509.

Green, P.C. and Gullone, E. (2005) Knowledge and attitudes of Australian veterinarians to animal abuse and human interpersonal violence. *Australian Veterinary Journal* 83(10), 619–625.

Gullone, E. (2009) A lifespan perspective on human aggression. In: Linzey, A. (ed.) *The Link Between Animal Abuse and Human Violence*. Sussex Academic Press, Eastbourne, UK.

Gullone, E., Johnson, J. and Volant, A. (2004) The link between animal abuse and family violence: a Victoria-wide study. In: *Australian Veterinary Association Welfare and Ethics group, Australian Veterinary Association Conference Proceedings*, AVAWE, Canberra, Australia.

Hensley, C. and Tallichet, S.E. (2005) Animal cruelty motivations: assessing demographic and situational influences. *Journal of Interpersonal Violence* 20, 1429–1443.

Hewitt, B., Harms, J. and Stewart, B. (1997) The avenger. *People*, 3 November, vol. 48, no. 18. Available at: http://www.people.com/people/archive/article/0,20123633,00.html (accessed 9 November 2011).

Hickey, E.W. (2006) *Serial Murderers and Their Victims*, 4th edn. Thomson Wadsworth, Belmont, California.

Horvath, M. (2011) cited in 'Multiple perpetrator rape a "National and international problem" warn experts', Middlesex University. Available at: http://www.mdx.ac.uk/aboutus/news-events/news/seminars.aspx (accessed 2 April 2012).

HSUS (2012) End Dogfighting – Preventing dogfighting by strengthening bonds between people and dogs. Humane Society of the United States, March 21. Available at: http://www.humanesociety.org/issues/dogfighting/end_dogfighting.html (accessed 21 April 2012).

Kellert, S.R. (1980) American attitudes toward and knowledge of animals: an update. *International Journal for the Study of Animal Problems* 1(2), 87–119.

Kellert, S.R. and Felthous, A.R. (1985) Childhood cruelty toward animals among criminals and noncriminals. *Human Relations* 38, 1113–1129.

Levin, J. (2008) *Serial Killers and Sadistic Murderers: Up Close and Personal*. Prometheus Books, Amherst, New York.

Loar, L. and Colman, L. (2004) *Teaching Empathy: Animal Assisted Therapy Programs for Children and Families Exposed to Violence*. The Latham Foundation, Alameda, California.

Mckean, B. (2009) Maximum term for torture of dog. *Daily Mercury* 4 September. Available at: http://www.dailymercury.com.au/story/2009/09/04/maximum-term-torture-familys-pet-dog/ (accessed 13 May 2011).

McLaughlin, E.C. (2011) From 'privileged' youth to afternoon of carnage. *CNN World*, July 27. Available at: http://articles.cnn.com/2011-07-27/world/norway.breivik.chronology_1_muslim-gangs-street-gangs-manifesto/2?_s=PM:WORLD (accessed 26 May 2012).

Metropolitan Police Service (n.d.) Dangerous dogs – get the facts. Available at: http://safe.met.police.uk/dangerous_dogs/get_the_facts.html (accessed 21 April 2012).

Miller, K.S. and Knutson, J.F. (1997) Reports of severe physical punishment and exposure to animal cruelty by inmates convicted of felonies and by university students. *Child Abuse & Neglect* 21(1), 59-82.

Mirabelli, J. (2012) cited in 'Man, teen arrested for animal cruelty, torture videos on YouTube', FOX Chicago News and Sun-Times Media Wire, 9 March. Available at: http://www.myfoxchicago.com/dpp/news/crime/joshua-moore-animal-cruelty-torture-videos-youtube-arrested-teen-boy-20120309 (accessed 11 April 2012).

Munro, H.M.C. (1999) The battered pet – signs and symptoms. In: Ascione, F.R. and Arkow, P. (eds) *Child Abuse, Domestic Violence and Animal Abuse*. Purdue University Press, West Lafayette, Indiana.

Munro, H.M.C. and Munro, R. (2008) *Animal Abuse and Unlawful Killing – Forensic Veterinary Pathology*. Saunders Elsevier, London.

Patronek, G.J. (2004) Animal cruelty, abuse, and neglect. In: Miller, L. and Zawistowski, S. (eds) *Shelter Medicine for Veterinarians and Staff*. Blackwell Publishing, Ames, Iowa, pp. 427–452.

Patterson-Kane, E.G. and Piper, H. (2009) Animal abuse as a sentinel for human violence: a critique. *The Journal of Social Issues* 65(3), 589–614.
Pet-abuse.com (2012) Animal abuse statistics. Available at: www.pet-abuse.com (accessed 2 April 2012).
Raphael, P., Colman, L. and Loar, L. (1999) *Teaching Compassion: a Guide for Humane Educators, Teachers, and Parents.* The Latham Foundation, Alameda, California.
Reitzel-Jaffe, D. and Wolfe, D.A. (2001) Predictors of relationship abuse among young men. *Journal of Interpersonal Violence* 16, 99–115.
SCAS (2010) Status dogs. Society for Companion Animal Studies. Available at: http://www.scas.org.uk/1931/status-dogs.html (accessed 21 April 2012).
Singer, P. (1995) *Animal Liberation.* Pimlico, London.
Steele, J. (2002) Horses injured in Millwall mob's attack. *The Telegraph*, 4 May. Available at: http://www.telegraph.co.uk/news/uknews/1393137/Horses-injured-in-Millwall-mobs-attack.html (accessed 21 April 2012).
Taylor, N. and Signal, T. (2006) Community demographics and the propensity to report animal cruelty. *Journal of Applied Animal Welfare Science* 9(3), 14–20.
Thompson, K.L. and Gullone, E. (2006) An investigation into the association between the witnessing of animal abuse and adolescents' behavior toward animals. *Society & Animals* 14(3), 221–243.
Tingle, D., Barnard, G.W., Robbins, L., Newman, G. and Hutchinson, D. (1986) Childhood and adolescent characteristics of pedophiles and rapists. *International Journal of Law and Psychiatry* 9, 103–116.
Verlinden, S. (2000) Risk factors in school shootings. Unpublished doctoral dissertation, Pacific University, Forest Grove, Oregon. Cited by Ascione, F.R. in Animal Abuse and Youth Violence. *Juvenile Justice Bulletin*, US Department of Justice, Office of Juvenile Justice and Delinquency Prevention, September 2001. Available at: https://www.ncjrs.gov/pdffiles1/ojjdp/188677.pdf (accessed 26 April 2012).
Wright, J. and Hensley, C. (2003) From animal cruelty to serial murder: applying the graduation hypothesis. *International Journal of Offender Therapy and Comparative Criminology* 47(1), 71–88.

4 Why Some People Care for Animals

Catherine Tiplady

Why are Some People Kind to Animals?

Fortunately, many people have compassion for animals. This chapter discusses people's empathy for animals, the nature of the human–animal bond and ways in which animal advocates may act to protect animals from abuse.

Human–Animal Bond

The emotional attachment between humans and animals is often referred to as the 'human–animal bond'. Knowledge of the human–animal bond helps us to understand the role animals play in people's lives and how we can encourage a positive, healthy relationship. It can also help us identify a failure to bond, which, in some cases, could lead to animal neglect and abuse.

Both veterinary students and practising veterinarians believe understanding the human–animal bond is important yet most feel they are not adequately trained in this area (Williams *et al.*, 1999; Martin and Taunton, 2005).

A number of researchers have studied emotional bonds and prominent among them is Bowlby, whose attachment theory describes the nature of emotional attachment in relationships (Bowlby, 1969, 1973, 1980). Applying Bowlby's attachment theory to a veterinary clinic setting, Meehan (n.d.) describes behaviours that people may show (via verbal or non-verbal behaviours) toward their pet:

1. Proximity seeking – seen in a veterinary client who wishes to stay in close proximity to their pet and when the pet wants to climb on the owner's lap and be close to them.
2. Separation distress – seen in a client who becomes distressed when away from their pet and shows grief when the animal is ill or euthanized.
3. Secure base – the pet is regarded as providing unconditional support, giving the client a feeling of security.
4. Safe haven – the pet is considered a source of support and safety when the client is experiencing personal stress such as divorce or a death in the family.

Some of the questions developed by Lago *et al.* (1988) that could be used to assess the strength of the human–animal bond in veterinary clients include the following:

- Do you buy your pet a birthday present?
- Do you think of him/her as a member of the family?
- Do you miss your pet when you are away?
- Is your pet up to date with his/her vaccinations?
- Do you enjoy playing with/exercising/grooming your pet?

Although a strong human–animal bond has benefits for animal welfare (by motivating owners to devote time and money to treat their animals), it is also a potential source of compromised welfare if highly bonded owners are reluctant to euthanize on humane grounds or if they allow behavioural problems and obesity to develop (Wensley, 2008).

Therapeutic Applications of the Human–Animal Bond

There are a range of programmes where the human–animal bond is used for therapeutic purposes, such as pets visiting hospitals and nursing homes, to warn owners of impending health problems such as seizures and as assistance animals for those with a disability. Prison programmes for young offenders to train shelter dogs benefit both humans and animals – they help the dogs find new homes and are successful in building people's self-esteem and reducing re-offending rates (discussed by Jacobs, 2011). Clinical applications and techniques for conducting animal assisted therapy are discussed further by Arkow (2011).

Application of the human–animal bond in pet therapy for children from violent homes is described by Zoe Hinds and Jenna Ooi in Chapter 13.

Compassion and Empathy

Compassion is defined as 'suffering together with another' and empathy as 'the power of projecting one's personality into, and so fully understanding, the object of contemplation' (Britannica, 1962). Empathy is often used synonymously with compassion, sympathy, kindness and sentimentality (Daly and Morton, 2003) and has been described as 'an innate, hardwired response connecting us as social beings to the emotional plights of others' (Zahn-Waxler and Radke-Yarrow, 1990 p. 111). As a social species we are biologically prepared to recognize and attend to the emotional needs of other humans (Hoffman, 1975).

Children and Empathy

Children have been described as having a 'natural connection' with animals (Randour and Davidson, 2008), and animals (both real animals and toys and story characters) play prominent roles in their lives. Part of animals' appeal is the emotional support they provide to children. It has been suggested that children feel an affinity to animals due to the common feeling of vulnerability within the family and, as such, may be observers or victims of abuse and neglect (Loar and Colman, 2004).

Parents widely believe that pet ownership is beneficial for children and often encourage their child's interest in animals. Perceived benefits include (Serpell, 1999):

- teaching a child responsibility;
- encouraging caring attitudes and behaviour;
- providing companionship, security and comfort;
- as a source of amusement; and
- as an outlet for affection.

These benefits of pet ownership may persist into adulthood. Paul (2000) has reported a positive relationship between human-oriented and animal-oriented empathy, finding that adults who owned pets in childhood, or currently owned pets, demonstrated greater empathy than non-pet-owners.

Some people choose to act on their empathy for animals by becoming members of advocacy groups, becoming vegetarian or vegan, purchasing 'cruelty-free' products or performing actions such as signing petitions. It has been found that those in the animal protection community (e.g. members of animal welfare and rights organizations) are significantly more likely to be pro-welfare than people in the general community (Signal and Taylor, 2006). A survey of over 2000 people aged 15 and over in the UK found that: 7% had been a member of an animal welfare organisation; 8% of respondents had been a vegetarian or vegan; 20% had signed a petition on an animal welfare issue; and 32% had bought 'cruelty-free' cosmetics, not tested on animals (Ipsos/MORI, 1999).

Although many people who wish to help abused animals are conservative in their approach and will limit their involvement to legal activities such as volunteering, fundraising and signing petitions, others are willing to take 'direct action' in their desire to protect animals. In some cases this may involve threats and damage to property and people. The next section will cover animal activism.

Animal Activists Who Take Direct Action

An animal activist is defined as 'a person who engages in different actions to bring about changes to the treatment and/or status of animals' (Olsson, 2010, p. 16). Although activism can include a wide range of positions and actions, activists are considered to hold 'more radical' positions than others (Olsson, 2010, p. 16). Some animal activists commit illegal acts such as arson, theft, burglary and breaking into laboratories to release or steal the animals (Bailey *et al.*, 2010) and may also threaten or harm those employed in animal experimentation (Paton, 1993).

Such events are quite common – according to the Foundation for Biomedical Research (2011), most states in the USA have experienced 'criminal activities in the name of "animal rights"' in the years 1997–2011. The actions of these activists cause anxiety to those who have been confronted with them, particularly if the targeted person's family members are also harmed or threatened (Kordower, 2007). A particularly upsetting example occurred during a 6-year campaign to close down a guinea pig breeding unit in the UK – the owners of the laboratory animal company reportedly were threatened and the body of their 82-year-old family member removed from her grave by activists (Cooper and Cooper, 2007). The activities of animal rights activists have been widely discussed in the media and scientific journals, with the latter warning that 'Anyone involved with animal research faces some degree of risk and can become a target of extremists' (Bailey *et al.*, 2010, p. 139).

Several scientific organizations offer guidelines to assist those believed to be vulnerable to such crimes. According to the Applied Research Ethics National Association and the Office of Laboratory Animal Welfare (ARENA/OLAW 2002, p. 71), there are four key elements to an institution's preparedness for 'anti-animal research' crises such as break-ins, vandalisms, threats and harassment:

- an animal care and use programme of impeccable integrity;
- a security programme, which is based on risk assessment;
- an integrated communication plan with descriptions of research projects in lay person's terminology, spokespersons and a telephone tree;[1] and
- an internal and external community outreach programme that includes legislators and funding agencies.

Many would regard activists who go to illegal lengths for animal rights as 'extremists' or even 'terrorists'. Others, however, may wonder who the real extremists are. In one well-known case of animal 'liberation' or theft, the Animal Liberation Front raided the University of California and seized hundreds of animals, among them 'Britches', a stump-tailed macaque monkey (ALF, n.d.(a)). Britches had been part of a sensory deprivation experiment in which he was born in the dark, removed from his mother and placed alone in a cage with his eyelids stitched together to simulate blindness (Fig. 4.1).

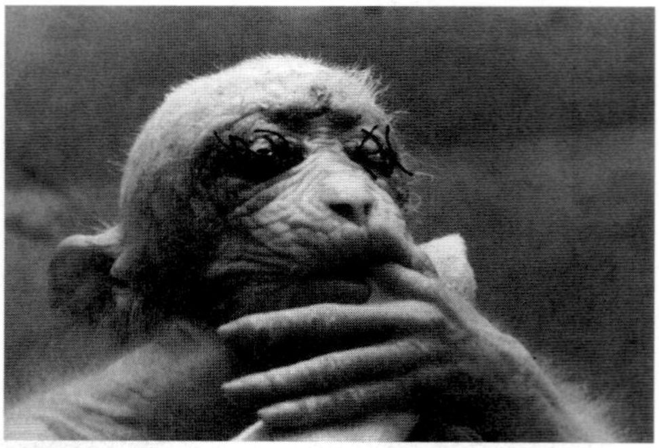

Fig. 4.1. This infant monkey, known as 'Britches', had his eyelids crudely stitched together as part of a sensory deprivation experiment. (Photograph courtesy of PETA.)

[1] A 'telephone tree' involves people taking a message and passing it on via telephone to a number of other people, who each pass on the message to a number of other people and so on. It enables a large group of people to be quickly contacted (Department of Sustainability and Environment, 2011).

A journal article written by the scientists involved in this research described the preparation for these experiments (Strelow *et al.*, 1987):

> Animals 2 and 3 had eyelids sutured, with additional bandages placed over the facial region. A capsule weighing 35 g, containing sonar transducers, eartubes and some of the electronics, was fixed over the eyes and snout with elastic straps and bandages.

Britches was removed from the laboratory by the Animal Liberation Front and taken to a veterinarian for examination and treatment. According to Ingrid Newkirk of PETA (ALF, n.d.(a)), the report by veterinarian Dr Bettina Flavioli stated:

> Beneath the bandages are two cotton pads, one for each eye . . . Both pads are filthy and soaked with moisture. Bilaterally upper eyelids are sutured to lower eyelids. The sutures are grossly oversized for the purpose intended. Many of these sutures have torn through lid tissue resulting in multiple lacerations of the lids. There is an open space between upper and lower lids of both eyes of about one quarter inch, and sutures are contacting corneal tissue resulting in excessive tearing . . .

Britches had his stitches removed and, when well enough, he was later transported to a monkey sanctuary for rehabilitation with other monkeys (Fig. 4.2).

If the lives of blind children could be improved by the sonar navigational study of which Britches was a part, is the suffering of monkeys justified? The president of the American Council of the Blind, Dr Grant Mack, reportedly called the experiment 'one of the most repugnant and ill-conceived boondoggles that I've heard about for a long time' (Britches, n.d.).

The Role of the Internet in Raising Public Awareness

Public involvement and education in animal abuse issues is increasingly achieved via Internet sites, as well as by traditional methods of posters,

(a) (b)

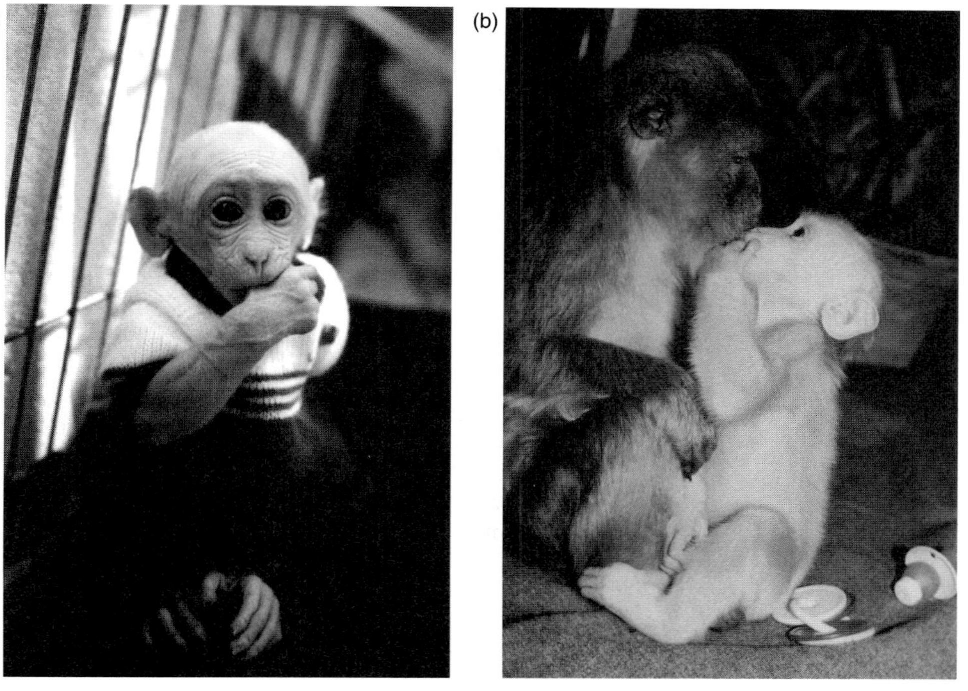

Fig. 4.2. (a) Britches was taken to a monkey sanctuary after being removed from the laboratory. (b) He is pictured gazing up at another monkey he met at the sanctuary. Britches lived until he was about 20 years old (ALF, n.d.(a)). (Photographs courtesy of PETA.)

brochures and exposés in the mainstream media. Such confrontation with images and descriptions of animal cruelty can be distressing to members of the public, yet many report feeling pleased that the media inform them of these issues (C. Tiplady *et al.*, 2012, unpublished results).

Stop Huntingdon Animal Cruelty (SHAC) is an international group that aims to close down Huntingdon Life Sciences, an organization that performs testing of a range of products and chemicals on animals (SHAC, n.d.(a)). SHAC, like many other activist groups, relies on the Internet to display powerful images, descriptions and video footage of animal abuse to inform the public, gain support for campaigns and drive change. Regardless of the country or setting (e.g. farm, abattoir, research laboratory, circus), the common feature of undercover videos by activists is animals being repeatedly physically and verbally abused by the people who are meant to protect their welfare.

Occasionally, co-workers are seen standing nearby ignoring or seemingly indifferent to the abuse. Are these isolated incidents? The frequency of animal cruelty exposés from around the world indicates that such abuse is a global problem, which would not reach the public eye if it were not for the work of activists. Undercover investigation is a feature of many animal advocacy campaigns, with supporters feeling this is the only way the public will learn about animal cruelty. The senior investigator of Compassion in World Farming has stated, 'Going undercover, often in dangerous situations, is the only way that the truth about intensive farming can be exposed' (CIWF, n.d.).

Activist groups emphasize that there is a range of activities that can be undertaken to help in a campaign against animal cruelty, both in the 'frontline' (such as attending protests) and behind the scenes (e.g. letter-writing campaigns) (SHAC, n.d.(a); PETA, 2012). Books have also been published that detail the various ways people can get involved to stop animal cruelty (Singer *et al.*, 1991; Stallwood, 2001; Hawthorne, 2008). Some activists train as animal attendants, veterinarians and scientists and work undercover within animal industries to document animal abuse. One such worker at Huntingdon Life Sciences reports being upset by seeing the dogs being abused (SHAC, n.d.(b)):

> Some dogs were not happy to be bled and they would struggle and not sit still. The licence holder would pull them around by the scruff, shout at them, and sometimes even used to pick the dog up off the chair by its scruff and have it dangling whilst they shouted at it. It could be a very disturbing time.
>
> I saw co-workers grab them by the scruff, shout and swear at them, swing them by the scruff and slap them. I was told I was 'too close' to my dogs because when I carried them to and from procedures I would hold them tight to me and cuddle and kiss them.

Common to many animal activist websites are guidelines to help people campaign against animal abuse, images and video footage of animal abuse, requests for donations, goods for sale (such as campaign T-shirts and stickers), options to sign up for email updates or become a member and links to research articles, publications and updates to recent news events in animal activism. Also on the SHAC website are contact details for those wishing to write to animal rights prisoners, a list of suppliers and customers of Huntingdon Life Sciences that are 'current targets' and a list of recommended criminal and civil lawyers who are experienced in defending activists (SHAC, n.d.(a)). Despite encouraging people to take action to stop animal cruelty, the SHAC newsletter carries a disclaimer that it is 'not intended to encourage illegal activity of any kind' (SHAC, 2011, p. 11).

The website of global group Animal Defenders International (ADI, 2012) covers a range of issues, including animals in circuses, laboratories and farms. Information about animal rescues and rehabilitation, links to the National Anti-Vivisection Society and scientific information on alternatives to animal testing are also included (ADI, 2012). Some animal advocacy groups also have a section of their website specifically aimed at young people, such as Animals Australia's 'Unleashed' (Animals Australia Unleashed, n.d.).

The successful use of the Internet and social media such as Facebook and Twitter to promote animal activism is particularly concerning to those supportive of animal testing, with some researchers stating (Bailey *et al.*, 2010, pp. 142–143):

> The AR [animal rights] movement no longer must depend on traditional media for publicity – propaganda and misinformation about animal

> research can be spread rapidly without interference from responsible, fact-checking journalists. On the web, AR organizations are free to create their own spin and use their own 'experts' to assert that animal research is cruel, 'bad,' or 'outdated' science and unnecessary because valid alternatives are available for every type of research.

Actually, animal rights groups often include reference to peer-reviewed scientific research on their websites and links to scientific organizations. Humane Research Australia (2012a) asks people to complain to the ethics committee and university that approved research in which pigs were given 'breast implants' (mammoplasty), some of which were deliberately infected with *Staphylococcus epidermidis*. A summary of this study, by Tamboto *et al.* (2010), is included on the website. Another study mentioned on the Humane Research Australia (2012b) website is that by Finnie *et al.* (2012), which involved anaesthetized lambs being shaken to death by researchers to replicate the effects of the child abuse 'shaken baby syndrome'. The National Anti-Vivisection Society (2004) has a 'Science Corner' and links to sites such as the Fund for the Replacement of Animals in Medical Experiments (FRAME), John Hopkins Center for Alternatives to Animal Testing and the UC Davis Center for Animal Alternatives as well as the Office of Laboratory Animal Welfare and US government animal welfare sites.

Similary, the American Association for Laboratory Animal Science (n.d.) includes links to websites promoting alternatives to animal testing, as well as animal adoption forms for those wishing to adopt healthy animals that were used for non-invasive research at several universities in the USA.

Veterinarian and animal advocate Dr Andrew Knight, on the topic of animal activism, argues that intelligent, strategic activism is needed, stating (Knight, n.d.):

> Truly ending animal experimentation requires awareness by governments, ethics committee members, scientists and the public of the poor human clinical and toxicological predictivity and utility of animal experiments, and of their burdensome cost:benefit ratio when compared to other means of protecting and advancing human health.

Public Attitudes to Animal Rights Groups and Animal Research

Most people oppose animal cruelty. A US study of over 1000 households found that 85% of respondents thought it was either 'very important' or 'important' to protect animals from cruelty (Lockwood, 2006).

Those who feel strongly about animal protection may take action by contacting politicians to outline their concerns and request change.

In the European Parliament, 'intergroups' have been formed to unite different political groups on specific issues, with one of the largest intergroups being dedicated to animal welfare. Neil Parish, the Chair of this intergroup, has said that 'animal welfare is the issue raised most frequently in my mailbag ... the intergroup is a powerful tool with which to fight the corner for animals' (European Parliament, 2007). Despite the strong feelings from the public about animal welfare, public demand for change may not be successful. UK politician Zac Goldsmith said although he had received 'a huge number of letters' supporting a ban on lions, tigers and elephants performing in circuses, the Government rejected introduction of a ban (Hickman, 2011).

One Australian politician with an interest in animal welfare believes the level of interest and concern for animal welfare issues amongst some politicians has declined (Bartlett, 2009). UK Member of Parliament Frank Field questions the government's lack of time devoted to the licensing of animal experiments. This is described in the following excerpt of his speech at the House of Commons (Field, 2011):

> Last year, 3.6 million experiments were licensed in this country to be performed on animals. Only three of those licences were referred to the Animal Procedures Committee for consideration. The others were decided by Home Office civil servants. If we tally up the number of experiments on animals that the House has agreed to since the establishment of the current system in 1986, we get a total of 65 million. I want to contrast the care that the House took over possible cruelty in hunting with dogs with the care we have taken in our supervisory role for those 65 million experiments. The House spent 700 hours considering changing the law on hunting with

> dogs. We spent only 7 hours committing our country to the war in Iraq. We did not spend 1 second on those 65 million experiments.

A UK political party 'Animals Count' was formed in 2006 with the mission (Animals Count, n.d.):

> To establish a voice for the animals through a dedicated political party that focuses on respect and compassion for all living beings.

Among their key policies were to (Animals Count, 2010):

- phase out farming practices with poor welfare consequences for animals;
- educate children about the importance of compassion and respect towards all living beings; and
- eliminate the failed practice of animal experimentation.

A survey of adults in Britain conducted by Ipsos/MORI (2011) found that one in three people do not support the use of animals in any experimentation because of the importance they place on animals, and one in six (17%) agree that the government should ban all experiments on animals for any form of research.

Most people surveyed supported activities by animal rights groups such as:

- handing out leaflets (81%);
- writing letters (76%);
- asking people to put a sticker or poster in their window (71%); and
- organizing petitions (70%).

Most feel it is not acceptable to use terrorist methods (85%), use physical violence (82%) or destroy or damage property (82%), and less than half feel that demonstrating outside research laboratories is acceptable (48%) (Ipsos/MORI, 2011).

It is worthwhile learning more about the beliefs of activists who are willing to take direct action in their desire to protect animals.

Who Are the Animal Activists?

Animal activists come from all professions and age groups, although the majority are female (Groves, 1997; Galvin and Herzog, 1998; Munro, 2001) and only a small minority report being involved with groups that take direct action (Herzog, 1993). Not surprisingly, activists prefer to describe themselves as 'compassionate' and 'determined' rather than 'misguided' or 'extremists' (SHAC, n.d.(c)). Some activists may harm their own health in their desire to help the animals and highlight their suffering. Barry Horne, a UK animal activist, undertook several lengthy hunger strikes and died while serving a sentence for crimes against companies involved in vivisection (Barry Horne Animal Liberationist, n.d.). Guidance on how to care for yourself while working with animal abuse is provided in Chapter 14.

Typically, those who use animals in their work (e.g. farmers and those using animals for experiments) are viewed with suspicion by animal activists. The feeling of distrust appears to be mutual and is not helped by the apparent secrecy in the way many animals are housed and used in laboratories and farms. Members of the scientific community may be fearful of activists. When one researcher told scientist colleagues he would be interviewing activists for a research paper, he received negative responses such as 'those people are just crazy' and 'aren't you afraid of talking to them?' (Herzog, 1993, p. 118). Herzog reports that he actually found the activists to be 'intelligent, articulate, and sincere' and that most were surprised and pleased that a scientist was interested in hearing their views (Herzog, 1993, p. 118).

Other researchers have surveyed activists for their views on the effectiveness of their campaign tactics. They found that 'disruptive' tactics (harassment of researchers and liberation of laboratory animals) were considered by activists to have been the least effective methods of activism and company boycotts, setting personal examples, attending marches (Fig. 4.3) and demonstrations as having been the most effective (Galvin and Herzog, 1998). Education of school students to the importance of ethical issues was deemed as the most important future tactic, and none of the respondents surveyed advocated physically harming their opponents (Galvin and Herzog, 1998).

Although numerous activist organizations exist around the world, the Animal Liberation Front is one of the best known due to their direct

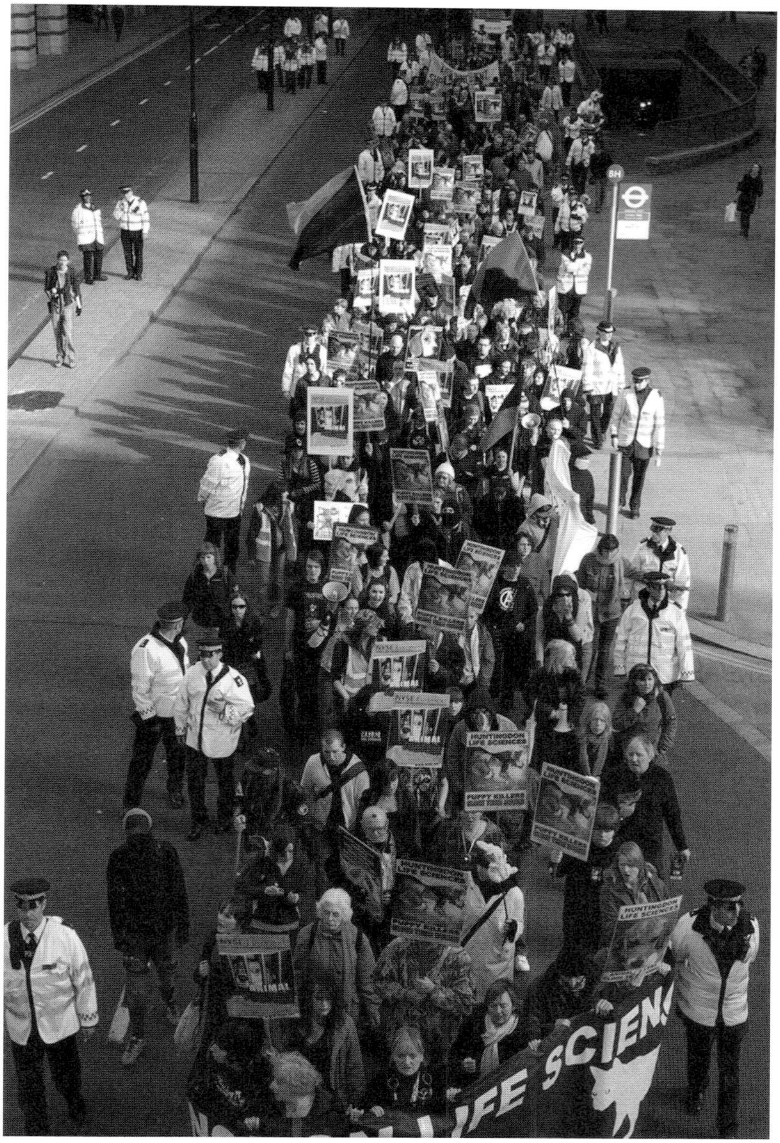

Fig. 4.3. Supporters of SHAC ('Stop Huntingdon Animal Cruelty') in a protest march. (Photograph courtesy of SHAC.)

action – the letters 'ALF' are often written on walls to indicate that they were responsible. To understand more about how they operate, their credo is included here (Animal Liberation Front, n.d.(b)):

> The Animal Liberation Front (ALF) carries out direct action against animal abuse in the form of rescuing animals and causing financial loss to animal exploiters, usually through the damage and destruction of property.
>
> The ALF's short-term aim is to save as many animals as possible and directly disrupt the practice of animal abuse. Their long term aim is to end all animal suffering by forcing animal abuse companies out of business.

It is a nonviolent campaign, activists taking all precautions not to harm any animal (human or otherwise).

Because ALF actions may be against the law, activists work anonymously, either in small groups or individually, and do not have any centralized organization or coordination.

The Animal Liberation Front consists of small autonomous groups of people all over the world who carry out direct action according to the ALF guidelines. *Any group of people who are vegetarians or vegans and who carry out actions according to ALF guidelines have the right to regard themselves as part of the ALF.*

Clearly, although most people oppose animal abuse, the ways in which they choose to act are diverse.

A series of interviews with people who work to prevent and raise awareness of animal abuse is included in Part 6 of this book.

References

American Association for Laboratory Animal Science (n.d.) The Institutional Animal Care and Use Committee. Available at: http://www.iacuc.org/aboutus.htm (accessed 13 May 2012).

Animal Defenders International (ADI) (2012) About us. Available at: http://www.ad-international.org (accessed 14 May 2012).

Animal Liberation Front (ALF) (n.d.(a)) Britches' story. Available at: http://animalliberationfront.com/ALFront/Actions-USA/BritchesStory.htm (accessed 12 December 2011).

Animal Liberation Front (ALF) (n.d.(b)) The ALF credo and guidelines. Available at: www.animalliberationfront.com (accessed 21 January 2012).

Animals Australia Unleashed (n.d.) Animals Australia Unleashed. Available at: http://www.unleashed.org.au (accessed 7 April 2012).

Animals Count (n.d.) Aims and principles. Available at: http://www.animalscount.org/manifesto/aims (accessed 12 April 2012).

Animals Count (2010) 2010 General Election manifesto. Available at: http://www.animalscount.org/manifesto/2010-ge-manifesto (accessed 1 October 2012).

ARENA/OLAW (2002) Institutional Animal Care and Use Committee Guidebook, 2nd edn. Available at: http://grants.nih.gov/grants/olaw/GuideBook.pdf (accessed 13 May 2012), p. 71.

Arkow, P. (2011) *Animal-assisted Therapy and Activities: A study and research resource guide for the use of companion animals in animal-assisted interventions*, 10th edn. AnimalTherapy.net, Stratford, New Jersey.

Bailey, M.R., Rich, B.A. and Bennett, B.T. (2010) Crisis planning to manage risks posed by animal rights extremists. *Institute for Laboratory Animal Research Journal* 51(2), 138–148.

Barry Horne Animal Liberationist (n.d.) Barry Horne – animal liberationist. Available at: http://www.barryhorne.org (accessed 19 April 2012).

Bartlett, A. (2009) Animal welfare in a federal system: a federal politician's perspective. In: Sankoff, P. and White, S. (eds) *Animal Law in Australasia*. The Federation Press, Annandale, New South Wales, Australia, pp. 376–388.

Bowlby, J. (1969) *Attachment and Loss*, Vol. 1. *Attachment*. Basic Books, New York.

Bowlby, J. (1973) *Attachment and Loss*, Vol. 2. *Separation: Anxiety and Anger*. Basic Books, New York.

Bowlby, J. (1980) *Attachment and Loss*, Vol. 3. *Loss: Sadness and Depression*. Basic Books, New York.

Britannica (1962) *Britannica World Language Edition of the Oxford Dictionary*. Oxford University Press, London.

Britches (n.d.) Britches' story. Available at: http://www.britches.org.uk/story.asp (accessed 6 April 2012).

Compassion in World Farming (CIWF) (n.d.) Going undercover to expose cruelty to farm animals. Available at: http://www.ciwf.org.uk/what_we_do/investigations/672 default.aspx (accessed 6 August 2011).

Cooper, J.E. and Cooper, M.E. (2007) *Introduction to Veterinary and Comparative Forensic Medicine*. Blackwell Publishing, Oxford, UK.

Daly, B. and Morton, L.L. (2003) Children with pets do not show higher empathy: a challenge to current views. *Anthrozoös* 16(4), 298–314.

Department of Sustainability and Environment (2011) Telephone trees. Available at: http://www.dse.vic.gov.au/effective-engagement/toolkit/tool-telephone-trees (accessed 6 April 2012).

European Parliament (2007) Intergroups: MEPs unite on single issues across party lines. Available at: http://www.europarl.europa.eu/sides/getDoc.do?pubRef=-//EP//TEXT+IM-PRESS+20070314STO04219+0+DOC+XML+V0//EN (accessed 8 September 2011).

Field, F. (2011) 'House of Commons main chamber debates', 5 April. Available at: http://www.theyworkforyou.com//debates/?id=2011-04-05c.979.1&s=speaker%3A10197#g993.0 (accessed 11 May 2012).

Finnie, J.W., Blumbergs, P.C., Manavis, J., Turner, R.J., Helps, S., Vink, R., Byard, R.W., Chidlow, G., Sandoz, B., Dutschke, J. and Anderson, R.W.G. (2012) Neuropathological changes in a lamb model of non-accidental head injury (the shaken baby syndrome). *Journal of Clinical Neuroscience: Official Journal of The Neurosurgical Society of Australasia* 19(8), 1159–1164.

Foundation for Biomedical Research (2011) Illegal incidents 1997 – present. Available at: http://fbresearch.wsol.net/OneColumnWireframe.aspx?pageid=169 (accessed 6 April 2012).

Galvin, S.L. and Herzog, H.A. (1998) Attitudes and dispositional optimism of animal rights demonstrators. *Society and Animals* 6(1), 1–11.

Groves, J.M. (1997) *Hearts and Minds: The Controversy over Laboratory Animals.* Temple University Press, Philadelphia, Pennsylvania.

Hawthorne, M. (2008) *Striking at the Roots – a practical guide to animal activism.* O-Books, Winchester, UK.

Herzog, H.A. (1993) 'The movement is my life': the psychology of animal rights activism. *Journal of Social Issues* 49(1), 103–119.

Hickman, M. (2011) Zac Goldsmith attacks refusal to outlaw wild animals in circuses. *The Independent,* 8 June. Available at: http://www.independent.co.uk/news/uk/politics/zac-goldsmith-attacks-refusal-to-outlaw-wild-animals-in-circuses-2294697.html (accessed 19 September 2011).

Hoffman, M.L. (1975) Developmental synthesis of affect and cognition and its interplay for altruistic motivation. *Developmental Psychology* 11, 607–622.

Humane Research Australia (2012a) Breast implants on pigs. Available at: http://www.humaneresearch.org.au/case-studies/porcine-implants (accessed 14 May 2012).

Humane Research Australia (2012b) Shaking baby lambs to death. Available at: http://www.humaneresearch.org.au/case-studies/shaking-baby-lambs-to-death (accessed 13 July 2012).

Ipsos/MORI (1999) Attitudes Towards Experimentation on Live Animals. Available at: http://www.ipsos-mori.com/researchpublications/researcharchive/poll.aspx?oItemId=1883 (accessed 13 May 2012).

Ipsos/MORI (2011) Attitudes towards the activities of animal rights organisations. In: Views on Animal Experimentation (BIS research)/Alternatives to Animal Experimentation (NC3R research) vol. 1. Available at: http://www.ipsos-mori.com/Assets/Docs/SRI_HEALTH_BIS_NC3Rs_combined_animal_experimentation_2011_FINAL_report_PUBLIC_110411.pdf (accessed 14 May 2012).

Jacobs, C. (2011) Benefits of animal-assisted interventions to young offenders. *Veterinary Record* 169, 115–117.

Knight, A. (n.d.) Campaigning to end animal experimentation. Available at: http://www.andrewknight.info/presentations/presentations/animal_expt_campaigns.html (accessed 10 April 2012).

Kordower, J. (2007) In: Miller, G.: Animal extremists get personal. *Science* 318(5858), 1856–1858.

Lago, D., Kafer, R., Delaney, M. and Connell, C. (1988) Assessment of favorable attitudes toward pets: development and preliminary validation of self report pet relationship scales. *Anthrozoös* 1(4), 240–254.

Loar, L. and Colman, L. (2004) *Teaching Empathy: animal-assisted therapy programs for children and families exposed to violence.* A Latham Foundation Publication, Alameda, California.

Lockwood, R. (2006) *Animal Cruelty Prosecution: Opportunities for Early Response to Crime and Interpersonal Violence.* American Prosecutors Research Institute, Alexandria, Virginia.

Martin, F. and Taunton, A. (2005) Perceptions of the human-animal bond in veterinary education of veterinarians in Washington State: structured versus experiential learning. *Journal of Veterinary Medical Education* 32(4), 523–530.

Meehan, M.P. (n.d.) Human-animal bond part 1. Bayer Accelerate course notes. Available at: http://www.bayeraccelerate.com.au (accessed 23 April 2012).

Munro, L. (2001) Caring about blood, flesh, and pain: women's standing in the Animal Protection Movement. *Society & Animals* 9, 43–61.

National Anti-Vivisection Society (2004) The NAVS resource center. Available at: http://navs.convio.net/site/PageServer?pagename=ResourceCenter (accessed 10 April 2012).

Olsson, A. (2010) Animal Activist. In: Marchant-Forde, J.N., McGreevy, P.D., Mills, D.S., Morton, D.B. and Nicol, C.J. (eds) *The Encyclopedia of Applied Animal Behaviour and Welfare.* CAB International, Wallingford, UK, p. 16.

Paton, W. (1993) *Man and Mouse – animals in medical research.* Oxford University Press, Oxford, UK.
Paul, E.S. (2000) Empathy with animals and with humans: are they linked? *Anthrozoös* 13(4), 194–202.
PETA (2012) Join PETA's action team and help animals. Available at: http://www.peta.org/action/action-team/default.aspx (accessed 5 April 2012).
Randour, M.L. and Davidson, H. (2008) *A Common Bond: maltreated children and animals in the home, guidelines for practice and policy.* American Humane, Englewood, Colorado.
Serpell, J. (1999) Guest editor's introduction: Animals in children's lives. *Society and Animals* 7(2), 87.
SHAC (n.d.(a)) Introduction to SHAC. Available at: http://www.shac.net/SHAC/shac_intro.html (accessed 14 May 2012).
SHAC (n.d.(b)) Inside HLS. Available at: http://www.shac.net/HLS/exposed/inside_hls/Inside_HLS_Full_Report.html (accessed 18 April 2012).
SHAC (n.d.(c)) Campaigners. Available at: http://www.shac.net/SHAC/campaigners.html (accessed 14 May 2012).
SHAC (2011) SHAC newsletter 56. Available at: http://www.shac.net/resources/newsletters/Newsletter56.pdf (accessed 18 April 2012).
Signal, T. and Taylor, N. (2006) Attitudes to animals within the animal protection community compared to a normative community sample. *Society & Animals* 14(3), 265–274.
Singer, P., Dover, B. and Newkirk, I. (1991) *Save the Animals! 101 Easy things you can do.* Collins Angus & Robertson, North Ryde, New South Wales, Australia.
Stallwood, K.W. (ed.) (2001) *Speaking Out For Animals.* Lantern Books, New York.
Strelow, E.R., Warren, D.H., Sonnier, B.J., Riesen, A.H., Kay, L. and Sinton, J. (1987) Behavioral observations of sensory substitution in neonate macaques (*Macaca arctoides*). *Behavioural Neuroscience* 101(5), 738–741.
Tamboto, H., Vickery, K. and Deva, A.K. (2010) Subclinical (biofilm) infection causes capsular contracture in a porcine model following augmentation mammoplasty. *Plastic and Reconstructive Surgery* 126(3), 835–842.
Wensley, S.P. (2008) Animal welfare and the human-animal bond: considerations for veterinary faculty, students, and practitioners. *Journal of Veterinary Medical Education* 35(4), 532–539.
Williams, S., Butler, C. and Sontag, M.A. (1999) Perceptions of fourth-year veterinary students about the human-animal bond in veterinary practice and in veterinary college curricula. *Journal of the American Veterinary Medical Association* 215(10), 1428–1432.
Zahn-Waxler, C. and Radke-Yarrow, M. (1990) The origins of empathic concern. *Motivation and Emotion* 14, 107–130.

Part II

Animal Abuse in Culture and Society

Although animals are abused for a range of reasons and in a range of situations, some abuse is accepted and defended by certain cultures, groups and societies. Understanding how religion, philosophy and ethics affect our treatment of animals is essential to help us comprehend different people's treatment of animals. This section covers contentious topics of animal use and abuse in food and fibre production as well as in hunting, sport, entertainment, art and veterinary education. Feminist aspects of animal abuse are also included here, drawing comparisons between the abuse of animals and the abuse of women and describing how animals are sexually abused in pornography.

5 Animal Abuse in Food and Fibre Production

Catherine Tiplady

Although some people consider that any use of animals for food and fibre production is inherently cruel others find it acceptable under certain conditions, such as free-range farming. Along with increasing intensification of livestock production, people are becoming increasingly concerned about the welfare of farmed animals.

Many people live in urban areas and do not know how animal products are produced and may rely on the media rather than farmers to learn about farming. Opportunities to visit intensive farms are few, probably due to a combination of biosecurity concerns and a deliberate attempt by farmers to conceal certain farming methods (e.g. sow stalls, caged hens) from the public. Distancing of consumers in this way is widely criticized among animal advocates who describe a 'veil of silence' surrounding animal production (Gellatley and Wardle, 1996).

This section will focus on the issue of abuse in intensively farmed animals, using the primary examples of poultry and pigs. It is acknowledged, however, that abuse also occurs among many other species as well as in extensively farmed animals.

Industrialization of agriculture began after the Second World War to supply food for a growing and increasingly urbanized population. Human labour was replaced by machinery and farm animals were moved into intensive housing systems, as described in Ruth Harrison's book *Animal Machines* (1964). In 1965, a committee (the Brambell Committee) was established by the UK Ministry of Agriculture to investigate the welfare of intensively housed farm animals. This committee developed 'The Five Freedoms', a set of guidelines that could be used to evaluate the welfare of farm animals (Brambell Committee, 1965). The Five Freedoms (Freedom from hunger and thirst; Freedom from discomfort; Freedom from pain, injury or disease; Freedom to express normal behaviour; Freedom from fear and distress) can be applied to all animal species and have since been widely adopted by animal welfare organizations, such as the RSPCA.

The egg industry was one of the first areas of agriculture to experience industrialization and with this intensification has come welfare concerns and allegations of abuse.

Abuse of Poultry

Egg-laying chickens

Osteoporosis is a major predisposing factor for bone fractures and is increased in layer hens kept in cages where they have restricted movement (Whitehead, 2004). Researchers have found that hens are highly motivated to perform dust-bathing behaviour (Lindberg and Nicol, 1997) and will work harder to gain access to a nest box in which to lay eggs than they will to have access to food (Cooper and Appleby, 2003). Beak trimming is commonly practised (without anaesthesia or analgesia) in an attempt to minimize feather pecking (Fig. 5.1) and cannibalism between hens – around a third of the young chick's beak is removed and the resulting nerve and tissue damage can cause both acute and chronic pain (Cheng, 2006).

Forced moulting is a method used by some egg producers to keep hens laying eggs for longer and improve shell quality – hens are deliberately starved until they have lost approximately 30% of their body weight (Duncan, 2001; Fraser *et al.*, 2001). This causes extreme distress and the formation of stereotyped pacing (Mench, 1992; Duncan, 2001).

Hens suffer foot injuries from constantly standing on wire. As they are not able to use their claws for natural behaviours of scratching and foraging, the claws grow overly long and may become deformed (Fig. 5.2).

Despite the obvious welfare concerns, millions of hens remain in cages. Is this animal abuse on a massive scale? Clearly the conventional cage systems supply virtually no behavioural needs of the hen. Supporters of the cage system could argue that cages provide shelter, food, water and contact with their co-specifics (albeit in a very confined manner). It could be argued that the entire system of egg production is ethically wrong, killing the vast majority of unwanted male chicks (often by maceration or carbon dioxide gas) and denying chickens the opportunity to live in a natural way in small family groups, hatching and raising their chicks.

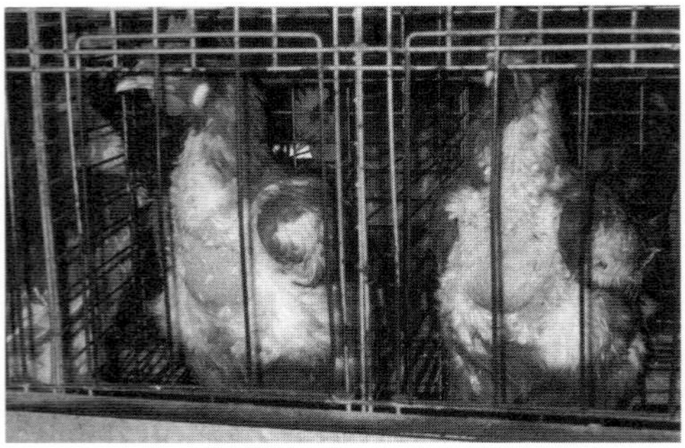

Fig. 5.1. Caged hens suffer due to the way they are housed and feather pecking is a common problem. Beaks are often trimmed (without analgesia or anaesthesia) while the birds are chicks. The birds in this photograph have not had their beaks trimmed. (Photograph courtesy of Catherine Tiplady.)

Meat chickens

Many meat (broiler) chickens (Fig. 5.3) suffer greatly. Bred to rapidly gain weight, they are usually killed at less than 40 days of age. During their short lives they may endure pain from lameness, heart disease and collapse on the floor of the sheds in which they are kept and be unable to access food and water. These birds are also at risk of injury during capture, transportation and slaughter. Standards of care for meat chickens vary greatly depending on the country in which the chickens live.

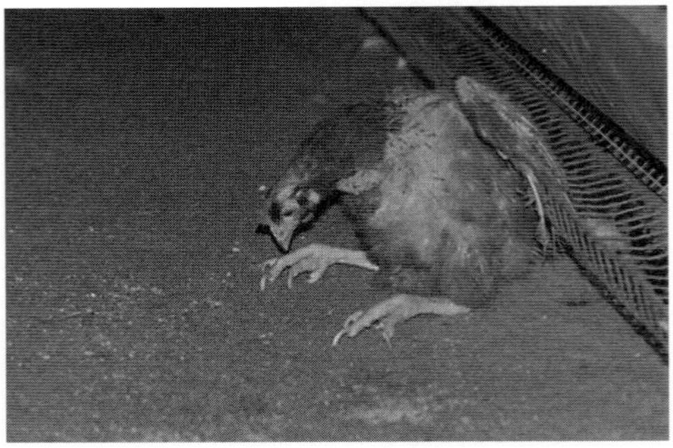

Fig. 5.2. Lame hen removed from her cage. (Photograph courtesy of Animals Australia.)

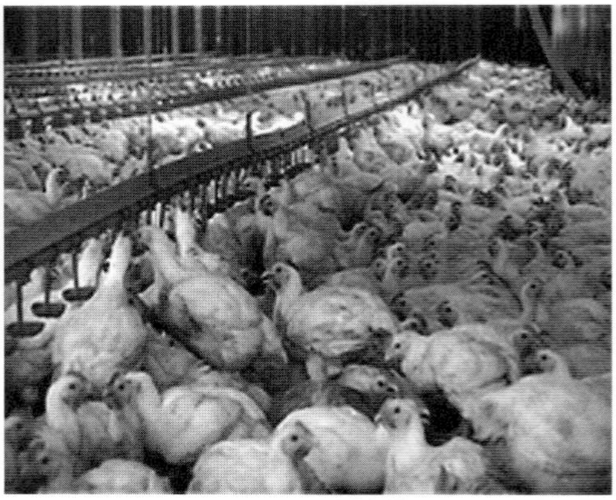

Fig. 5.3. Chickens in intensive farm. (Photograph courtesy of WSPA.)

Foie gras

Foie gras production is inherently cruel, yet is considered a delicacy to many. To produce pâté de foie gras, geese and ducks are force fed by inserting a funnel into the bird's oesophagus and feeding a wet mash through it, after which the bird goes into a torpor for up to 5 hours (Gregory, 2004). The birds are housed in very confined cages and just before liver failure occurs they are killed, although some will die during the force-feeding process (Broom and Fraser, 2007). Birds used for foie gras production are denied the ability to express natural behaviours important to them, such as flying, swimming and feather preening.

Ortolan

The eating of the ortolan, a small wild bird, in France has historically been considered a great delicacy, yet the preparation has involved extreme cruelty. The birds were traditionally blinded with a knife, kept in a dark box to be fattened on millet and, finally, drowned in brandy and cooked in their own fat 'until they sing' (Paterniti, 1998). The ortolan is then eaten whole, the diner covering their head with a large, white napkin before they chew and swallow the beak, bones, skull, feathers and internal organs.

Although ortolan hunting is now banned in France, poachers kill up to 50,000 of these birds per year – if caught, poachers are fined, yet most are only given a verbal warning (Mount, 2010).

Abuse of Pigs

Intensive housing of pigs in dry sow/gestation stalls and farrowing crates (Figs 5.4 and 5.5) is considered a major welfare concern and is widely condemned as cruel. Supporters of the intensive systems defend the practice, pointing out benefits for the pigs in being kept this way (protection from the weather and predators, preventing sows from crushing piglets and enhanced ability of the stockpeople to closely monitor the sow and piglets' health).

Piglets are often subjected to a range of painful procedures early in life (including castration, tail docking, teeth clipping), all without any analgesia or anaesthesia.

Lameness, skin sores, gastric ulceration and stereotypic behaviour are a few of the issues seen among intensively farmed pigs. Abusive handling during husbandry procedures and slaughter has also been reported. A video filmed at an abattoir in England shows pigs being beaten with a bat, kicked, punched in the head, dragged by their ears and burned by cigarettes (Caba, 2011).

Dogs and Cats as Meat Animals

Dog meat is considered a delicacy in places including southern China, Korea, the northern Philippines, Cambodia, Laos and Nigeria (Gregory, 2007). Dog meat is believed by some South Koreans to have medicinal properties (Gerges, 2012) and eating dogs seems to be linked to national identity (Podberscek, 2009). While the idea of eating dogs and cats may shock some people, particularly Westerners who tend to view cats and dogs as pets, it is really no more shocking than eating a pig or sheep. Eating a dog is not necessarily an abusive act; however, the manner in which the animal was kept, transported and slaughtered can certainly involve cruelty.

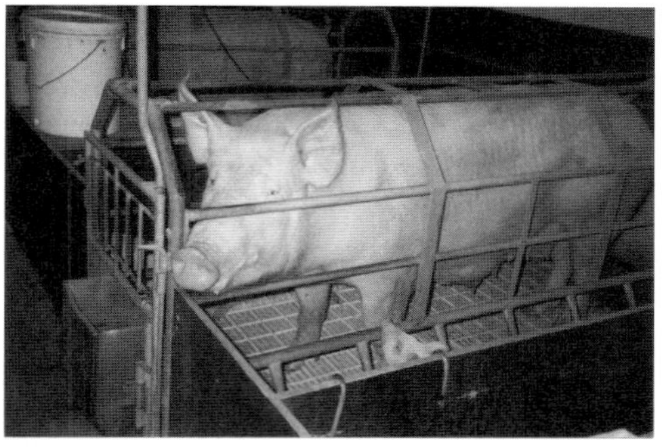

Fig. 5.4. A sow in farrowing crate with her piglet looking up at her. Intensively housed sows in stalls or crates are denied the ability to walk, turn, interact with their young (other than suckling), nest build, wallow or play. They do, however, have shelter, food, water and are easy to examine by the farmer. Do the advantages of such intensive housing outweigh the disadvantages? (Photograph courtesy of Catherine Tiplady.)

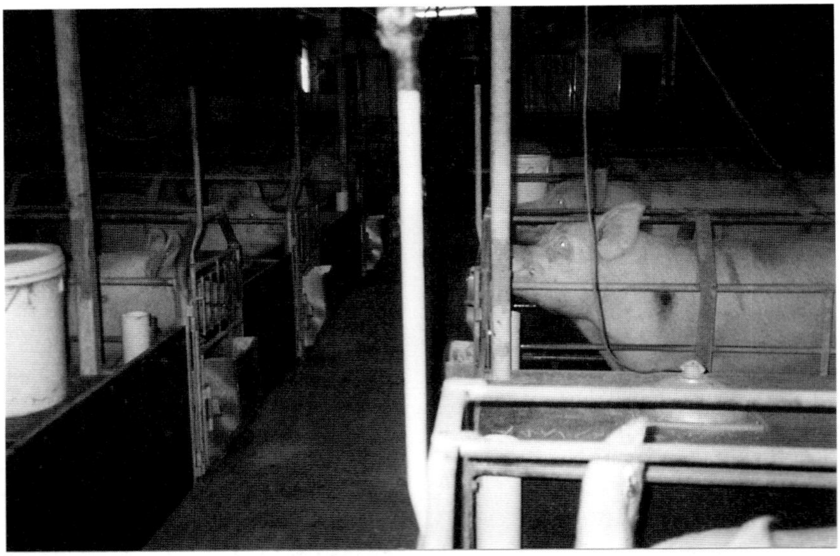

Fig. 5.5. Sows in farrowing crates. The sow on the right side of the photograph has a skin sore on her shoulder. Intensively housed sows are typically kept on concrete or slatted floors without any bedding, and pressure sores and lameness often develop. (Photograph courtesy of Catherine Tiplady.)

The pet status of dogs and subsequent criticism of dog eating has led to it being performed in secrecy (Gregory, 2007). This undercover approach may have a negative welfare impact as by removing an activity from the public gaze it can become difficult to monitor.

Dogs used for meat are usually not grown specifically for this purpose but may be stolen, old, sick, semi-feral or feral and taken to markets by walking with them or transporting them in trucks, which may be confined and unhygienic (Gregory, 2007).

Various methods of slaughter are mentioned by Gregory (2007):

- In the Ogun region of Nigeria, some dogs are sacrificed by killing with an iron object to appease Ogun, the god of iron. Dogs may be killed by stabbing with a knife or running them over with a car, a method that is gaining in popularity.
- In some rural areas of the Philippines it is customary to beat dogs before they are killed. This may be performed by tying or suspending the dog and beating it with a cane. Dogs may also be beaten to death with a heavier stick. The aim is to pulverize the muscle, cause bruising and tenderize the meat.
- Dogs used for meat in South Korea were traditionally hanged and beaten to death with sticks – this was believed to tenderize the meat and increase its aphrodisiacal qualities (Podberscek, 2009). Electrocution is reported to be another method of killing dogs for meat (Corrall, 2002).

Educating people in humane methods of dog euthanasia may help the welfare of dogs used for human consumption, but is unlikely to be accepted if there are entrenched cultural beliefs that live dogs must be beaten and bruised to improve the quality of the meat. Video footage of dogs and puppies transported in Asia (Gerges, 2012) shows puppies crammed into tiny cages on a truck, the animals vocalizing and in very poor condition (Gerges, 2012). It is possible, if dogs are to be eaten, to raise them and slaughter them in a much more humane manner than the appalling methods of beating them to death or driving over them. Use of barbiturates is not an option in animals destined for food consumption. One idea for killing these dogs is shooting through the skull by highly skilled operators – according to the AVMA euthanasia guidelines (AVMA, 2007, p. 13), 'A properly placed gunshot can cause immediate insensibility and humane death'. Considering the way many 'farm' animals are kept and slaughtered in other cultures, it is not acceptable simply to condemn and ignore people who choose to kill and eat other animals as part of their culture.

Abuse in Animals for Production of Fibre – Feathers, Fur and Skins

Feathers, skins, leather, silk, wool and fur production can involve abuse, and these are often by-products of the meat industry. Although feather plucking from live birds is 'likely to be painful' (Gentle and Hunter, 1991), manual plucking of down and feathers from live geese may be performed every 6–7 weeks from 10 weeks of age until slaughter (Rosinski, n.d.).

Silk production involves baking the cocoons of the silkworms or dropping them into vats of boiling water while they are undergoing metamorphosis – approximately 3000 silkworm pupae are killed to make 1 pound of silk (PETA Asia Pacific, 2012). Does this cause pain and is it animal abuse? It is advised that we should assume invertebrates feel pain 'unless it can be proved to the contrary' (Cooper, 2006, p. 215). Silk can be produced in a way that does not harm the silkworm pupae, although it is unlikely that this will replace the large-scale, conventional methods of silk production.

Wool production

Merino sheep originated in Spain and are commonly used for wool production, particularly in Australia. To prevent these wrinkly-skinned sheep from getting fly-strike or cutaneous myiasis (maggots burrowing into the urine- or faecal-soaked perineal skin), they are 'mulesed'. Mulesing involves cutting off loose skin around the hindquarters of a sheep to result in hairless scar tissue, which is less likely to attract dampness and flies. Typically, mulesing has been practised without providing any analgesic or anaesthetic. Research has found that mulesed lambs show behavioural changes (reduced feeding, resting and abnormal gait) for 3 weeks after the procedure (Hemsworth *et al.*, 2009).

Fine-wool sheep

Fine-wool sheep are those that produce fleece of a very fine micron. They are kept individually penned in enclosures as small as 0.9 m^2 (Code of Practice for the Welfare of Sheep, 2008).

These sheep wear nylon coats and are housed in pens 24 hours a day for up to 5 years, to supply 'Ultra-fine' wool to the international fashion market (Animals Australia, n.d.). Stereotypic behaviours are a problem in many chronically confined animals. The sheep in Fig. 5.6 is chewing on the wire of the enclosure.

Fur farming

Farming of animals for fur is widely condemned as cruel, yet leather from cattle is generally accepted by Western society. Animals used specifically for fur production include ferrets, foxes, raccoons, mink, coypu, chinchillas and sable, as well as dogs and cats (Broom and Fraser, 2007). Cages are often small and barren with bare wire floors (Fig. 5.7), which do not satisfy

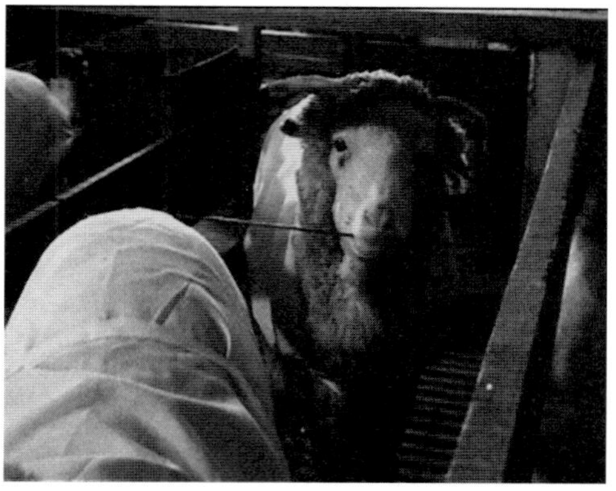

Fig. 5.6. Fine-wool sheep. (Photograph courtesy of Animals Australia.)

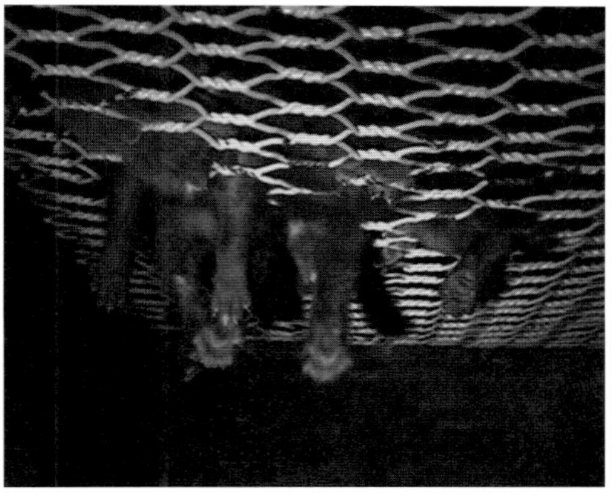

Fig. 5.7. Fox cubs' legs protruding through wire of cage in a fur farm. (Photograph courtesy of Animal Defenders International.)

the animals' requirements to perform natural behaviours such as swimming (mink), and self-mutilation and stereotypic behaviours can occur at high levels (Broom and Fraser, 2007). Many animals farmed for fur are allegedly killed in a cruel way (Fig. 5.9), such as electrocution and live skinning (WSPA, n.d.(a)) and the animals can suffer poor health, which is exacerbated by their environment (such as eye problems, Fig. 5.8).

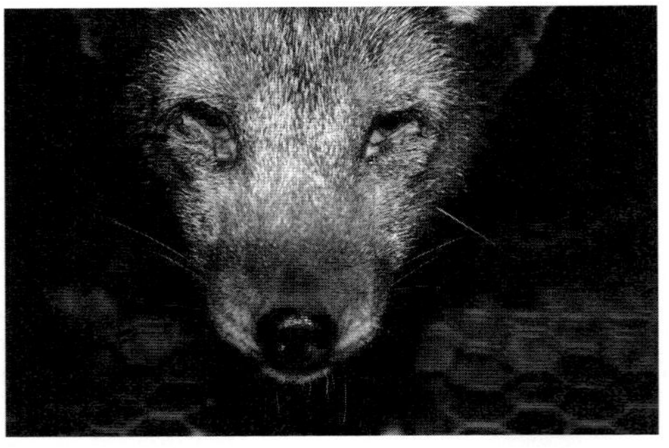

Fig. 5.8. A fox in a fur farm. This fox has discharges, staining and crusting around both eyes. Eye problems are reportedly common on fur farms (ADI, 2010). This can be secondary to entropion, a painful condition where the eyelids roll in, causing chronic irritation and pain. A dirty, dusty environment would exacerbate this. (Photograph courtesy of Animal Defenders International.)

Animals Abused for Medicinal Reasons

Animals may be abused to supply humans with traditional medicines. An example of this is farming bears for their bile, a cruel industry that involves bears being confined to small cages so the bile can be harvested (Fig. 5.10). These bears may also have their paws cut off while alive for inclusion in bear paw soup (Thorne and Boniface, 2008). Bile is removed from bears in a number of ways (WSPA, n.d.(b)):

- A tube leading to the gall bladder is inserted and the abdominal wound constantly reopened to stop the tube closing up.
- A needle and syringe are inserted into the gall bladder.
- The bear is killed and bile extracted after death.

Farming horses for urine

Pregnant mares are farmed for their urine in parts of the USA and Canada and their urine used in some brands of medication for menopausal

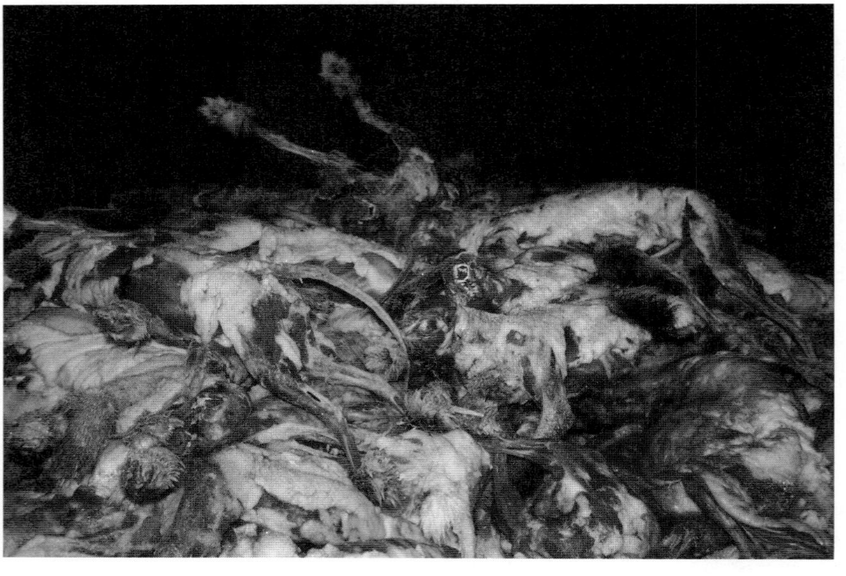

Fig. 5.9. A pile of animals that have been skinned for their fur. (Photograph courtesy of Animal Defenders International.)

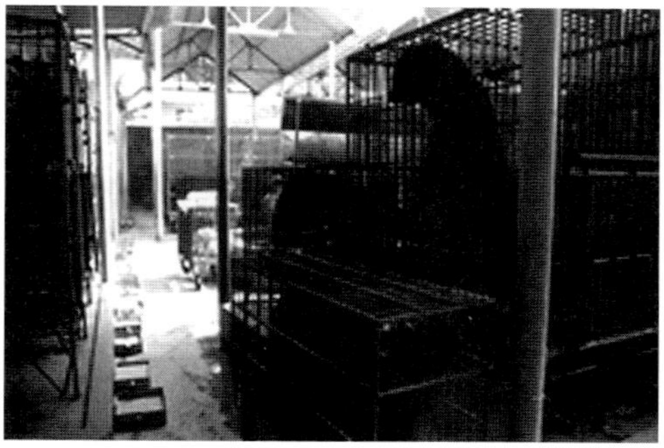

Fig. 5.10. Bears caged at a bear bile farm near Hanoi, Vietnam. (Photograph copyright WSPA.)

women. These mares are housed in stalls for up to 24 hours a day without exercise (Houpt *et al.*, 2001) and continually wear a harness for collection of the urine – most of the foals born at urine farms in the USA and Canada are transported to feed-lots and then to slaughterhouses (Williams, 1994). People who rescue and rehabilitate horses from urine farms have commented on the animals having a 'skittish fear of people' (Bechman, 2008).

Animals are also vulnerable to abuse in entertainment and in hunting, art and sport. The next chapter will discuss these issues further.

References

ADI (2010) *Bloody Harvest – the real cost of fur.* Animal Defenders International, London.

Animals Australia (n.d.) Ultra-fine wool. Available at: http://www.animalsaustralia.org/issues/ultra_fine_wool.php (accessed 19 May 2012).

AVMA (2007) AVMA guidelines on euthanasia. American Veterinary Medical Association. Available at: http://www.avma.org/issues/animal_welfare/euthanasia.pdf (accessed 16 March 2012).

Bechman, A. (2008) A second chance – rescuers save horses from slaughterhouse. *Payson Roundup* 24 October. Available at: http://www.paysonroundup.com/news/2008/oct/24/second_chance/ (accessed 21 May 2012).

Brambell Committee (1965) *Report of the Technical Committee to Enquire into the Welfare of Animals Kept Under Intensive Livestock Husbandry Systems.* Her Majesty's Stationery Office, London.

Broom, D.M. and Fraser, A.F. (2007) *Domestic Animal Behaviour and Welfare*, 4th edn. CAB International, Wallingford, UK.

Caba, J. (2011) Secret footage allegedly shows pigs abused at abattoir. *The Telegraph*, 29 July. Available at: http://www.telegraph.co.uk/earth/agriculture/batteryfarming/8670309/Secret-footage-allegedly-shows-pigs-abused-at-abattoir.html (accessed 19 September 2011).

Cheng, H. (2006) Morphological changes and pain in beak trimmed laying hens. *World's Poultry Science Journal* 62, 41–52.

Code of Practice for the Welfare of Sheep (2008) Code of practice for the welfare of sheep housed for wool production. Available at: http://www.woolproducers.com.au/uploads/Final%20COP%20Housed%20Sheep%20Version%206.pdf (accessed 19 September 2011).

Cooper, J.E. (2006) Insects. In: Lewbart, G.A. (ed.) *Invertebrate Medicine.* Blackwell Publishing, Oxford, UK.

Cooper, J.J. and Appleby, M.C. (2003) The value of environmental resources to domestic hens: a comparison of the work-rate for food and for nests as a function of time. *Animal Welfare* 37, 39–52.

Corrall, S. (2002) Dog meat matters. *Animal Life,* Autumn, 14–15.

Duncan, I.J.H. (2001) Animal welfare issues in the poultry industry: is there a lesson to be learned? *Journal of Applied Animal Welfare Science* 4, 207–221.

Fraser, D., Mench, J. and Millman, S. (2001) Farm animals and their welfare in 2000. In: *State of the Animals.* Humane Society Press, Washington, DC, p. 90.

Gellatley, J. and Wardle, T. (1996) *The Silent Ark.* Thorsons, London.

Gentle, M.J. and Hunter, L.N. (1991) Physiological and behavioural responses associated with feather removal in *Gallus gallus* var *domesticus. Research in Veterinary Science* 50(1), 95–101.

Gerges, D. (2012) Truck full of dogs crammed into tiny cages and bound for Chinese restaurants is intercepted by animal lovers. *Daily Mail,* 19 January. Available at: http://www.dailymail.co.uk/news/article-2088309/Truck-dogs-crammed-tiny-cages-bound-Chinese-restaurants-rescued-animal-lovers.html (accessed 19 May 2012).

Gregory, N.G. (2004) *Physiology and Behaviour of Animal Suffering.* Universities Federation for Animal Welfare, Blackwell Science, Oxford, UK.

Gregory, N.G. (2007) *Animal Welfare & Meat Production*, 2nd edn. CAB International, Wallingford, UK.
Harrison, R. (1964) *Animal Machines*. Ballantine Books, New York.
Hemsworth, P.H., Barnett, J.L., Karlen, G.M., Fisher, A.D., Butler, K.L. and Arnold, N.A. (2009) Effects of mulesing and alternative procedures to mulesing on the behaviour and physiology of lambs. *Applied Animal Behaviour Science* 117, 20–27.
Houpt, K., Houpt, T.R., Johnson, J.L., Erb, H.N. and Yeon, S.C. (2001) The effect of exercise deprivation on the behaviour and physiology of straight stall confined pregnant mares. *Animal Welfare* 10(3), 257–267.
Lindberg, A.C. and Nicol, C.J. (1997) Dust-bathing in modified battery cages: is sham dust-bathing an adequate substitute? *Applied Animal Behaviour Science* 55, 113–128.
Mench, J. (1992) The welfare of poultry in modern production systems. *Poultry Science Review* 4, 112.
Mount, H. (2010) The songbirds slaughtered for a Frenchman's supper. *Mail Online*, 7 September. Available at: http://www.dailymail.co.uk/femail/food/article-1309634/The-songbirds-slaughtered-Frenchmans-supper.html#ixzz1YMCPxWfS (accessed 19 September 2011).
Paterniti, M. (1998) The last meal. *Esquire*, 1 May. Available at: http://www.esquire.com/features/The-Last-Meal-0598#ixzz1KKiGU36R (accessed 23 April 2011).
PETA Asia Pacific (2012) Animals are not ours to wear. Available at: http://www.petaasiapacific.com/issues-nottowear.asp#silk (accessed 20 May 2012).
Podberscek, A.L. (2009) Good to pet and eat: the keeping and consuming of dogs and cats in South Korea. *Journal of Social Issues* 65(3), 615–632.
Rosinski, A. (n.d.) *Goose Production in Poland and Eastern Europe*. Department of Poultry Science, Agricultural University of Poznan, Poznan, Poland.
Thorne, F. and Boniface, S. (2008) Brit saves rare bears from being eaten. *The Sunday Mirror*, 24 February. Available at: http://www.mirror.co.uk/sunday-mirror/2008/02/24/bear-soup-98487-20329369/ (accessed 23 September 2011).
Whitehead, C.C. (2004) Skeletal disorders in laying hens: the problem of osteoporosis and bone fractures. In: Perry, G.C. (ed.) *Welfare of the Laying Hen. Poultry Science Symposium Series*. CAB International, Wallingford, UK.
Williams, L.S. (1994) Canada's huge pregnant-mare-urine industry faces growing pressure from animal-rights lobby. *Canadian Medical Association Journal* 151(7), 1009–1012.
WSPA (n.d.(a)) Be fur free – a consumer guide. Available at: http://www.wspa-international.org/helping/animalfriendlyliving/befurfree.aspx (accessed 22 September 2011).
WSPA (n.d.(b)) Inside the Bear Farms. Available at: http://www.wspa.org.au/wspaswork/bears/bearfarming/insidebearfarms.aspx (accessed 23 September 2011).

6 Animal Abuse in Hunting, Sport, Entertainment and Art

Catherine Tiplady

This chapter will discuss some of the common and less common ways animals may be abused as part of hunting, sport, entertainment and art.

Abuse of Show and Performance Animals

Horses and abuse

Animals abused in racing

There are many concerning welfare issues in the use of horses for sport and work animals. These include the use of the whip in racing horses, the use of very young animals in racing and the risk of harm during training and performance, particularly during jumps racing.

Although use of the whip is widespread and jockeys claim it is needed for control, analysis of whip use during racing has shown that the horses hit the most frequently do not win races (Arthur, 2011). The Grand National jumps race in the UK has received a lot of criticism from animal advocates because of the number of horses injured and killed during the race. In response to this, organizers made some changes prior to the 2012 event, including: reducing the height of one jump by 2 inches (down to 4 foot 10 inches), only allowing experienced horses aged 7 years and over to participate and providing water and fans to horses after the race (Wilson, 2012). Despite these 'safety measures', in the 2012 Grand National two horses had to be euthanized due to injuries and only 15 of 40 horses actually finished the race (Delgado, 2012).

Show horses and abuse

Some show animals may be abused in order to increase the owner's chances of winning a ribbon or trophy. In the USA, some gaited horses (for example, Tennessee Walking Horses) have had their forelegs deliberately injured to produce the exaggerated high-stepping gait desired in the show ring. This practice is known as 'soring' and is achieved by injuring a horse's forelegs with blistering chemicals or mechanical devices (USDA, 2010). Sored horses can develop permanent scars in the pasterns due to the application or injection of painful chemicals (USDA, 2009).

These horses may also endure 'pressure shoeing', where the hoof is cut almost to the quick and a shoe nailed tightly to deliberately cause discomfort, placing chains around the horses' pasterns or fitting hooves with large stacks of pads to force the horse to stand at an unnatural angle (HSUS, 2009). Sored horses may exhibit tissue damage, swelling, pain, abrasions and a bloody or serous discharge (USDA, 2009).

The United States Department of Agriculture enforces the Horse Protection Act, prohibiting sored horses from participating in shows, sales, exhibitions and auctions – methods of detecting soring include evaluating the horse's gait, physically examining the forelegs from knee to hoof and the use of gas chromatography/mass spectrometry and thermography (USDA, 2009).

Other horse breeds may also be abused to increase their chances of winning. Arabian horses may have a piece of ginger inserted into their anus so the tail is lifted higher and be struck with a whip during training, so they learn to arch their neck and look 'alert' when later threatened with a whip in the show ring (Heird, 2011).

Many of these cruel training practices are being addressed by the breed associations and show organizations (Heird, 2011).

Breeding purebred animals that suffer

The breeding of purebred (or any other) animals that are known to be beset by congenital physical ailments is a major welfare concern. To willingly continue this without attempts to rectify it is abuse. The breeding of purebred dogs with inherited diseases is concerning to many veterinarians and has been investigated by the British Broadcasting Corporation's 'Pedigree Dogs Exposed Documentary' (BBC, 2012). Some purebred animals are deliberately inbred and may suffer painful congenital conditions and deformities. Puppy farming (also known as puppy mills or factories) is a major cause of animal abuse and suffering among companion animals and can involve purebred dogs or so-called 'designer' cross-breeds. This is discussed further in Chapter 18.

Animal Abuse, Hunting and Wildlife

Animals may be abused in hunting and fishing, primarily if the animal's death is not immediate and there is prolonged suffering. This section will briefly cover a few of the many species that are hunted, whether for food, 'pest' control or as sport.

Feral animals

Introduced or 'feral' animals such as free-living domestic cats, dogs and pigs may cause massive environmental damage, compete for resources and kill native and domestic species. The term feral has various meanings, such as 'wild', 'untamed', 'uncultivated' or 'brutal' (*The Concise Oxford Dictionary*, 1974, p. 446), but more recently has entered common parlance to describe criminal behaviour in humans (Pash, 2011). In this book, 'feral' refers to a free-living domestic animal.

'Pest' animals can include introduced or native animals, and consideration of what constitutes a pest varies between people and countries. Cats are popular pets, yet it is estimated that feral cats in Australia eat 2 million native animals every day just in the top one-sixth of the continent (Lloyd, 2011). In various countries animals considered feral include foxes, dogs, pigs, donkeys, camels, some species of birds, fish and amphibians. Wildlife or livestock may be protected from predation by feral and pest animals using a range of techniques, some of which are cruel and cause high levels of suffering, for example steel jaw leg traps. Strychnine poisoning is an unacceptable method of euthanasia as it causes painful muscle contractions and violent convulsions (AVMA, 2007).

Kangaroo culling in Australia

Kangaroos (Fig. 6.1) are an Australian icon, a popular animal with tourists and culturally important to Indigenous Australians. In 2010, the Australian government set a quota for just over 4 million kangaroos to be commercially

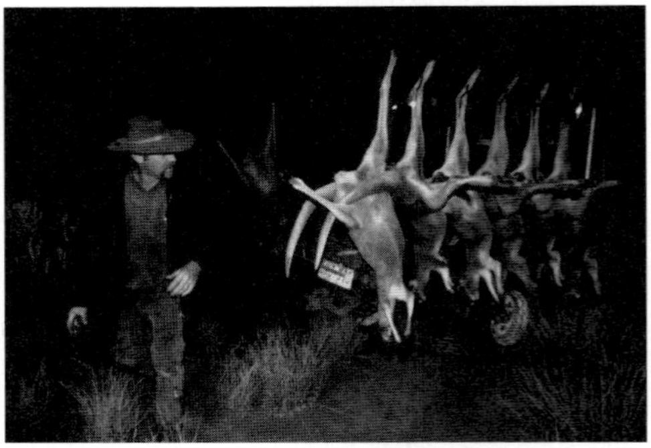

Fig. 6.1. Millions of kangaroos are shot in Australia each year. Non-commercial shooters are not required to undergo competency testing to ensure the kangaroos and joeys are humanely killed. (Photograph copyright IFAW.)

killed (Australian Government, 2011a), of a population of approximately 25 million (Australian Government, 2011b).

Kangaroos are killed for their meat (for human and pet consumption) and also made into leather goods and novelty souvenir items such as kangaroo paw back-scratchers and kangaroo scrotum money-bags.

Free-living kangaroos are killed in Australia by either trained professionals killing for commercial reasons, by recreational shooters, for scientific research or as damage mitigation in the case of pastoralists – all shooters are required to comply with the relevant Codes of Practice (Australian Government 2008a,b); however, non-commercial shooters are allowed to shoot kangaroos without undergoing any competency testing (Australian Government, 2008b).

Cruelty concerns centre around the method of killing, the competency of the killer and the fact that orphaned joeys may disperse and suffer after their mother is shot (RSPCA, 2009). The Code recommends joeys are killed by a forceful blow to the skull to destroy the brain, by stunning and decapitation or shooting the brain or heart (Australian Government 2008a,b), but without training and supervision of all shooters there is the probability of animals suffering. Euthanasia by a blow to the head can be a humane method of euthanasia, providing operators are 'properly trained and monitored for proficiency' (AVMA, 2007, p. 13).

Rodent/Insect Abuse

Rodents and insects are frequently vilified as vermin and poisoning methods often involve the animals suffering for several days (Mason and Littin, 2003).

Glue traps are flat trays coated with a non-drying adhesive in order to trap small animals such as rodents. Rodents caught in glue traps experience enormous distress and pain while trapped – they may suffocate in the glue or squeal, tear at their hair and skin, break their limbs or bite their own legs off as they try to escape (Mason and Littin, 2003). Insects are not covered in the Prevention of Cruelty to Animals legislation in Australia so glue traps for insects are freely available (Department of Primary Industries, 2009). There is no reason to believe that an insect would not suffer as a mammal would when caught in a glue trap.

Trapping and relocation of some unwanted wild animals, such as possums, from suburban areas has resulted in possums dying in stressful circumstances soon after they were released (Pietsch, 1994). Depending on the species, it may be possible to provide an alternate nest box in a more desirable (according to humans) place. Knowledge about the target species' natural behaviour and home range will assist with management of wild or feral animals, and people interested in humane pest control are advised to speak to an expert on the health and behaviour of the species.

Humane rodent traps and rodent-proofing houses and sheds are alternatives to poisons and glue traps.

Animal Abuse and Hunting/Fishing

There is great potential for animal suffering in hunting and fishing, particularly if the hunter/fisher is inexperienced or unwilling to humanely kill animals. Hunting and fishing are generally viewed as male pursuits but women are also involved. Pro-hunting Internet sites are overwhelmingly male, with endless photographs of grinning men holding guns and crouching next to a bleeding animal.

Trophy hunting often involves wealthy people paying great sums of money to travel the world shooting animals. For an extra cost they get to take home their 'trophy' of a stuffed cadaver or decapitated head. Hunters may argue that trophy hunting is actually 'conservation' and will go to great lengths to extol the beauty of nature and their vital role within it as hunters.

Animal Abuse and Tourism

Animal abuse and tourism are intrinsically linked in some countries and while many people will accept this as the culture of the place they are visiting (e.g. bullfighting in Spain), others may want to get involved to help prevent suffering (Fig. 6.3).

Case study: Cruelty to wild animals

A badger was found dead in a cage trap (Fig. 6.2). Expert veterinary evidence showed that it had been drowned. The defendant admitted he had previously tried to shoot at badgers using an air rifle because they had damaged his garden and eaten his bird food, but the pellets had just bounced off the animal.

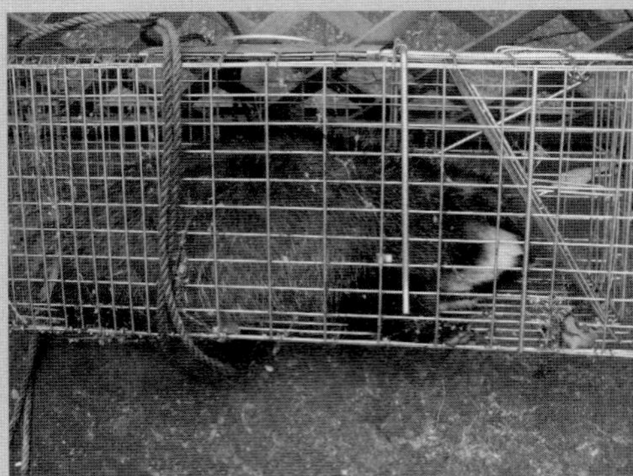

Fig. 6.2. This badger had been caught in a trap and drowned. (Photograph copyright RSPCA England and Wales.)

At court the defendant pleaded guilty to taking a badger, contrary to the Badgers Act 1992, and causing it to suffer by its confinement in a cage trap. The magistrates said they found the matter to be a serious one, but giving the defendant credit for his guilty pleas they decided to sentence him to a conditional discharge for the maximum period of 3 years, and ordered him to pay the RSPCA's costs of £2800. An order was made for confiscation and destruction of the trap.

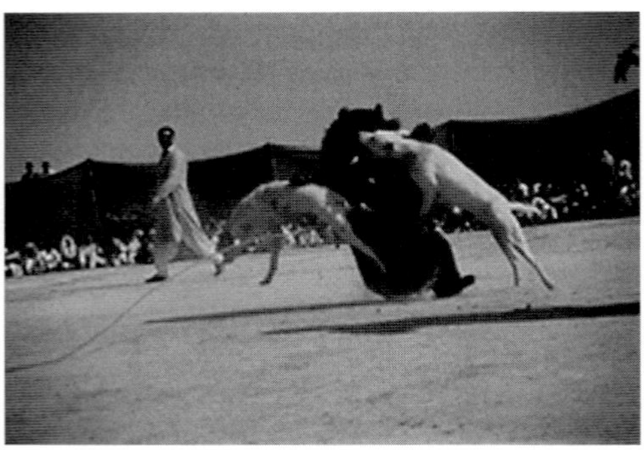

Fig. 6.3. Bear-baiting is popular is some regions of the world, with thousands of spectators gathering to watch the tethered, clawless bears being attacked by trained dogs. (Photograph courtesy of WSPA.)

Awareness of how animals are trained and kept would be expected to make tourists less supportive of animal cruelty, but without an alternative means of making money, the local operators and their families will suffer.

Snake charming, where snakes such as cobras appear to dance to the music of a flautist, has traditionally been seen on the streets of India. It is believed that training is done by physical abuse (Hodge, 2011) and it is fear of the moving flute and self defence that cause snakes to sway to the music, resulting in exhaustion (*The Times of India*, 2010). Prior to being used for charming, a snake's venom glands are pierced with a hot needle, their mouths are sewn shut and they may only be offered milk – as a result, the snakes suffer severe allergic reactions and die of dysentery and dehydration (*The Times of India*, 2010). Removal of fangs and venom sacks can cause infection, pain and death (Hodge, 2011).

Snake charming is now banned in India. This has deprived 800,000 members of Bengal's Bedia community, who have worked as snake-charmers for generations, of their only source of income, with an estimated 20,000 serving jail terms for defying the ban (Nelson, 2009).

The Bedia snake-charming community has now formed a union and is campaigning for an exemption from the ban and state support for retraining (Nelson, 2009).

Suggestions for alternative employment for snake charmers, such as employing them to remove snakes from people's homes, in conservation education or selling venom to the pharmaceutical industry, have not been successful, apparently because the caste-cultural differences and education gap were too great (Magnier, 2012).

A similar problem exists for the owners of dancing bears in India. These bears are taken from their mothers at less than 4 weeks of age and, without anaesthetic, have a rope inserted through their muzzle, have their canines removed and are castrated (Humane Society International, n.d.). Pulling on the rope makes the bears 'dance'.

The Kalandars are a semi-nomadic group who use bears to make money for their families, but now the capture and keeping of bears is prohibited and they take the bears to rural areas to dance for money (WSPA, n.d.(a)). Groups such as WSPA and the Wildlife Trust of India are attempting to help both the bears and the owners by the following steps (WSPA, n.d.(a)):

- educating the public;
- preventing cubs being poached;
- striving to provide lifetime care for confiscated bears; and
- helping the owners find new, cruelty-free ways to earn money.

Groups such as The Brooke equine welfare organization and SPANA are similarly involved with educating owners and providing healthcare for horses, donkeys and mules in Africa, Asia and Latin America, as well as educating tourists who visit these countries (The Brooke, n.d.).

In rural Pakistan up to 2000 spectators will gather to watch tethered, clawless bears being attacked by trained dogs (WSPA, n.d.(b)). Animal fighting has been popular for centuries and involves cruelty to both the victor and the loser – baiting of bears is banned by the Pakistan Wildlife Act and contravenes Islamic teachings (WSPA, n.d.(b)).

Abuse of Circus and Performance Animals

> It is not usually a pretty sight to see the big cats trained.
>
> Ringling North and Hatch (2008, p. 299)

Circus animals, like many domesticated animals, live lives far removed from their natural habitat and social grouping. For circus animals this is combined with constant travelling, confinement and training methods that may involve cruelty, pain and suffering. A member of the Ringling circus described animals working from fear, chained to their pedestals with 'ropes around their necks to choke them down and make them obey' (Ringling North and Hatch, 2008, p. 299). Tamed elephants may suffer abuse as they are rarely trained or ridden without use of a dagger, which can be stabbed into the elephant's neck (Broom and Fraser, 2007). Numerous undercover videos have repeatedly shown incidents of cruelty to circus and performance animals around the world.

Animal Abuse in Entertainment

Animals are often used for human entertainment in the advertising, film and television industries. This may be monitored on-set by groups such as the American Humane Association (AHA). The AHA formed in response to complaints after a horse was ridden off a 70-foot cliff in the 1939 film *Jesse James*, resulting in the animal's death (The Fifth

Case study: Circus animal cruelty

Anne, a 58-year-old circus elephant in Britain, endured ongoing and severe abuse from her keeper as seen in footage secretly filmed over a three and a half week period by Animal Defenders International (Greenwood and Elicott, 2011). The footage shows Anne being repeatedly stabbed, kicked and beaten with a pitchfork as she stands helplessly chained by the legs (Fig. 6.4). Circus owner Bobby Roberts insisted he didn't know the groom was abusing the elephant, saying Anne is 'part of the family' and to separate her from him and the circus would cause her to 'pine away and die' (Greenwood and Elicott, 2011).

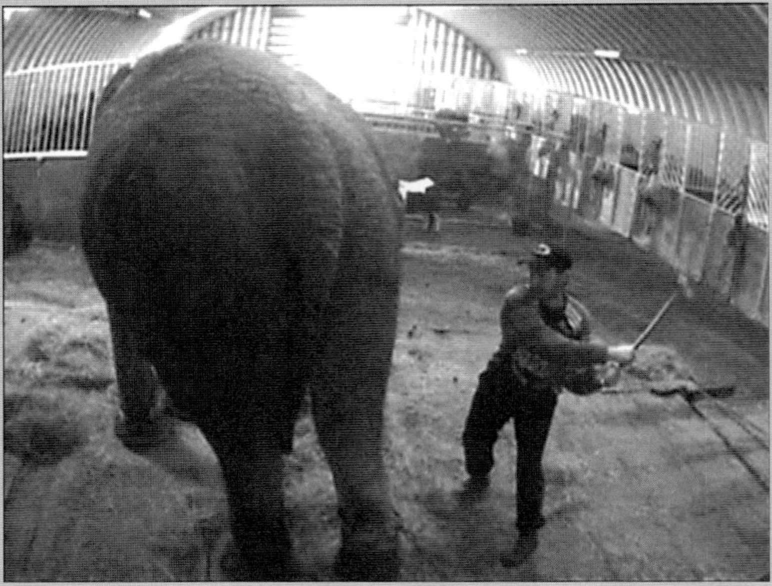

Fig. 6.4. This image from an investigation by Animal Defenders International shows Anne being beaten with a pitchfork. (Photograph copyright Animal Defenders International.)

In April, 2011 the Bobby Roberts Super Circus handed Anne over for rehabilitation and veterinary care at Longleat Safari Park (Animal Defenders International, 2011).

Estate, 2010). People for the Ethical Treatment of Animals (PETA, n.d.), however, have criticized the AHA's 'No Animals Were Harmed' seal of approval saying animals are not monitored off-set, during pre-production training or during the separation of young animals from their mothers. PETA (n.d.) believes that animatronics, animation and computer-generated imagery should replace animal actors. Undercover filming of a Las Vegas animal trainer allegedly showed him beating orang-utans with a metal bar, pinching them, pulling their hair and punching them in the face before they went on stage (Newkirk, 1999).

Early examples of animals being harmed and filmed include the 1903 film *Electrocuting an Elephant*, made by Thomas Edison's film-makers at Coney Island, USA. Topsy, a captive elephant at the Coney Island theme park, had killed her keeper after he reportedly fed her a lighted cigarette (Vanderbilt, 2003). Over a thousand people gathered to watch the actual execution and it became a popular film in cinemas, showing Topsy twitching and her skin smoking before she finally collapses (The Fifth Estate, 2010).

Many animals were killed by electrocution in experiments, some of them conducted in public to show the safety or otherwise of electricity. These animal electrocutions were instrumental in developing the electric chair for killing humans (Moran, 2002).

Animal Abuse and Art

There is a difference between animal abuse *in* art and animal abuse *as* art. In the former, art may educate viewers about the moral issues surrounding abuse, while in the latter, the spectator may become the perpetrator of abuse.

One of the most famous depictions of animal abuse in art is the series of pictures by English artist William Hogarth in 1751. The series of four etchings is entitled 'The Four Stages of Cruelty', and focuses on the exploits of a male character named Tom Nero. Nero is initially depicted as a child pushing an arrow into a dog's anus as the struggling dog is held by two other children (Fig. 6.5). In the second picture, Nero has become a young man beating his horse, which has collapsed on a London street. The third picture depicts Tom Nero being arrested for murder, his pregnant girlfriend lying dead at his feet with her throat slit. The final picture shows Tom Nero's body being dissected for anatomy teaching, after his execution by hanging. A dog is seen in the foreground of the picture, licking at Nero's intestines which spill on to the floor.

Quite clearly, the moral message of Hogarth's series of pictures is to present in graphic detail the link between childhood cruelty to animals and progression to violence against humans. The underlying theme appears to warn that violence against humans could have been prevented if the issue of animal cruelty was dealt with when Nero was a child.

Hogarth described the series of works:

> The Four Stages of Cruelty were done in hopes of preventing in some degree that cruel treatment of poor animals which makes the streets of London more disagreeable to the human mind than anything whatever, the very describing of which gives pain.
>
> (Quoted in Porter, 1991, p. 269)

Several modern artists and performers are using art to raise awareness of animal cruelty, sentience and exploitation issues, such as Sue Coe, Yvette Watt and poet Benjamin Zephaniah.

Animals may also be abused as 'art'. A famous example of this is the 2000 work *Helena* by Marco Evaristti, in which the artist installed live goldfish in ten plugged-in food blenders (Hibbert, 2005). The audience was provided with the opportunity to grapple with their morals – would they choose to blend and kill the goldfish or leave it to live in its blender aquarium (Hibbert, 2005). Evaristti's idea was to divide visitors to the exhibition into three groups, 'The idiot, who pushed the button, the voyeur, who loves to watch and the moralist' (Buchhart and Hofbauer, 2002). The artist regarded the media and the public as the voyeurs, and complainers such as the Animal Protection League as the moralists, his website stating 'it is not Evaristti who comes over as irresponsible and spineless, but where he passes on the ethical and moral issues to the observer' (Evaristti, 2011). More than one person chose to blend the fish and two fish died (BBC, 2003). As a result, the artist was briefly arrested (Hibbert, 2005); however, a judge found that the fish had been killed humanely after a veterinarian told the court the fish would have died 'painlessly' (BBC, 2003).

In 2008, Parisian artist Adel Abdessened opened an exhibition of 'art', which included six video screens continually depicting animals being beaten to death with a sledgehammer (described by Moussaieff Masson, 2011). These scenes of animal cruelty masquerading as 'art' are sadly an example of an even lower form of human entertainment – animal abuse pornography. This will be described further in Chapter 9, with a section on first aid treatment, case studies and rehabilitation of sexually abused animals in Chapter 18.

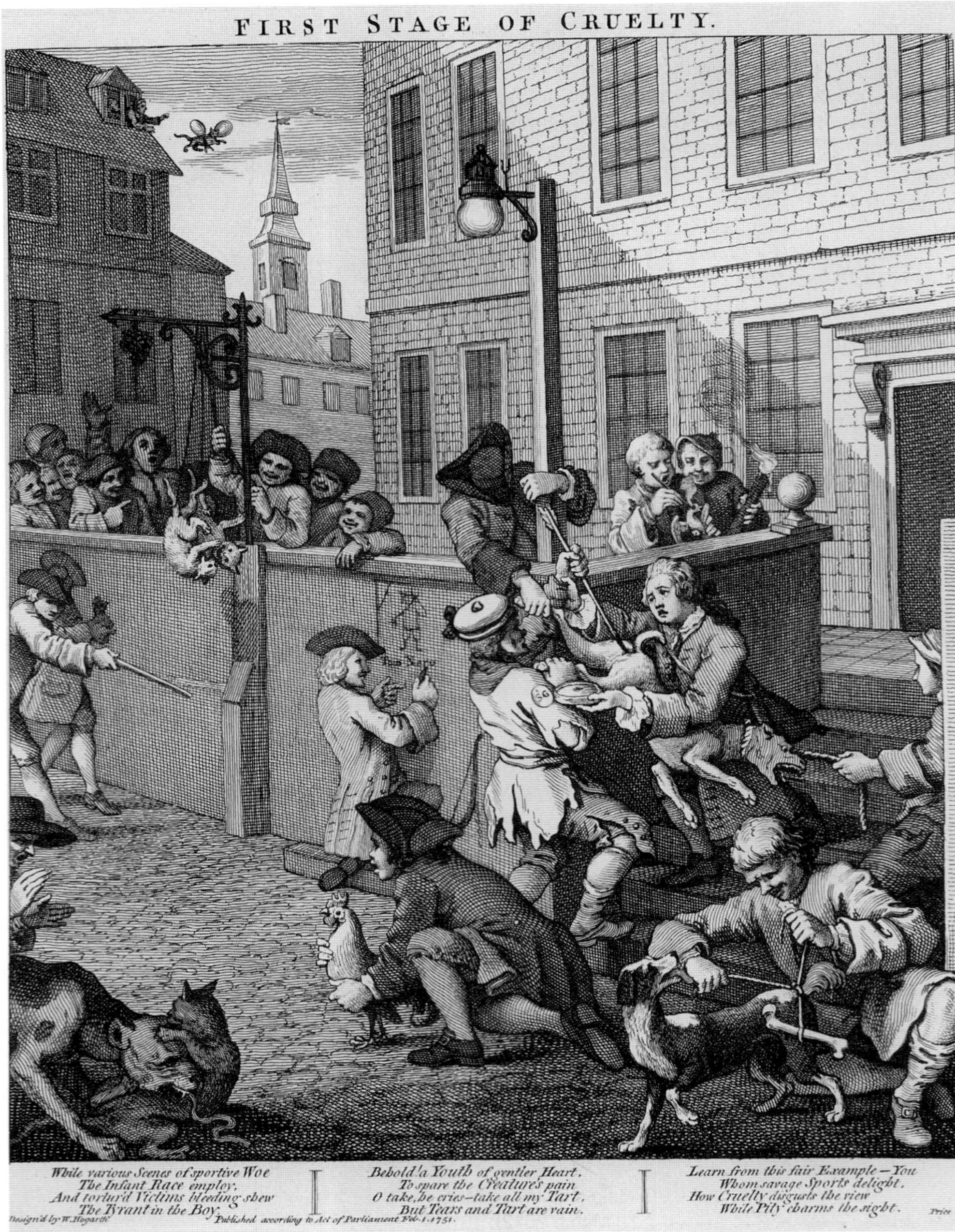
FIRST STAGE OF CRUELTY.
While various Scenes of sportive Woe
The Infant Race employ,
And tortur'd Victims bleeding shew
The Tyrant in the Boy.
I
Behold! a Youth of gentler Heart,
To spare the Creature's pain
O take, he cries–take all my Tart,
But Tears and Tart are vain.
I
Learn from this fair Example–You
Whom savage Sports delight,
How Cruelty disgusts the view
While Pity charms the sight.
Design'd by W. Hogarth
Published according to Act of Parliament Feb. 1. 1751.
Price 1s

Fig. 6.5. *First Stage of Cruelty*, 1751 (engraving) by William Hogarth (1697–1764). William Hogarth's 'The Four Stages of Cruelty' etchings in 1751 illustrated how childhood animal abuse could progress to human interpersonal violence. This picture, the first of the series, shows the young Tom Nero pushing an arrow into a dog's anus. (Private Collection/The Bridgeman Art Library/out of copyright.)

References

ADI (Animal Defenders International) (2011) Anne the elephant safe at last. 3 April. Available at: http://www.ad-international.org/animals_in_entertainment/go.php?id=2088&ssi=10 (accessed 22 September 2011).

Arthur, R.M. (2011) Welfare issues in horse racing. In: McIlwraith, C.W. and Rollin, B.E. (eds) *Equine Welfare*. UFAW/Blackwell Publishing, Chichester, UK, pp. 229–244.

Australian Government (2008a) *National Code of Practice for the Humane Shooting of Kangaroos and Wallabies for Commercial Purposes*. Australian Government, Canberra, Australia.

Australian Government (2008b) *National Code of Practice for the Humane Shooting of Kangaroos and Wallabies for Non-Commercial Purposes*. Australian Government, Canberra, Australia.

Australian Government (2011a) Commercial kangaroo harvest quotas in 2010. Available at: http://www.environment.gov.au/biodiversity/wildlife-trade/wild-harvest/kangaroo/quota/2010.html (accessed 27 May 2012).

Australian Government (2011b) Kangaroo population estimates. Available at: http://www.environment.gov.au/biodiversity/wildlife-trade/wild-harvest/kangaroo/population.html#2010 (accessed 27 May 2012).

AVMA (2007) AVMA guidelines on euthanasia. American Veterinary Medical Association. Available at: http://www.avma.org/issues/animal_welfare/euthanasia.pdf (accessed 16 March 2012).

BBC (2003) Liquidising goldfish 'not a crime'. 19 May. Available at: http://news.bbc.co.uk/2/hi/3040891.stm (accessed 7 April 2011).

BBC (2012) Pedigree dogs exposed – three years on. Available at: http://www.bbc.co.uk/programmes/b01cqp75 (accessed 7 May 2012).

Broom, D.M. and Fraser, A.F. (2007) *Domestic Animal Behaviour and Welfare*, 4th edn. CAB International, Wallingford, UK.

Buchhart, D. and Hofbauer, A.K. (2002) Sollen wir alle Menschen verklagen, die Meeresfrüchte essen? *Kunstforum International* 162, 270–279.

Delgado, M. (2012) Another National tragedy: Despite public outcry after last year's carnage at Aintree, two more horses die at notorious jump – including the Gold Cup winner. *Mail Online*, 14 April. Available at: http://www.dailymail.co.uk/news/article-2129727/Grand-National-2012-horse-deaths-notorious-Aintree-jump-included-Gold-Cup-winner.html (accessed 5 May 2012).

Department of Primary Industries (2009) Glue traps. Department of Primary Industries, August 2009, Victorian Government, Melbourne, Australia.

Evaristti, M. (2011) Marco Evaristti and the open work. Available at: http://www.evaristti.com/index.php/essays/1-essays/5-open-work (accessed 7 April 2011).

Greenwood, C. and Elicott, C. (2011) Anne's agony: Battered, kicked and stabbed, the desperate plight of Britain's last circus elephant. *Daily Mail* online, 28 March. Available at: http://www.dailymail.co.uk/news/article-1370050/Britains-circus-elephant-Anne-Battered-kicked-stabbed.html#ixzz1l4jE9geP (accessed 2 April 2011).

Heird, J. (2011) Abusive treatment and subsequent policy development within various breeds of show horses in the USA. In: McIlwraith, C.W. and Rollin, B.E. (eds) *Equine Welfare*. UFAW/Blackwell Publishing, Chichester, UK, pp. 245–254.

Hibbert, A. (2005) *Cruelty to Animals*. Franklin Watts, London.

Hodge, A. (2011) Brief reprieve for diehard snake charmers. *The Australian*, 13 April, p. 10.

HSUS (2009) What is soring? Humane Society of the United States, 2 October. Available at: http://www.humanesociety.org/issues/tenn_walking_horses/facts/what_is_soring.html (accessed 9 January 2011).

Humane Society International (n.d.) Help stop the misery of the dancing bears. Available at: http://www.hsi.org.au/?catID=164 (accessed 18 March 2012).

Lloyd, G. (2011) Bringing beasties back from the brink. *The Australian*, 7 May. Available at: http://www.theaustralian.com.au/national-affairs/bringing-beasties-back-from-the-brink/story-fn59niix-1226051432090 (accessed 27 May 2012).

Magnier, M. (2012) India snake charmers have identity crisis. *Los Angeles Times*, 21 February. Available at: http://articles.latimes.com/2012/feb/21/world/la-fg-india-snakes-20120222/2 (accessed 18 March 2012).

Mason, G. and Littin, K. (2003) The humaneness of rodent pest control. *Animal Welfare* 12, 1–38.

Moran, R. (2002) *Executioner's Current – Thomas Edison, George Westinghouse and the invention of the electric chair*. Alfred A. Knopf, New York.

Moussaieff Masson, J. (2011) Pornography and animals. In: Tankard Reist, M. and Bray, A. (eds) *Big Porn Inc.* Spinifex Press, North Melbourne, Victoria, Australia, pp. 63–68.

Nelson, D. (2009) India's snake charmers form union to defy ban. *The Telegraph*, 12 February. Available at: http://www.telegraph.co.uk/news/worldnews/asia/india/4601043/Indias-snake-charmers-form-union-to-defy-ban.html (accessed 18 March 2012).

Newkirk, I. (1999) *You Can Save the Animals – 251 simple ways to stop thoughtless cruelty.* Prima Publishing, California.

Pash, C. (2011) Cliché of the week. *The Australian*, 12 September, p. 31.

PETA (n.d.) Animal actors. Available at: http://www.peta.org/issues/animals-in-entertainment/animal-actors.aspx (accessed 28 May 2012).

Pietsch, R.S. (1994) The fate of urban Common Brushtail Possums translocated to sclerophyll forest. In: Serena, M. (ed.) *Reintroduction Biology of Australian and New Zealand Fauna.* Surry Beatty and Sons, Sydney, Australia, pp. 239–246.

Porter, R. (1991) *English Society in the Eighteenth Century (The Penguin Social History of Britain)*, 2nd edn. Penguin, London.

Ringling North, H. and Hatch, A. (2008) *The Circus Kings – our Ringling family story.* University Press of Florida, Gainesville, Florida, p. 299.

RSPCA (2009) What happens to joeys when female kangaroos are shot? RSPCA Knowledgebase. Available at: http://kb.rspca.org.au/What-happens-to-joeys-when-female-kangaroos-are-shot_76.html (accessed 18 September 2011).

The Brooke (n.d.) Brooke. Available at: http://www.thebrooke.org/ (accessed 18 March 2012).

The Concise Oxford Dictionary (1974) Oxford University Press, 5th edn. Oxford, UK.

The Fifth Estate (2010) Cruelty on Film. Available at: http://www.cbc.ca/fifth/cruelcamera/cruelty.html (accessed 26 December 2010).

The Times of India (2010) This Nag Panchami, save snakes from atrocities. 14 August. Available at: http://articles.timesofindia.indiatimes.com/2010-08-14/pune/28298757_1_snake-charmers-nag-panchami-reptile (accessed 13 April 2011).

USDA (2009) Animal care – the Horse Protection Act. United States Department of Agriculture Animal and Plant Health Inspection Service. Available at: http://www.aphis.usda.gov/publications/animal_welfare/content/printable_version/faq_rev_horsep.pdf (accessed 20 March 2011).

USDA (2010) United States Department of Agriculture Horse Protection Act Information, June 24. Available at: http://www.aphis.usda.gov/animal_welfare/hp/ (accessed 9 January 2011).

Vanderbilt, T. (2003) City lore: They didn't forget. *New York Times*, 13 July. Available at: http://www.nytimes.com/2003/07/13/nyregion/city-lore-they-didn-t-forget.html?src=pm (accessed 23 May 2012).

Wilson, J. (2012) Grand National: Aintree aims for safer race. BBC Sport Horseracing. Available at: http://www.bbc.co.uk/sport/0/horse-racing/17619996 11 April (accessed 5 May 2012).

WSPA (n.d.(a)) Dancing bears. Available at: http://www.wspa.org.au/wspaswork/bears/dancingbears/default.aspx (accessed 18 March 2012).

WSPA (n.d.(b)) Bear baiting. Available at: http://www.wspa.org.au/wspaswork/bears/bearbaiting/default.aspx (accessed 21 April 2011).

7 Education and Animal Abuse

Catherine Tiplady

> When the long, miserable week (of frog dissection) was over, all the class was allowed to 'do as you wish' with the remainders of the bodies. So all of the boys broke bones, tore off body parts, tossed them around – it was absolutely horrible. I can still hear the bones of those poor souls breaking and cracking. I had nightmares.
>
> (Student quoted in Balcombe, 1997, p. 14)

Animal abuse may feature in teaching in two ways. First, animal abuse may be spoken about in teaching, in order to raise awareness of animal abuse, prevent cruelty and encourage compassion. This teaching can happen informally, for example a parent speaking to their child or formally in classes for children and adolescents at school, or for adults in tertiary education or continuing professional development. Unfortunately, animals may be abused during teaching. Dead animals may also have their bodies handled in a disrespectful way, which some would consider 'abusive', as seen in the quote above.

This section will first consider the potential for animal abuse in teaching, before outlining the way compassion for animals may be encouraged by educators and how veterinarians and veterinary students can be involved.

Animals Abused in Teaching

> It was wonderful to hold the dog's heart in my hand as it died!

Veterinary student after participating in terminal resuscitation practical class on live, anaesthetized pound dogs. These dogs are repeatedly resuscitated and overdosed with anaesthetic before having their chest cut open for students to perform open heart massage on.

The quote above shows that one person's idea of 'wonderful' is not necessarily another's. Many would see the quote as callous, not to mention alarming when spoken by a future veterinarian, despite the context of an educational experience. But is it 'abuse'? Isn't it essential that future veterinarians know how to resuscitate an animal? These students may later graduate and save the lives of much-loved pets. Are owned animals more important and worthy of care than an 'unwanted' pound animal or ex-racing greyhounds? If animals are destined to die whether students use them or not, should we at least be using them to help others in the future? Or, could students learn by use of mannequins, videos and computer programs to minimize use of live animals that results in harm or death? Tackling these issues involves understanding animal welfare and ethics and appreciating the need for graduating veterinarians to have achieved competencies in a range of clinical procedures prior to entering practice.

To find out whether there is a way veterinarians can be trained without harming animals it is necessary to examine how animals are used in teaching.

Animal use in teaching and research – the potential for abuse

Primum non nocere

First, do no harm.

Laws and codes of practice outline the way in which the animals are to be treated in teaching and research and, typically, this must follow the 3 Rs which were first devised by Russell and Burch in 1959 (Russell and Burch, 1992). The 3 Rs are: Reduction of the number of animals used, Replacement of animals with non-animal alternatives and Refinement (designing experiments to avoid/alleviate animal suffering and with the animal's welfare as the primary concern). Even when permission is granted from an animal ethics committee prior to conducting such a class, animal abuse can still occur. Some teachers fail to closely monitor how animals are being treated and, in doing so, inadvertently provide students with an opportunity for cruelty. Some researchers may regard animals as mere tools they can use and discard in pursuit of scientific achievement rather than sentient beings.

It is most disturbing when animals are misused by future veterinarians who appear to show no compassion or respect towards them. Cattle used for teaching purposes have had obscenities written on their bodies by veterinary students who used livestock marking crayons to deface the animals and ridicule them. Students have laughed while watching a video of a dog having seizures after being given strychnine. One student suggested that the university's herd of dairy cows be culled as 'The Final Solution'. Other veterinary students photographed themselves playing with pieces of animal cadavers and posted the images on the Internet with comments about sexually abusing animals.

Why would they do this? It has been found that people working in stressful occupations often use humour as a coping mechanism (Moran and Roth, 2006; Roth and Vivona, 2010) – although inappropriate, such humour could indicate that these students are not coping with the rigours of veterinary training. One author describes her experiences as a student in one veterinary school (Woon, 2011, p. 382):

> It is not uncommon to witness or hear of students using dissection specimens in practical jokes, indicating a resistance to the usual sensitivity and repulsion elicited by these materials. The notoriously high alcohol consumption by veterinary students is further testament to this macho bravado culture.

'Conscientious' or 'ethical' objection

Some students have ethical objections to the ways in which animals are used in their education, and a number of universities now allow humane teaching alternatives to students with these beliefs (New England Anti-Vivisection Society, 2012).

In Australia, the Code of Practice for the Care and Use of Animals for Scientific Purposes, referring to animal use, states that institutions must ensure 'that personnel and students may voice their concerns without jeopardizing their employment, careers, or coursework' (Australian Government National Health and Medical Research Council, 2004, pp. 9–10).

Rather than announce their beliefs, some students remain quiet about their feelings, fearing a loss of grades (Langley, 2003). Some people who are strongly motivated to work in animal care will choose to avoid education that involves animals being killed for dissection and live clinical training (Martinsen and Jukes, 2005).

It has even been suggested that veterinary training can have a detrimental effect on some students. One author believes that when students are forced to use animals in ways that they view as harmful, painful, stressful or lethal, several reactions may occur: students may suffer psychological trauma, their cognitive abilities may become impaired, resulting in less learning and they may withdraw and lose interest in their training (Capaldo, 2004).

Euthanasing animals specifically for teaching purposes can lead to the desensitization toward harmful animal use of those involved (Jukes and Chiuia, 2003), and progression through veterinary training can affect student attitudes toward animal sentience (Paul and Podberscek, 2000), affect moral development (Self *et al.*, 1991, 1996) and even cause hardening or detachment (O'Farrell, 1990; Blackshaw and Blackshaw, 1993). Vet student preference for 'ethically sourced' cadavers (animals that have been euthanized due to medical reasons and donated by the owners for teaching purposes) is highest prior to undertaking the initial dog dissection classes and lowest among the cohort of final year students (Tiplady *et al.*, 2011).

Students of veterinary or animal science can be marked on how enthusiastically they participate in practical classes. Those students who have ethical objections toward activities such as castrating and tail docking of unanaesthetized piglets and lambs may join in purely due to fear their grades will suffer. Some students may also have religious objections to the way some animal species are used in teaching (Phillips, 2007).

There are now many alternatives available to minimize or eliminate harmful animal use in teaching (Fig. 7.1). Companies such as Rescue Critters (2012) have a range of animal mannequins available, including synthetic models of skulls and skeletons and resuscitation mannequins for practising cardiopulmonary resuscitation techniques. Some veterinary schools have established Ethical Memorial Programmes, in which owners choose to donate the body of pets euthanized for medical reasons for teaching purposes (Knight, 2002), thereby minimizing or eliminating reliance on pound animals.

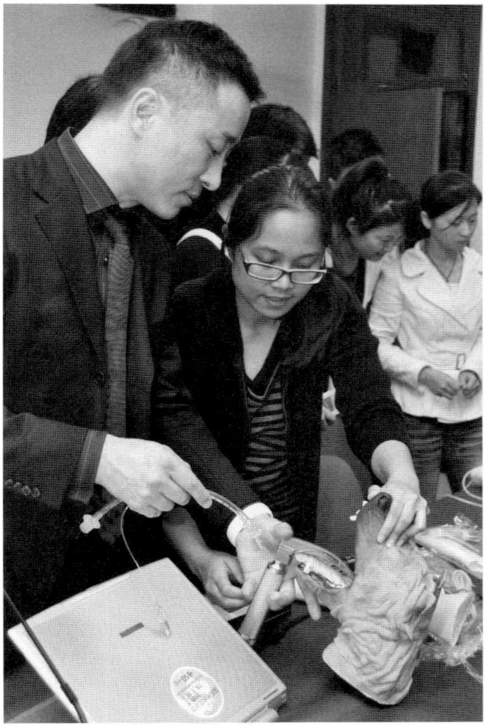

Fig. 7.1. WSPA conducted a lecturer training workshop in Beijing, China for animal welfare educators from veterinary and agriculture schools in 2009. The workshop focused on tertiary-level concepts in animal welfare, including using alternatives to live animal use in teaching. This photograph shows a demonstration of intubating a model of a dog's head. (Photograph courtesy of Natasha Lee.)

Education to Prevent Animal Abuse

Around the world, there are numerous animal welfare, humane and veterinary organizations working to educate people of all ages about animal abuse. Veterinarians and nurses are regularly invited to volunteer for these programmes. Many of these programmes are aimed at young children (Fig. 7.3) rather than adolescents and involve veterinarians visiting schools to talk about safety around animals, how to care for them and treat them with respect (AVA PetPEP, 2010).

Education programmes for children

Children who participated in a humane education programme demonstrated statistically significant increases in humane attitudes toward animals compared to a control group (Hein, 1987). Another researcher found human-directed empathy to be higher in the group of children who received humane education compared to a control group (Paul, 2000). These elevated empathy levels were also present in a follow-up study a year later.

Education programmes for children from violent homes is discussed in Chapter 13.

Education for adults

Education programmes for adults who work with animals are an effective method of disseminating practical methods of improving

Case study: Use of cattle for learning rectal palpation

Veterinary students often learn cow pregnancy diagnosis via rectal examination of dairy cows confined in a crush (Fig. 7.2). In some cases, excessive or rough palpation has led to rectal bleeding.

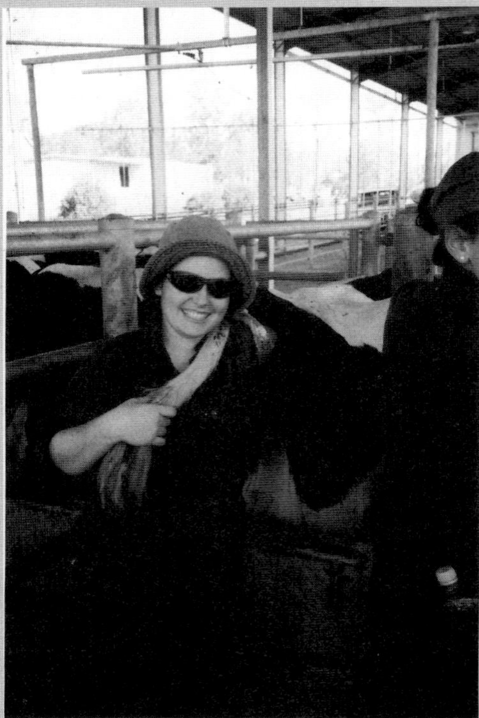

Fig. 7.2. Veterinary students may commence learning rectal palpation for pregnancy diagnosis using live cattle, although mannequins are available. Close supervision is needed for these types of invasive practical classes to avoid animals being harmed. (Photograph courtesy of Catherine Tiplady.)

Excessive use of the same individual animal for invasive practical classes must be avoided. Applying the principles of the 3 R's to the example of rectal palpation in cattle, we can make the following humane changes:

1. Replace use of live cattle (in the initial stages of learning at least) by commencing training using mannequins and computer-assisted learning.
2. Reduce the number of students performing rectal palpation per animal and reduce the number of times each animal is used.
3. Refine the practical, using adequate lubricating gel for the cattle, placing gloves on inside-out to prevent the seam irritating the rectal mucosa, and ensuring adequate supervision. Pain relief or sedation may be advisable for the cattle.

Use of a cow mannequin would enable students to learn the basics of rectal examination technique before using a live animal and would supplement, rather than replace, live animal use. Students who received supplementary training using a virtual reality-based teaching tool – the Bovine Rectal Palpation Simulator – showed significantly better performance when examining cows for the first time, compared with a group of traditionally trained students ($P < 0.001$) (Baillie *et al.*, 2005).

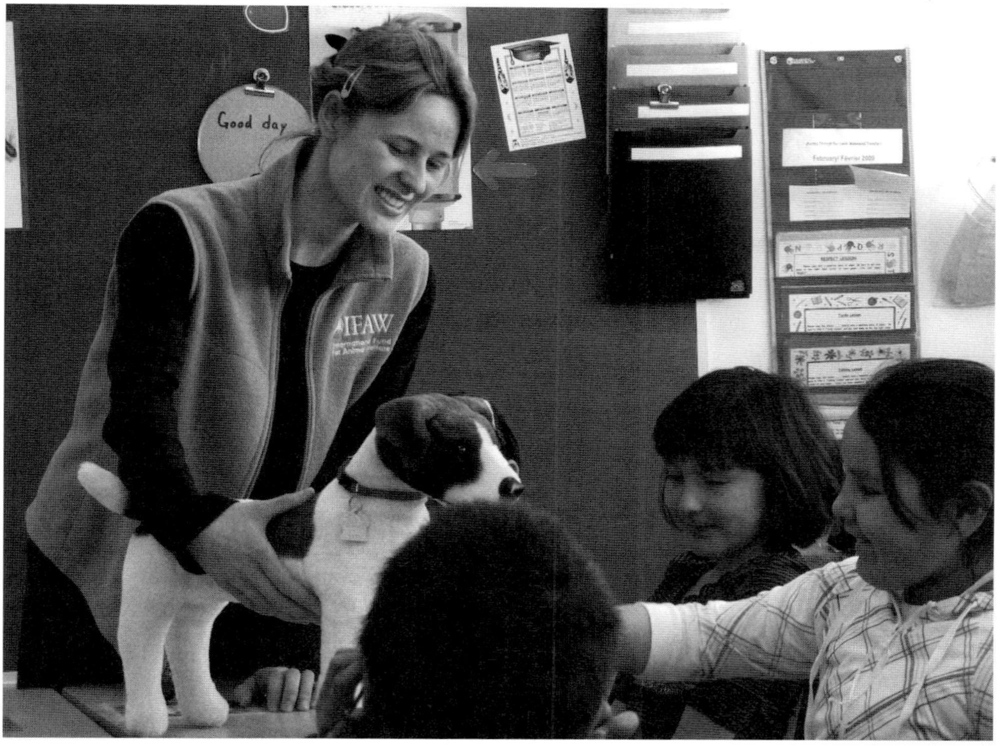

Fig. 7.3. Humane education programmes in schools are helpful in teaching children about animal welfare and how to approach animals safely. (Photograph courtesy of IFAW.)

animal welfare (Figs 7.4, 7.5 and 7.6). This training can have far-reaching impacts on both the participant and their colleagues as the knowledge is passed on. A veterinarian who works in an animal protection organization in Asia describes her experiences of conducting training workshops to vets and animal workers (Natasha Lee, personal communication, 18 January 2012):

> The most rewarding aspects of my work are seeing people change their attitudes and my training being passed on to others. I not only organize training workshops for people working in the field. If I find them to have potential, I like to give them the opportunity to travel abroad, spread their knowledge and influence others (many local people who work with animals in developing countries never had the opportunity to travel abroad). It is nice to see them change their behaviour after getting this exposure and even better when they themselves start teaching others to change too.

> An example: during a neutering training, I included some lessons on welfare and assessment to the local vets. Sometime later, I find that that lesson has been passed down to the other staff in the organization and those staff are then passing on that knowledge to the community. And when one of the vets left to join the government, he brought that knowledge and passion with him.

> Another example is at an animal control officer training. Usually dog catching is one of the lowest ranking jobs in this region. And because a lot of these dogs are considered as 'pests' and are meant to be killed in the end, many workers do not see the need to use humane methods to handle these animals. So the training not only focuses on the technical aspects of animal handling, but touches on many aspects to give a more comprehensive training for this profession. This includes the animal–human bond and how the animal control officer benefits the community. At the end of the workshop there are many participants who indicate their

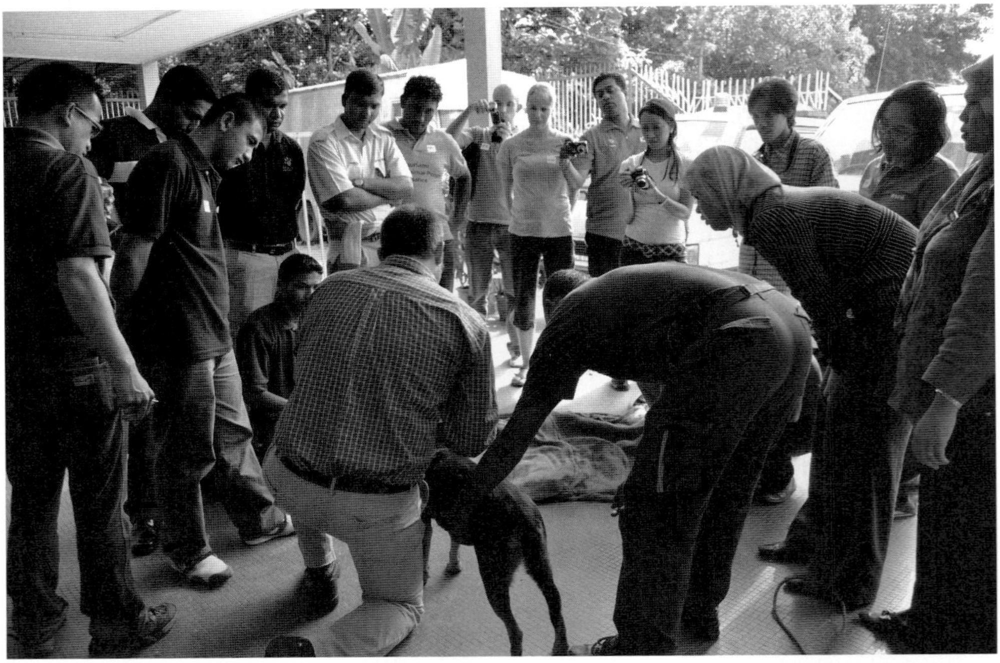

Fig. 7.4. A comprehensive Animal Control Officer workshop was conducted in Kuala Lumpur, Malaysia in 2009. This workshop was attended by animal handlers from seven Asian countries. Practical classes are invaluable in teaching humane animal handling. Some animal abuse may happen because people do not know how to handle the animals or are afraid of them. (Photograph courtesy of Natasha Lee.)

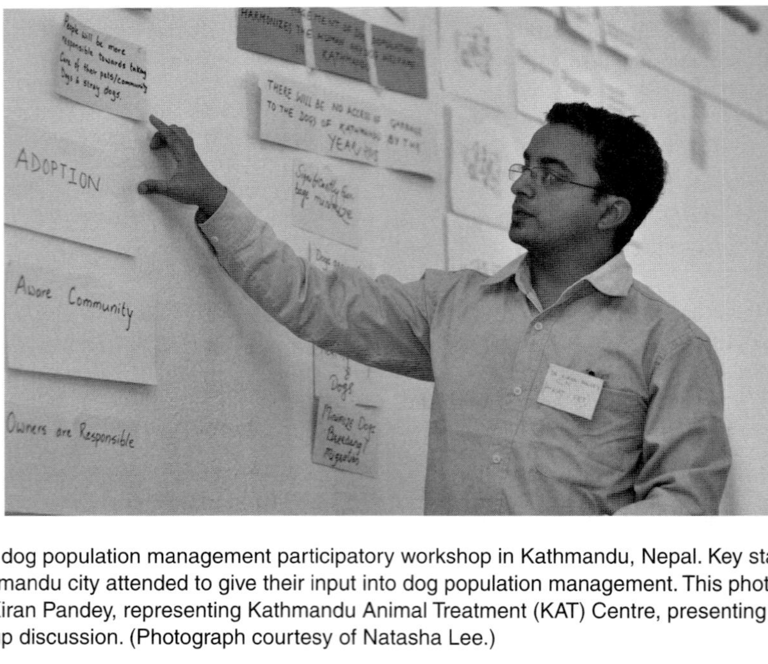

Fig. 7.5. A dog population management participatory workshop in Kathmandu, Nepal. Key stakeholders within Kathmandu city attended to give their input into dog population management. This photograph shows Dr Kiran Pandey, representing Kathmandu Animal Treatment (KAT) Centre, presenting the results from a group discussion. (Photograph courtesy of Natasha Lee.)

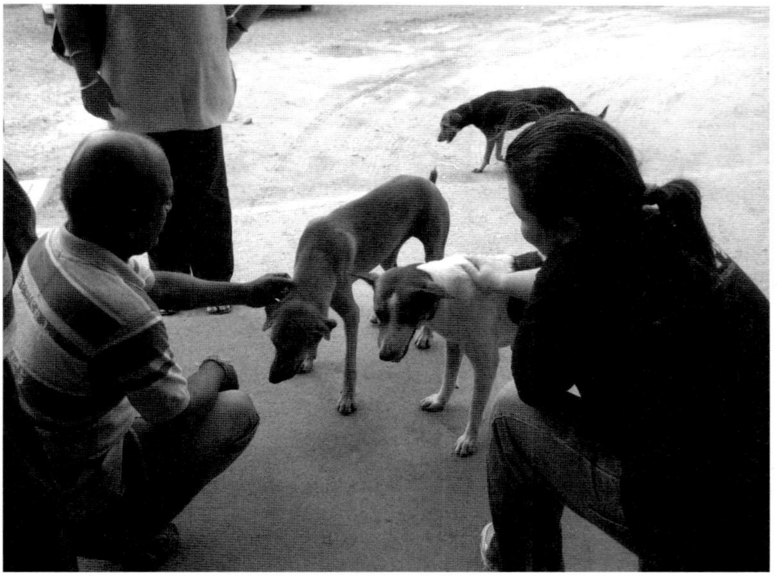

Fig. 7.6. A comprehensive Animal Control Officer workshop was conducted in Colombo, Sri Lanka in 2010 for government and non-governmental organization animal handlers in the country. Understanding basic dog behaviour and how to approach dogs were included in the training. (Photograph courtesy of Jutamart Jattuchai.)

willingness to change to a more humane method of handling animals. An outstanding student from India has not only performed better at his role, he has also had a change in his attitude. He became more enthusiastic to learn and has voluntarily taken up more responsibilities including record keeping, an incredible feat for someone who only learnt to write not too many years ago.

Education of veterinarians in animal abuse and human interpersonal violence

A survey of Australian veterinarians assessed their knowledge about and attitudes towards human and animal abuse (Green and Gullone, 2005).

Over half the respondents agreed with the statements 'People who abuse animals are more likely to abuse their spouses', 'People who abuse their animals are more likely to abuse their children' and 'Veterinarians have a moral responsibility to intervene where they suspect animal abuse'; however, less than 10% felt that veterinary schools provided adequate training in animal abuse prevention (Green and Gullone, 2005).

Similarly, a study in Indiana, USA found that only 7% of veterinarians reported having received instruction in handling animal abuse and none reported having received instruction in handling human abuse (Landau, 1999).

It is concerning that training in animal abuse prevention is inadequately dealt with by those teaching the veterinarians of the future. It has been suggested that lack of training is a major reason why vets do not report abuse (Sharpe and Wittum, 1999). Further training has been recommended both by Australian (Green and Gullone, 2005) and American (Sharpe and Wittum, 1999) researchers. The Australian Veterinary Association 'supports education of the profession and community in recognizing cases of potential animal abuse and its relevance' (AVA, 2010).

Not all countries and regions have legally mandated reporting by veterinarians of suspected cases of animal abuse.

In Australia, veterinarians are not legally mandated to report suspected cases of animal abuse, the Australian Veterinary Association (AVA) believing it may 'discourage people from bringing their animals to the veterinarian if they believe they may be reported' (AVA, 2010).

Even mandatory reporting of animal abuse is unlikely to guarantee all cases being reported – in the medical profession, where doctors are legally mandated to report child abuse, 43% of surveyed doctors have at some stage decided not to report a suspected case of child abuse or neglect (Van Haeringen *et al.*, 1998).

Rollin (1994) believes legally mandated reporting would remove any dilemma for the veterinarian – the veterinarian in this case is not betraying any confidence as they are reporting by the ethic of social consensus.

Absence of mandatory reporting laws should not be an excuse for veterinarians to fail to report suspected cases of animal abuse. Similarly, lack of education in human/animal abuse should not be a reason to turn your back on victims of abuse but rather serve as an incentive to learn more and become a proactive member of your profession.

References

Australian Government National Health and Medical Research Council (2004) *Code of Practice for the Care and Use of Animals for Scientific Purposes*, 7th edn. NHMRC, Canberra, Australia.

Australian Veterinary Association (AVA) (2010) Policy 1.2 Animal abuse. Available at: http://ava.test.ava.com.au/policy/12-animal-abuse (accessed 18 February 2011).

AVA PetPEP (2010) Australian Veterinary Association PetPEP. Available at: http://petpep.ava.com.au/ (accessed 22 February 2012).

Baillie, S., Crossan, A., Brewster, S., Mellor, D. and Reid, S. (2005) Validation of a bovine rectal palpation simulator for training veterinary students. *Studies in Health Technology and Informatics* 111, 33–36.

Balcombe, J. (1997) Animals and values in education. Can we dissect one without rejecting the other? *HSUS News* 42, 4, Washington, DC.

Blackshaw, J. and Blackshaw, A.W. (1993) Student perceptions of attitudes to the human–animal bond. *Anthrozoös* 6, 190–198.

Capaldo, T. (2004) The psychological effects on students of using animals in ways that they see as ethically, morally or religiously wrong. *Alternatives to Laboratory Animals* 32 (Suppl. 1), 525–531.

Green, P.C. and Gullone, E. (2005) Knowledge and attitudes of Australian veterinarians to animal abuse and human interpersonal violence. *Australian Veterinary Journal* 83, 619–625

Hein, G.E. (1987) *Massachusetts Society for the Prevention of Cruelty to Animals Outreach Program Evaluation: Final report.* Boston SPCA, Massachusetts.

Jukes, N. and Chiuia, M. (2003) *From Guinea Pig to Computer Mouse: Alternative methods for a progressive, humane education*, 2nd edn. International Network for Humane Education (InterNICHE), Leicester, UK.

Knight, A. (ed.) (2002) Learning without killing: A guide to conscientious objection. Available at: http://www.interniche.org/system/files/public/Conscientious_Objection/akcoguide.pdf (accessed 30 April 2012).

Landau, R.E. (1999) A survey of teaching and implementation: the veterinarian's role in recognizing and reporting abuse. *Journal of the American Veterinary Medical Association* 215(3), 328–331.

Langley, G. (2003) Foreword. In: Jukes, N. and Chiuia, M. (eds) *From Guinea Pig to Computer Mouse: Alternative Methods for a Progressive, Humane Education.* InterNICHE, Leicester, UK, pp. ix–x.

Martinsen, S. and Jukes, N. (2005) Towards a humane veterinary education. *Journal of Veterinary Medical Education* 32, 454–460.

Moran, L. and Roth, G.L. (2006) Humor in context: fire service and joking context. In: Ismail, M., Osman Gani, A., Ahmad, S., Abdullah, A., Ismail, I. and Othman, J. (eds) *Human Resource Development in Asia: Thriving on dynamism and change.* Universiti Putra Malaysia, Putrajaya, Malaysia, pp. 120–127.

New England Anti-Vivisection Society (2012) Alternatives in education. Available at: http://www.neavs.org/alternatives/in-education (accessed 30 April 2012).

O'Farrell, V. (1990) Students' stereotypes of owners and veterinarians. *Veterinary Record* 125, 625.

Paul, E.S. (2000) Love of pets and love of people. In: Podberscek, A.L., Paul, E.S. and Serpell, J.A. (eds) *Companion Animals and Us: Exploring the relationships between people and pets.* Cambridge University Press, Cambridge, pp. 168–186.

Paul, E.S. and Podberscek, A.L. (2000) Veterinary education and students' attitudes towards animal welfare. *Veterinary Record* 146, 269–272.

Phillips, C.J.C. (2007) Veterinary education – more than just science is needed. In: Tulloch, G. and de Fraga, C. (eds) *Humane Education: a compassionate ethic for animals. Inaugural Australian Symposium on Humane Education*, Brisbane, Australia, 5–6 October 2007, pp. 99–106.

Rescue Critters (2012) Rescue Critters Brand. Available at: http://www.rescuecritters.com/ (accessed 1 May 2012).

Rollin, B. (1994) An ethicist's commentary on whether veterinarians should report cruelty. *Canadian Veterinary Journal* 35, 408–409.

Roth, G.L. and Vivona, B. (2010) Mirth and murder: crime scene investigation as a work context for examining humor applications. *Human Resource Development Review* 9(4), 314–332.

Russell, W.M.S. and Burch, R.L. (1992) *The Principles of Humane Experimental Technique*, 2nd edn. Methuen, London.

Self, D.J., Schrader, D.E., Baldwin, D.C., Root, S.K., Wolinsky, F.D. and Shadduck, J.A. (1991) Study of the influence of veterinary medical-education on the moral development of veterinary students. *Journal of the American Veterinary Medical Association* 198, 782–787.

Self, D.J., Olivarez, M., Baldwin, D.C. and Shadduck, J.A. (1996) Clarifying the relationship of veterinary medical education and moral development. *Journal of the American Veterinary Medical Association* 209, 2002–2004.

Sharpe, M.S. and Wittum, T.E. (1999) Veterinarian involvement in the prevention and intervention of human violence and animal abuse: a survey of small animal practitioners. *Anthrozoös* 12(2), 97–104.

Tiplady, C., Lloyd, S. and Morton, J. (2011) Veterinary science student preferences for the source of dog cadavers used in anatomy teaching. *Alternatives to Laboratory Animals* 39(5), 461–469.

Van Haeringen, A.R., Dadds, M. and Armstrong, K.L. (1998) The child abuse lottery – will the doctor suspect and report? Physician attitudes towards and reporting of suspected child abuse and neglect. *Child Abuse and Neglect* 22(3), 159–169.

Woon, S.-Y. (2011) A veterinary student's perspective on educational animal use and the potential for humane alternatives. *Alternatives to Animal Experimentation, Proceedings of the 8th World Conference*, Montreal, Canada, 21–25 August 2011, pp. 377–385.

8 Religion, Philosophy and Ethics – How These Affect Our Treatment of Animals

Catherine Tiplady

Animal Abuse and Religion

Throughout history, religions of the world have played an influential role in how humans and animals are treated and several books have been published on the topic of religion and animals (e.g. Linzey, 1994, 2009; Webb, 1998; Wennberg, 2003).

People's interpretation of religious guidelines for how animals should be treated may lead to improved animal care for some animals whereas others may suffer for the same reason. Followers of each faith may also vary in the extent of their adherence to religious guidelines. Major religions in the world include Buddhism, Christianity, Hinduism, Islam and Judaism. This section will briefly consider each of these religions and how they may impact on their followers' attitudes toward animal abuse or protection. It will then cover ethics and philosophy of our treatment of animals.

Buddhism

> All living things fear being beaten with clubs.
> All living things fear being put to death.
> Putting oneself in the place of the other,
> Let no one kill or cause another to kill.
>
> (Dhammapada 129)

Buddhism began in the 6th century BCE when a prince, Siddhartha Gautama, left his privileged life and learned of the suffering in the world, eventually reaching enlightenment to become the Buddha, or 'enlightened one' (Rock, 2004).

Buddhists believe that suffering is at the heart of everything and follow guidelines to reach enlightenment, promising not to harm or kill any living thing and choosing work that does not cause harm (Rock, 2004). The doctrine of karma implies that misdeeds cause souls to be reincarnated as animals and this is considered a serious spiritual setback (BBC Religions, 2011). In artistic representation of the Buddhist Wheel of Life, the pig represents ignorance, the rooster denotes desire and the snake symbolizes anger (Meadows, 2003).

Because Buddhists follow the rule of Ahimsa, or non-violence, animal abuse is against their beliefs. Fishing, hunting, animal husbandry and use of animals in entertainment are forbidden (Phelps, 2004).

Hinduism

> Every living creature is the son of the Supreme Lord, and He does not tolerate even an ant's being killed.
>
> (Prabhupada, 2004, p. 487)

Hinduism began in India over 4000 years ago. Its followers believe in one God, Brahman, who represents absolute truth; however, there are numerous gods and goddesses that are part of the one Brahman (Rock, 2004). Some of the gods have animal features, such as Ganesha, the elephant god, who is the symbol of strength and wisdom and Hanuman, the monkey god, a symbol of strength and energy (Rock, 2004). These animal-like gods may increase people's empathy for the animals which the gods resemble. Hindus believe in reincarnation and the law of cause and effect (karma) ties the body to life on earth as a 'lowly' creature if misdeeds are performed (Rock, 2004, p. 26). Hinduism teaches non-violence and many Hindus are vegetarian.

A related faith of Hinduism is Hare Krishna and in both of these religions, cattle are considered holy. Lord Krishna was a cowherd and much is written in Krishna texts advocating cow protection. Krishna's followers, or 'devotees', are instructed never to steal, beat, chastise or kill a cow (Dasa, 2004) and the law of Karma and reincarnation dictates that those who abuse people or animals will be punished by experiencing the same violence and suffering in a future life (Prabhupada, 2001). The cow is considered auspicious as milk consumption is considered necessary for the human brain to attain transcendental knowledge (Prabhupada, 1977). Despite this emphasis on cow protection, welfare of cattle in India is considered poor by many who visit the country. Cattle may appear thin and unwell and roam the streets foraging in rubbish to find food to eat. Ingestion of rubbish can cause impactions and death.

Christianity

> Let them have dominion over the fish of the sea, over the birds of the air, and over the cattle, over all the earth and over every creeping thing that creeps on the earth.
>
> (Genesis 1, the Bible)

Christianity began about 2000 years ago and is based on the teachings of Jesus, a man who Christian followers believe to be the Son of God.

The dominionistic view of humans having control over animals could be viewed as a duty of care to protect animals or, conversely, giving humans the right to use and abuse animals as they see fit. Jesus is seen as a protector, a benevolent shepherd who watches over his flock (of people) and this may have encouraged some followers to care for their animals in a similar way.

The treatment of animals and people's responsibilities toward them features strongly in the Christian Bible although there are contradictions in the messages. Animal care is taken seriously in the story of Noah's Ark where animals are saved from a great flood and taken, in male and female pairs, on to a boat to safety. It could be argued that the rescue of animals was not purely altruistic – it would be in the best interests of surviving humans to have a supply of animals to breed, eat and use in the aftermath of a devastating flood.

Central to the Christian faith are the Ten Commandments, a set of guidelines by which Christians are expected to live, including 'Thou shalt not kill'. Some have interpreted this as an instruction to kill neither humans nor animals, arguing that if the intention had been to protect humans from being killed, the commandment would have been 'Thou shalt not *murder*' (Prabhupada, 2006).

Murder, killing and cruelty to animals are written about in Isaiah in the Bible. Despite warning that 'he who kills a bull is as if he slays a man; he who sacrifices a lamb, as if he breaks a dog's neck' (Isaiah 66:3), sacrificial animal killing is described elsewhere in the Bible in some technical detail, almost in a DIY fashion. 'Aaron and his sons laid their hands on the head of the bull for the sin offering, And Moses killed it. Then he took the blood and put some on the horns of the altar all around with his finger.' Moses is described killing animals, including calves, lambs, kids, rams and bulls and sprinkling their blood around an altar in acts of sin offerings apparently commanded by the Lord (Leviticus 8, 9).

A conservative Christian view may not correspond with increased empathy for animals. A sample of regular Christian churchgoers found a more humane attitude toward animals in those with a more liberal, rather than conservative theological position (Bowd and Bowd, 1989).

Islam

> There is not an animal on earth, nor a bird that flies on its wings – but they are communities like you.
>
> (The Qu'ran, 6:38)

Islam began in Arabia in 610 CE with the belief that Allah is the One True God and that a man named Muhammad was chosen to be Allah's prophet (Rock, 2004). Followers of Islam are called Muslims and follow the teachings of their holy book, the Qu'ran and the Hadith.

Muslims are required to consume 'Halal' meat, obtained from animals killed while conscious, the slaughterer blessing the animal as a sharp knife makes a single cut across the neck (Drum and Gunning-Trant, 2008).

Religious guidelines for Muslims do not allow animal cruelty and state: 'Verily Allah has prescribed proficiency in all things. Thus, if you kill, kill well; and if you slaughter, slaughter well. Let each of you sharpen his blade and let him spare sufferings to the animal he slaughter' (Halal Australia, 2004). Despite the guidelines to spare animal suffering, there are concerns from some that ritual slaughter for religious reasons is cruel.

Western methods of slaughter typically involve animals being stunned first, using a captive bolt stunner to render each animal unconscious before it is hung up and major blood vessels severed to exsanguinate the animal.

Defenders of Halal slaughter claim that a single incision to the throat of a conscious animal is not painful; however, it is argued that an animal choking on its own blood is likely to experience extreme suffering (Webster, 1994).

Judaism

> I will make a covenant on behalf of Israel with the wild beasts, the birds of the air, and the things that creep on hearths that all living creatures may lie down without living in fear.
>
> (Hosea 2:18)

Judaism began over 3000 years ago and the father of the Jewish faith is said to be Abraham (Rock, 2004). Within the Talmud (a set of laws and traditions) are specific instructions that Jews are not to cause pain to animals and should treat them with compassion (BBC Religions, 2009).

Jewish people are required to eat food that is Kosher. To satisfy the requirements for Kosher slaughter, a Rabbi who is specially trained in religious slaughter cuts the throat of a conscious animal. Although the animal must be killed so it feels little pain, this method of slaughter is considered 'cruel and inhumane' by the RSPCA (Tensen, 2009).

Philosophy, Ethics and Animal Abuse

Ethics refers to a whole field of moral science and rules of conduct (*Concise Oxford Dictionary*, 1974).

For centuries, philosophers provided people with ethical guidance about how they should treat animals. In the 17th century CE, philosopher Descartes argued that animals had no souls or feelings (Brown, 1974) and cruel vivisection experiments were practised by people who followed Cartesian principles. Later philosophers such as Kant and Schopenhauer denounced cruelty – Kant because he believed it would 'harden our hearts' against our fellow humans (Bernstein, 2009, p. 185) and Schopenhauer because he considered that anybody who is cruel to animals cannot be a good person (Schopenhauer, 1841).

Jeremy Bentham (1748–1832) proposed that 'The day *may* come, when the rest of the animal creation may acquire those rights which never could have been withholden from them but by the hand of tyranny' and prompted people to consider animals as sentient beings by asking 'The question is not, Can they *reason*? nor, Can they *talk*? but can they *suffer*?' (Bentham, 1989, pp. 25–26). This quote is often repeated by animal advocacy groups over two centuries later.

Ethical theory

Ethical decision making can be assisted by several different theoretical positions, some of which are listed by Palmer and Sandoe (2011) as:

- The contractarian view – only considers human interests.
- The utilitarian view – considers consequences to be important when we are making ethical decisions and that we

should consider not just the interests of humans but also all affected sentient beings.

- The animal rights view – considers that animals are sentient and have rights to life, liberty and respectful treatment.
- Contextual views – considers that a variety of factors are of significance, such as the emotional bond between humans and animals.
- Respect for nature view – considers the protection of species to be of moral significance.

Veterinarians and ethics

Veterinarians are bound by professional codes of ethics, societal ethics and by their personal ethics. Some, but not all veterinarians, take an oath at graduation, which includes a statement such as this example from Canada: 'I will practise my profession conscientiously, with dignity, and in keeping with the principles of veterinary medical ethics' (CVMA, 2004).

Knowledge of ethics is important as ethical dilemmas (cases where there appears to be no easy right or wrong way to proceed) are regularly encountered in veterinary practice – the decisions you make are crucial to protecting the animal's welfare, avoiding further suffering and enabling yourself to have peace of mind (and not be struck off from the veterinary profession). Despite the crucial role ethics plays in veterinary practice, some veterinary students try and avoid attending classes on ethics (Lane, 2002), and an optional summer course in ethics for veterinary students received few enrolments (Erde and Pollock, 1987).

The handling of ethical dilemmas connected with animal abuse and neglect can have major ramifications on your career and be very stressful. In these cases, seeking guidance from other professionals is always recommended.

Case Study: The cat hoarder

As a newly graduated veterinarian, you enter small animal practice and soon encounter a middle-aged woman, Ria, who runs her own cat rescue service. She lives alone, has no income other than her pension and seems like a very compassionate woman. Soon, Ria requests to see you specifically and, initially, you are quite flattered as it boosts your confidence. After a few months, however, you realize you have never seen the same cat twice and all of Ria's cats and kittens are introduced to you with a similar sad story of being dumped/abandoned/abused before being 'rescued'. Cat flu and cystitis are the main health complaints the cats present with during consultation. Ria is evasive about the exact number of animals owned yet admits that she is dividing your prescribed medication among other sick cats at home. You advise her not to do this and ask her to bring any sick cats in for examination. One day, Ria turns up demanding medication for a cat you have never seen. She tells you he obviously has a urinary tract infection as he is straining to urinate. You tell Ria that you must examine the animal immediately as he may have a blocked bladder, which could be life threatening, but she refuses and becomes verbally abusive. You are upset by this and worried the cat is suffering. You wonder if you should just dispense medication without question and telephone Ria later to try and gently encourage her to bring the cat in, even if you offer to pay for any treatment yourself.

What should you do?

First, do not be pressured by this client or anybody else to do anything such as hand out veterinary drugs without a prior examination and diagnosis. This is unethical, does not provide a high standard of patient care and can have serious repercussions for your reputation and career. In this case, it will only enable the hoarder to continue their hoarding and perpetuate animal suffering. It is recommended you discuss the case with other professionals, such as your manager and report this owner to the RSPCA or humane society as a suspected animal hoarder. Stress in your complaint the possible critical nature of the cat's condition. After investigation, it is likely the unwell cat/s will be removed from the owner and treated. Although this will provide much-needed assistance to the animals, without an interdisciplinary approach involving human mental health, animal welfare, legal and municipal agencies working together, there is a nearly 100% recidivism rate among hoarders (Patronek *et al.*, 2006). Dr Randall Lockwood of the ASPCA (2012) sums up the suffering inherent in hoarding cases: 'Being kept by a hoarder is a slow kind of death for the animal. Actually, it can be a fate worse than death.' Your veterinary association will be able to advise you of whether you are legally mandated to report suspected animal abuse and about confidentiality and legal issues.

When examining the ethics of animal treatment it is worthwhile trying to gain a perspective of all the parties involved before making an informed judgement.

Using an ethical matrix

An online ethical matrix system – developed by Nottingham University Centre for Bioethics – enables students and others to examine ethical issues surrounding the different ways animals are farmed and used (Mepham and Tomkins, 2003). Participants are encouraged to consider and apply ethical principles of well-being, autonomy and justice to farmers, consumers, animals and the environment in order to stimulate discussion and reach overall ethical judgements (Mepham and Tomkins, 2003).

The positive and negative consequences of the live export of animals

Live animal export is a contentious issue, which many animal advocates believe to be cruel.

Table 8.1 shows the positive and negative ethical consequences of transporting live animals via ship for slaughter overseas, considering the viewpoints of the farmers, the animals, the customers and the Australian public (Phillips, 2005).

Do any of the positive ethical consequences in Table 8.1 outweigh the animal abuse seen in Figs 8.1–8.4?

Table 8.1. Ethical consequences of live export of livestock (adapted from Phillips, 2005).

	Positive ethical consequences	Negative ethical consequences
Interests of the animals	Food and water is available on the journey (this may not be available to all farm animals in drought) Lives of some sheep and cattle are prolonged by the live export trade	Increased mortality compared to on-farm Subjected to on-board stresses including: high temperatures, high stocking density, motion sickness, rough handling, social disruption, noise, accumulation of excreta, neophobia Risk of disease transmission between countries (Kouba, 2003) Possibility of animal abuse during handling and slaughter post-embarkation (Sidhom, 2003)
Interests of the farmers/staff	Financial benefits (animals sold for live export command a higher price than those sold for local consumption) Value to Australian economy Provides a market for mature wool-producing wethers (male castrated sheep)	Estimated loss of jobs and money to Australia as local meat processing is impacted (Crawford, 2010) Stress in being part of trade in which animals face hardship Desensitization to seeing animal cruelty May perceive animals as objects rather than sentient beings
Interests of overseas customers	Meat available at affordable price Reduced pressure on grazing land If livestock not sourced from Australia, may obtain them from countries with less concern for animal welfare	Jobs of overseas customers may be lost due to live export (may have been able to produce own meat if they imported animal feed) Possibility that some Muslims (>98% of live exported sheep are exported to Muslim countries) object to supporting a largely Christian country (Australia)
Interests of Australian public	Maintenance of farmers' jobs Maintenance of rural environment Provision of meat to overseas public Possibility that the trade may help unite Muslim and Christian countries	Concern for animal welfare, e.g. animals slaughtered without prior stunning Australian abattoir jobs impacted by live export trade Grazing cattle and sheep industry may not be ecologically sustainable in long term

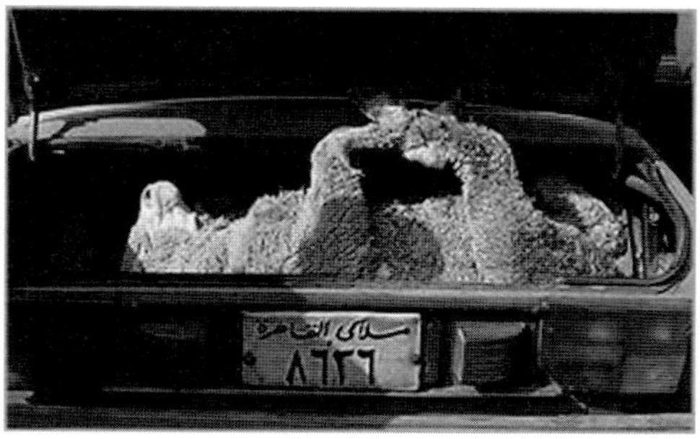

Fig. 8.1. Australian sheep in boot of car in Egypt. (Photograph copyright Animals Australia.)

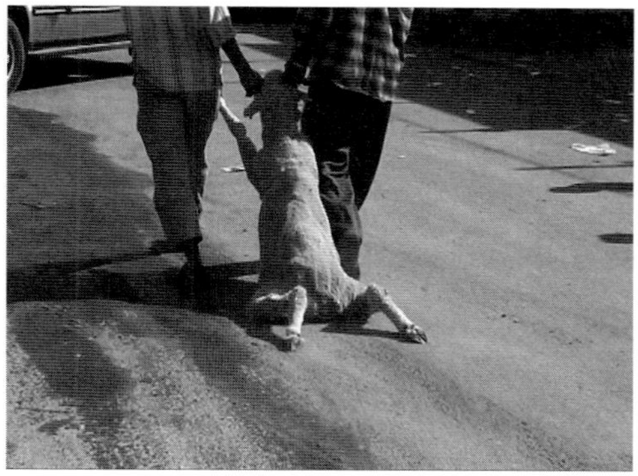

Fig. 8.3. Sheep being dragged by the horns to car in Kuwait. (Photograph copyright Animals Australia.)

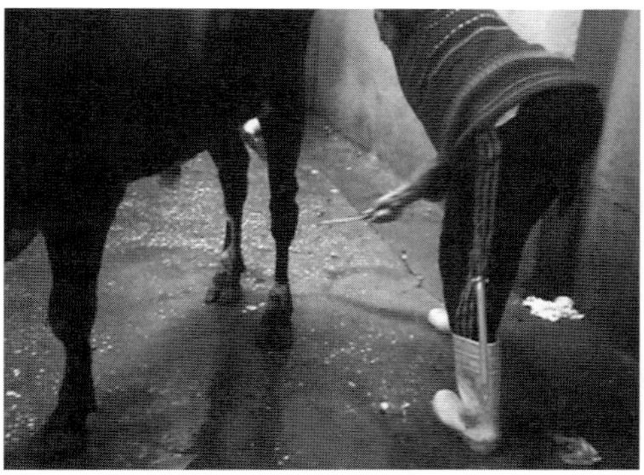

Fig. 8.2. Cow having leg tendon slashed in Egypt. (Photograph copyright Animals Australia.)

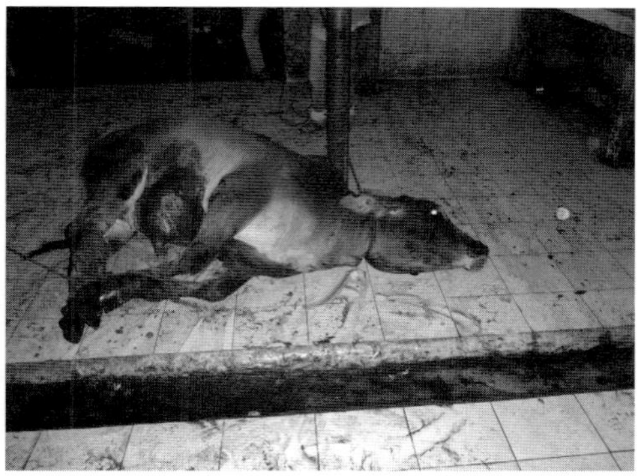

Fig. 8.4. Steer tied and beaten prior to slaughter in Indonesia. (Photograph copyright Animals Australia.)

References

ASPCA (2012) Animal hoarding. Available at: http://www.aspca.org/Fight-Animal-Cruelty/animal-hoarding (accessed 28 April 2012).

BBC Religions (2009) Treatment of animals. Available at: http://www.bbc.co.uk/religion/religions/judaism/jewishethics/animals_1.shtml (accessed 21 September 2011).

BBC Religions (2011) Buddhism and animals. Available at: http://www.bbc.co.uk/religion/religions/buddhism/buddhistethics/animals.shtml (accessed 11 September 2011).

Bentham, J. ([1789] 1989) A utilitarian view. In: Regan, T. and Singer, P. (eds) *Animal Rights and Human Obligations.* Prentice Hall, Englewood Cliffs, New Jersey, pp. 25–26.

Bernstein, M.H. (2009) Responding ethically to animal abuse. In: Linzey, A. (ed.) *The Link Between Animal Abuse and Human Violence.* Sussex Academic Press, Eastbourne, UK, pp. 184–189.

Bowd, A.D. and Bowd, A.C. (1989) Attitudes toward the treatment of animals: a study of Christian groups in Australia. *Anthrozoös* 3(1), 20–24.

Brown, A. (1974) *Who Cares for Animals?* William Heinemann Ltd, London.

Concise Oxford Dictionary (1974) Oxford University Press, London.

Crawford, B. (2010) Live export special report – an 'unlikely alliance' working together for a common goal. *The Meatworker* April, pp. 2–3.

CVMA (2004) Canadian veterinary oath. Canadian Veterinary Medical Association. Available at: http://canadianveterinarians.net/about-oath.aspx (accessed 28 April 2012).

Dasa, P. (ed.) (2004) *Sacred Cow* (translated by Bhumipati Dasa). Rasbihari Lal & Sons, Vrindavan, India.

Drum, F. and Gunning-Trant, C. (2008) Live animal exports: a profile of the Australian industry. In: *ABARE research report 08.1*. Department of Agriculture, Fisheries and Forestry, Canberra, Australia.

Erde, E.L. and Pollock, R.V.H. (1987) A course in ethics for veterinarians. *Journal of Veterinary Medical Education* 14, 26–29.

Halal Australia (2004) Halal Australia. Available at: http://www.halal-australia.com.au (accessed 22 June 2011).

Kouba, V. (2003) Globalization of communicable animal diseases – a crisis of veterinary medicine. *Acta Veterinaria Brno* 72, 453–460.

Lane, D.M. (2002) Veterinary ethics. *DVM* 33(9), 24–27.

Linzey, A. (1994) *Animal Theology*. University of Illinois Press, Chicago, Illinois.

Linzey, A. (2009) *Creatures of the Same God: Explorations in Animal Theology*. Lantern Books, New York.

Meadows, G. (2003) Buddhism and psychiatry: confluence and conflict. *Australasian Psychiatry* 11(1), 16–20.

Mepham, B. and Tomkins, S. (2003) *Ethics and Animal Farming*. Centre for Applied Bioethics, University of Nottingham, published by CIWF, Petersfield, Hampshire, UK. Available at: http://www.ethicalmatrix.net (accessed 3 May 2012).

Palmer, C. and Sandoe, P. (2011) Animal ethics. In: Appleby, M.C., Mench, J.A., Olsson, A.S. and Hughes, B.O. (eds) *Animal Welfare*, 2nd edn, CAB International, Wallingford, UK.

Patronek, G.J., Loar, L. and Nathanson, J.N. (eds) (2006) *Animal hoarding: Structuring interdisciplinary responses to help people, animals and communities at risk*. Hoarding of Animals Research Consortium, Boston, Massachusetts.

Phelps, N. (2004) *The Great Compassion: Buddhism and Animal Rights*. Lantern Books, New York.

Phillips, C.J.C. (2005) Ethical perspectives of the Australian live export trade. *Australian Veterinary Journal* 83(9), 558–562.

Prabhupada, A.C.B.S. (1977) *Srimad-Bhagavatam* 3.5.7. The Bhaktivedanta Book Trust, Los Angeles, California.

Prabhupada, A.C.B.S. (2001) *The Higher Taste*. The Bhaktivedanta Book Trust, Sydney, Australia.

Prabhupada, A.C.B.S. (2004) *Bhagavad-Gita As It Is*. 14.16. Bhaktivedanta Book Trust, Riverstone, New South Wales, Australia, p. 487.

Prabhupada, A.C.B.S. (2006) Factory farming and compassion. In: Dasi, K. (ed.) *The Higher Taste*. Bhaktivedanta Book Trust International, Watford, UK, pp. 23–34.

Rock, L. (2004) *Tell Me About the World's Religions*. Lion Hudson, Oxford, UK.

Schopenhauer, A. (1841) *On the Basis of Morality* (1841), trans. E. F. J. Payne (Indianapolis: Bobbs-Merrill/Library of Liberal Arts, 1965), sec. 17; cited in: Fox, M.A. (2006): 'Boundless Compassion': The Contemporary Relevance of Schopenhauer's Ethics, The European Legacy: Toward New Paradigms, 11:4, 369–387.

Sidhom, P. (2003) Welfare of cattle transported from Australia to Egypt. *Australian Veterinary Journal* 81(6), 364–365.

Tensen, M. (2009) In: Edwards L. 'Ministers allow ritual slaughter.' *The Age*, 10 November. Available at: http://www.halalmeat.com.au/halal-meat-articles/2009/11/10/ministers-allow-ritual-slaughter (accessed 22 June 2011).

Webb, S.H. (1998) *On God and Dogs: A Christian Theology of Compassion for Animals*. Oxford University Press, New York.

Webster, J. (1994) *Animal Welfare – a cool eye towards Eden*. Blackwell Science, Oxford, UK.

Wennberg, R.N. (2003) *God, Humans, and Animals: an invitation to enlarge our moral universe*. William B. Eerdmans Publishing Co., Grand Rapids, Michigan.

9 Feminist Aspects of Animal Abuse

Catherine Tiplady

Feminism, Racism and Animal Abuse

> The animals of the world exist for their own reasons. They were not made for humans any more than black people were made for whites or women for men.
>
> (Walker, 1996, p.14)

The issue of animal abuse has attracted attention by those seeing a connection between racism, violence against women and animal abuse. These types of abuse may occur concurrently, such as in domestic violence or in animal abuse/human abuse pornography.

In feminist theory, there is believed to be a link between the oppression of women and the eating of meat, for example, women reporting they feel like 'a piece of meat' after being raped (Adams, 2004). Female farm animals may be impregnated while restrained in a device some have 'jokingly' referred to as a 'rape rack' (Gellatley and Wardle, 1996, p. 7). An intensive piggery at an Australian veterinary school has 'Piggy Bordello' written on the wall of the enclosure where boars and sows are 'teased', perhaps in an ironic attempt to humorize the treatment of intensively housed pigs, most of which will never experience natural mating.

It has been argued by Adams (2004, p. 54) that 'sexual violence and meat eating, which appear to be discrete forms of violence, find a point of intersection in the absent referent... If animals are the absent referent in the phrase "the butchering of women", women are the absent referent in the phrase "the rape of animals"'. In *The Sexual Politics of Meat*, Adams (2004) provides disturbing examples of sexualization of animals, women and meat – a photograph of a sow dressed in lingerie and masturbating in 'Playboar' magazine and a picture entitled 'What's your cut?' shows a naked woman kneeling in blood, her body demarcated and labelled as meat portions (such as rump, loin and rib).

Is any of this really animal abuse though? Why would it upset women to see themselves and animals made fun of as sex/meat objects? Degrading animals in this way is a form of abuse and even though the animal victims may be unaware of the implications, many people find it offensive.

Some people have compared the suffering of animals with the suffering of groups of people. South African artist Ezrom Legae compared the struggles of the African people during Apartheid to animal abuse when describing his 'Chicken Series' of artworks created in the late 1970s (Legae, 1984):

> You see I used the chicken as a symbol of the black people of this country, because the chicken is a domestic bird. Now, one can maim a chicken by pulling out his feathers; one can crucify him and even kill him; but beware there will always be another egg and always another chicken.

Animal Abuse/Feminism in Language

> No woman who is called 'bitch' makes the mistake of thinking she is a man's best friend.
> (Grant, 1999, p. 165)

Comparing women/female animals unfavourably (such as 'stupid cow', 'silly bitch') is a common part of language. Comparisons of men to male animals are less common but when done, tend to be complimentary of a man's virility, for example 'he was a stallion', 'hung like a horse', 'a stud'.

Disturbingly, abuse of women and animals has historically been promoted in proverbs around the world, as seen in these examples (McEnroe and Ode, 1994):

- From Great Britain: 'A woman, an ass, and a walnut tree, bring the more fruit, the more beaten they be.'
- From Italy: 'As both a good horse and a bad horse heed the spur, so both a good woman and a bad woman need the stick.'
- From Nigeria: 'A woman is like a horse: He who can drive her is her master.'
- From China: 'A bride received into the home is like a horse that you have just bought; you break her in by constantly mounting her and continually beating her.'

Animal Abuse as 'Humorous'

Humour surrounding animal abuse and suffering is also commonly encountered, for example in the books *How to Kill Your Girlfriend's Cat* (Daphne, 1988), *The Book of Bunny Suicides* (Riley, 2003) and various video and online computer games featuring simulated animal killing. Jokes involving cruelty to animals are popular among many people, just as other vulnerable groups have been ridiculed throughout history. A reversal of animal-abusing computer games (but no less violent) is 'Polar Bear Payback', in which the player assumes the role of a polar bear, 'saving animals *and* the environment' by biting the heads off seal slaughterers and whalers (Bartlett, 2010).

Animal Abuse in Language

Animals are commonly referred to in a derogatory manner in everyday language and some may consider this to be a form of abuse to both animals and humans.

Phrases that suggest animal harm include:

- 'Kill two birds with one stone.'
- 'More than one way to skin a cat.'
- 'Flogging a dead horse.'
- 'Give a dog a bad name and hang him.'

Sexual Abuse of Animals and Animals in Pornography

Sexual abuse of animals is also known as 'bestiality' and 'zoophilia' and both male and female humans can be the perpetrators. Bestiality is defined as 'unnatural connexion with a beast' and a zoophile defined as 'a lover of animals' or one who opposes cruelty to animals (Britannica, 1962). In this section, the term 'animal sexual abuse' will be used to clarify the fact that this is a form of animal abuse rather than using the more ambiguous 'zoophilia'.

Animal sexual abuse has been part of civilization for millennia. Legends have described it, poets and authors have written about it and artists have depicted it. It is even warned against in religious guidelines, such as the Bible: 'Nor shall you mate with any animal, to defile yourself with it. Nor shall any woman stand before an animal to mate with it. It *is* perversion' (Leviticus 18:23). William Butler Yeats' poem 'Leda and The Swan' describes how Zeus (disguised as a swan) rapes a woman.

Animal sexual abuse is not as rare as people may think. Of the 448 cases of non-accidental injury in small animals in the UK, 6% were sexual in nature (Munro and Thrusfield, 2001), yet veterinarians are typically uncomfortable dealing with this issue, Munro (2006) describing it as 'the last taboo' of veterinary practice.

Sexual abuse of animals occurs where a human penetrates an animal's vagina, anus, mouth or cloaca with penis, finger or object or engages with or allows an animal to penetrate or stimulate them with the aim of human sexual gratification. Even in cases where the animal appears large enough or docile enough to cope with the physical aspects of sexual interaction it can never be considered an equal, consensual relationship and as such cannot be justified. Animals may be 'groomed' for sexual abuse just as paedophiles 'groom' children for sexual abuse

(Duffield *et al.*, 1998; Quayle and Taylor, 2002). Case studies of animal sexual abuse are discussed in Chapter 18.

Some animal sexual abuse is filmed and distributed as pornography. Beirne (2000) describes watching a pornographic film with a variety of animals in it. He comments that he is unsure whether the cattle or horses being sexually abused are experiencing boredom, indifference or calculated detachment to cope with the abuse. While some of the animal victims show apparent 'enthusiasm', Beirne (2000) also describes how some small animals have died as a result of sexual abuse.

Although all sexual abuse whether intraspecies (such as human rape) or interspecies (as in animal sexual assault by humans) is abhorrent, animal victims are at an even greater disadvantage compared to human victims. It is impossible for animals to seek help by communicating the facts of their abuse (Beirne, 2000) and should they wish to stop the abuse or complain later they have no redress.

Some people may satisfy their sexual fetishes for animal abuse by watching animals being slaughtered in an abattoir (Dekkers, 1994). Films where animals are killed are often known as 'crush' or 'squish' videos and may depict small animals being crushed to death by women as part of a sexual fetish. A woman who works as an animal sex prostitute believes she is empowered by taking part in animal pornography, stating it 'allows me to take charge of my own sexuality. I don't have to rely on a man' (Stray, 2011).

The seriousness of animal sexual abuse is summed up by Frank Ascione (2004, p. 167), who states that 'The domination of a helpless animal coupled with the perpetrator's sexual arousal and with injuries to, or the death of, the animal sexually assaulted is a terrible recipe for deviant sexual arousal'.

References

Adams, C.J. (2004) *The Sexual Politics of Meat.* Continuum International Publishing Group, New York.

Ascione, F.R. (2004) Afterword. In: Merz-Perez, L. and Heide, K.M. (eds) *Animal Cruelty – Pathway to Violence Against People.* AltaMira Press, Lanham, Maryland.

Bartlett, J. (2010) Polar Bear Payback: Slaughtering the Seal Slaughterers. The PETA Files. Available at: http://www.peta.org/b/thepetafiles/archive/2010/03/15/polar-bear-payback-slaughtering-the-seal-slaughterers.aspx (accessed 17 April 2012).

Beirne, P. (2000) Rethinking bestiality. In: Podberscek, A.L., Paul, E.S. and Serpell, J.A. (eds) *Companion Animals and Us – Exploring the Relationships Between People and Pets.* Cambridge University Press, Cambridge, UK.

Britannica (1962) *Britannica World Language Edition of the Oxford Dictionary.* Oxford University Press, London.

Daphne, R. (1988) *How to Kill Your Girlfriend's Cat.* Doubleday, New York.

Dekkers, M. (1994) *Dearest Pet: On Bestiality* (trans. Paul Vincent). Verso, New York.

Duffield, G., Hassiotis, A. and Vizard, E. (1998) Zoophilia in young sexual abusers. *Journal of Forensic Psychiatry* 9, 294–304.

Gellatley, J. and Wardle, T. (1996) *The Silent Ark.* Thorsons, London.

Grant, A. (1999) Resistance to the link at a domestic violence shelter. In: Ascione, F.R. and Arkow, P. (eds) *Child Abuse, Domestic Violence and Animal Abuse.* Purdue University Press, West Lafayette, Indiana.

Legae, E. (1984) Interview by Linda Given, 12 December. Goodman Gallery archives.

McEnroe, P. and Ode, K. (1994) A violent heritage in our homes – tradition has held that abuse of women is a lesser crime. *Minneapolis Star-Tribune*, 31 July, p. 01A.

Munro, H.M.C. (2006) Animal sexual abuse: a veterinary taboo? *The Veterinary Journal* 172, 195–197.

Munro, H.M.C. and Thrusfield, M.V. (2001) 'Battered pets': sexual abuse. *Journal of Small Animal Practice* 42, 333–337.

Quayle, E. and Taylor, M. (2002) Paedophiles, pornography and the Internet: assessment issues. *British Journal of Social Work* 32(7), 863–875.

Riley, A. (2003) *The Book of Bunny Suicides.* Penguin Group, New York.

Stray (2011) cited in: Moussaieff Masson, J. Pornography and animals. In: Tankard Reist, M. and Bray, A. (eds) *Big Porn Inc.* Spinnaker Press, North Melbourne, Victoria, Australia, pp. 63–68.

Walker, A. (1996) Foreword. In: Spiegel, M. *The Dreaded Comparison – Human and Animal Slavery.* Mirror Books/I.D.E.A., New York, p. 14.

Part III

Animal Abuse: the Human Aspect – Helping the People Involved

Veterinarians are in an ideal position to identify and support the human and animal victims of violence yet are often not adequately educated in how to assist in these cases or how to cope with seeing cases of abuse.

This section discusses the relationship between human and animal abuse and collaborates with interpersonal violence practitioners (Deborah Walsh and Moo Baulch) to provide practical guidance on how veterinarians can assist when confronted with cases of human/animal abuse in veterinary practice. Phil Arkow describes how human and veterinary medical professionals can unite to provide protection for human and animal victims of violence using an integrative 'One Health' approach.

The personal side of working with animal abuse is also included in this section, covering issues of self-care, avoiding compassion fatigue and safety when dealing with perpetrators. A case study from wildlife veterinarian Dr Howard Ralph is included to illustrate the risks and emotions he has experienced when rescuing shot waterbirds during the legal shooting season.

10 One Health

Phil Arkow

A 'One Health' Approach to Ending Family Violence: the Responsibilities of Veterinary Professionals in Recognizing and Reporting Animal Abuse, Domestic Violence, Child Abuse and Elder Abuse

In recent years, an innovative initiative that bridges the commonalities between veterinary and human medicine has emerged through a concept known as 'One Health'. This movement, whose origins lie largely in the veterinary community, is a collaborative effort among multiple health science professions to work locally, nationally and globally to attain optimal health for people, domestic animals, wildlife, plants and the environment. By building closer professional interactions, healthcare can transcend disciplinary and institutional boundaries and transform the way that human, animal, plant and ecosystem health professionals, and their related disciplines, work together.

Since its beginnings in an American Veterinary Medical Association (AVMA) task force in 2007, the One Health concept has resonated increasingly in academia and government, particularly in fields related to public health. A US National League of Cities resolution supports the concept and calls on the federal government to adopt legislation and practices that address human, animal and ecological health in an integrated fashion (National League of Cities, 2011). The concept is still somewhat novel to many veterinarians and physicians in private practice, although they may encounter zoonoses and other One Health examples where human and animal health overlap in their work (Burns, 2012).

The One Health concept is not new: an interdisciplinary approach has long been prevalent in such fields as comparative medical research, disease surveillance and food safety. Human and veterinary medicine, whether in research, clinical practice, public health or medical education, share many common interests in zoonotic disease prevention and health and wellness of patients.

More recently, One Health has included the human–animal bond, one aspect of which is the impact to public and individual health of animal cruelty, abuse and neglect. Although the prevention of cruelty to animals is linked historically with the child protection movement, humane work has long been marginalized outside the realm of community social services: human services and medical officials do not readily see a direct connection between animal maltreatment and the health and well-being of their clients and patients (Arkow, 1992). This perspective is changing with growing recognition of what is called 'The Link' between animal abuse and human violence (National Link Coalition, 2012). A One Health approach has the potential to bring human and veterinary medical professionals together in a common cause to protect all members of the family from violence.

Background: the Role of the Human Health Professional

The role of veterinarians and their staff today vis-à-vis the prevention of violence is analogous to that of human health professionals in the 1960s, at the dawn of the modern child protection movement, and in the 1970s, at the start of domestic violence awareness. Recognition of these forms of family violence as health issues resulted in widespread legislative, programmatic and policy changes that engaged the health community in systems of recognizing and reporting family violence.

Critical to the institutionalization of medical responses to child abuse and domestic violence was the resolution of many challenging ethical concerns and practice management issues. In many areas these remain unresolved, but the human medical fields today generally accept a responsibility to serve as sentinels for potential family violence, to receive training about the clinical indicators of non-accidental injuries (NAI) consistent with domestic violence and child abuse and neglect, and to include these scenarios in differential diagnoses (Arkow and Munro, 2008).

To achieve this, the human medicine fields first had to describe and disseminate diagnostic clinical indicators that differentiate child abuse and neglect from other traumas. Following publication of such indicators in the landmark 'Battered Child Syndrome' article (Kempe *et al.*, 1962), the USA launched one of its most rapid responses to a public health crisis, an institutional model of child maltreatment recognition and reporting that has been imitated worldwide. An earlier paradigm of what had been called 'accident-prone' children was replaced with a national system of mandatory child abuse prevention reporters and child protective services agencies.

Training manuals are now readily available to help medical personnel identify telltale spiral fractures, immersion or cigarette burns, characteristic bruises caused by slaps, electric cords or coat hangers, and other markers of child abuse (e.g. Kessler and Hyden, 1991). Similar publications provide guidance to identify intimate partner violence (e.g. Salber and Taliaferro, 1995; Schornstein, 1997; Jordan *et al.*, 2004) and elder abuse (e.g. National Center on Elder Abuse, 2005; Hildreth, 2011).

In contrast, practitioners of veterinary medicine have been largely excluded from reporting systems for child abuse, domestic violence, elder abuse and animal abuse. This exclusion occurs despite veterinarians being long recognized as having public health responsibilities, as caregivers who see more human clients than animal patients, and as having significant impact on clients' mental health (McCulloch, 1976). The failure to include veterinary medicine among its human medicine counterparts contradicts the One Health concept and is a barrier to achieving full community recognition of the seriousness of abuse and its implications for human health.

Animal Abuse as a Health Concern

Two US surgeons-general have called violence a matter best resolved through public health interventions rather than sociological or law enforcement approaches (Koop and Lundberg, 1992; Novello *et al.*, 1992). Whether victims of violence have two legs or four is often a matter of convenience or a means of emotional control to intimidate and coerce vulnerable women and children (Arkow, 2003). Abuse of animals, particularly household pets, is a common pattern in family violence and its early identification can save lives and protect the integrity of families (Randour, 2011).

Initial research into the links between animal abuse and interpersonal violence focused on the relationship between acts of animal cruelty committed in childhood and criminality in adulthood (Kellert and Felthous, 1985; Felthous and Kellert, 1987; Miller and Knutson, 1997). By 1987, cruelty to animals was added as a criterion for conduct disorder to the American Psychiatric Association's Diagnostic and Statistical Manual of Mental Disorders. Ascione (2001) reviewed psychiatric, psychological and criminological literature dating from 1809 linking juvenile animal cruelty to human violence and wrote (p. 1):

> Animal abuse has received insufficient attention ... as one of a number of 'red flags,' warning signs, or sentinel behaviors that could help identify youth at risk for perpetrating interpersonal violence ... and youth who have themselves been victimized.

Further studies continue to confirm this association (e.g. Ascione and Arkow, 1999; Becker and French, 2004; Merz-Perez and Heide, 2004; DeGue and DeLillo, 2009).

Increased awareness of this 'link' led to empirical research addressing other animal/human violence linkages of interest to the medical communities. Numerous studies, in the USA, UK, Canada, Australia, Japan, the Netherlands, Ireland, the Bahamas and elsewhere, have identified acts or threats of animal abuse as a controlling behaviour, one of many assaultive and non-assaultive tactics used by perpetrators of intimate partner violence and child sexual abuse to dominate, control and induce fear and/or subservience in their victims. These threats frequently prevent battered women and their children from leaving abusive situations (e.g. McIntosh, 2001; Fawcett *et al.*, 2002; Allen *et al.*, 2006; Goodman, 2006; Doherty and Hornosty, 2007; Maruyama and Ascione, 2008; Fielding, 2010; Tiplady *et al.*, 2012). Women living in domestic violence shelters were 11 times more likely to report that their partners had hurt or killed pets than a comparison group of non-abused women (Ascione, 2007). Domestic violence batterers who also abuse animals are more dangerous and use more forms of violence than those who do not harm animals (Simmons and Lehmann, 2007). A history of pet abuse is one of the four most significant indicators of who is at greatest risk of becoming a batterer (Walton-Moss *et al.*, 2005).

Additional research describes the impact of animal maltreatment on elders. Although empirical data are not yet widely available, it is surmised that animal welfare issues are associated with the four most commonly reported forms of elder abuse: self-neglect; caregiver neglect; financial exploitation; and emotional neglect (Cooke-Daniels, 1999; Boat and Knight, 2000; Lockwood, 2002; Ascione, 2009). A One Health issue of particular public health interest is the challenge of animal hoarders or collectors, a disproportionate number of whom are elderly, who have notoriously high rates of recidivism despite psychological, criminological and social services interventions. These individuals often live in situations clearly described as public health menaces (Hoarding of Animals Research Consortium, 2002).

Other studies have found not only extremely high rates of animal abuse in homes with physical and sexual child abuse, but also significant public health risks as these households report 11 times more dog bites than non-abusing families (DeViney *et al.*, 1983).

Veterinarians as Sentinels

With 99% of Americans perceiving animals as close companions or members of the family (American Veterinary Medical Association, 2012a), it is clear that animal abuse constitutes another form of family violence. Because the majority of clients in small-animal practice are women, many of whom and their children may have been abused, the potential for veterinarians to interact with dysfunctional families is considerable (Landau, 1999; Sharpe, 1999; Munro and Thrusfield, 2001a; American Humane Association, 2003; Kovacs *et al.*, 2004). Large-animal practitioners may see victims of child maltreatment or domestic violence while making 'house calls' (Lembke, 1999).

Veterinarians can fill critical roles in the prevention of family violence. They can act as counsellors to guide clients into proper husbandry to avert animal abuse, and as reporters of suspected abuse when educational efforts fail. Their specialized knowledge can aid in the collection of medically relevant evidence during an investigation, ranging from providing medical records detailing the condition of animals to performing necropsies and crime scene analyses. As recognized authorities on animal and public health, they may serve as expert witnesses and issue a professional opinion on whether an animal has been injured or is in pain (Benetato *et al.*, 2011). Because animal cruelty cases are notoriously difficult to prosecute, such knowledge can clarify the vague terminology that so frequently marks anti-cruelty statutes.

As a professional likely to interact with abused animal victims, the veterinarian is also in a unique position to hear about human abuse. Though veterinarians are not specifically trained in human health and actions in this area may be circumscribed, veterinarians, like physicians, have professional obligations to clients that require evaluation of human behaviours, particularly if these behaviours adversely impact the well-being of others (Arkow, 1994). Additionally, veterinarians are bound by codes of ethics, encouraged by professional organizations, and mandated by law in several jurisdictions to report various forms of family violence.

Veterinarians, much as their human medical counterparts, should be involved in the prevention of family violence because (Arkow and Munro, 2008):

- Intervention corrects public health problems and protects patients and others at risk.
- Participation in family violence prevention programmes builds bridges between veterinary medicine, other professions and the community.
- Positioning the veterinarian as a type of 'family practitioner' elevates the status of the profession on a par with human medicine and improves the status of animals as valued members of the family.

Integrating Veterinary Medicine into Violence Prevention

In order to create systems in veterinary medicine to recognize and respond to suspected abuse analogous to, and integrated with, processes already in place regarding child maltreatment and intimate partner violence, several issues must be addressed:

1. Materials and training must be made available to identify clinical conditions that indicate NAI, and to describe forensic evidence-gathering and record-keeping procedures that will withstand legal scrutiny should cases result in prosecution.
2. Practice management concerns must be resolved in such a way as to reduce the practitioner's exposure to civil and criminal liability while effectively balancing the interests of the practitioner, staff, client, patient and others in the patient's household.
3. Organizational systems must be developed in order that recognition and response to suspected violence becomes institutionalized as a normative practice with full peer support.

The veterinary profession has been somewhat sceptical of this concept and reluctant to proceed rapidly, due to numerous challenges:

- inadequate training in the recognition of and response to suspected maltreatment;
- underestimation of the prevalence of abuse cases seen;
- inconsistent systems of terminology, prevention and prosecution;
- ethical dilemmas as to whether one's primary responsibility is to the client or the patient;
- widely varying personal philosophies and a lack of universal standards supporting involvement;
- fear of litigation;
- fear of adverse economic impact;
- perception that no action will be taken;
- misperception that the practitioner's role is to prove a case of abuse; and
- fear of violating professional/client confidentiality.

Similar concerns were raised and largely resolved by the human medicine field in the early years of child abuse and domestic violence responsiveness. Strategies have been identified whereby veterinary medicine can replicate the work of human medicine in these areas, thereby facilitating a One Health approach to the prevention of family violence (Arkow and Munro, 2008).

Responses: Materials and Training

Munro (1996) first identified the term 'battered pets' in the professional literature, following the 'battered child syndrome' and 'battered women' nomenclature widely used to describe physical child abuse and intimate partner violence. Seminal papers (Munro and Thrusfield, 2001a–d, 2002) defined 'non-accidental injury' to animals as a clinical condition that should be considered in differential diagnoses.

Several textbooks now elucidate these conditions and assist the practitioner in recognizing diagnostic indicators of NAI (Leonard, 2004; Patronek, 2004; Reisman, 2004; Sinclair *et al.*, 2006; Cooper and Cooper, 2007; Merck, 2007; Munro and Munro, 2008). Veterinary forensics is becoming a speciality, with training through the University of Florida College of Veterinary Medicine, numerous continuing veterinary medical education opportunities, and veterinary college curricula. The International Veterinary Forensic Sciences Association (www.ivfsa.org) and the Association of Shelter Veterinarians (www.sheltervet.org) have been particularly active in this arena.

Responses: Resolving Practice Management Concerns

The diagnosis of NAI, neglect, or maltreatment is one of the most challenging in clinical work, requiring time, experience, emotional energy, sensitivity, tact and not a small measure of courage. Practitioners may be reluctant to admit that a client would present such animals for treatment. Nevertheless, most practitioners will be presented at some time with these cases (DeViney *et al.*, 1983; Donley *et al.*, 1999; Landau, 1999; Sharpe, 1999; Munro and Thrusfield, 2001a–d; Kuehn, 2002; American Humane Association, 2003; Gullone *et al.*, 2004; Kovacs *et al.*, 2004; Patronek, 2004; Enders-Slegers and Janssen, 2009). While such cases may not be seen regularly, they are invariably problematic and difficult to resolve (Crook, 2000).

When these cases occur, practitioners often face confounding dilemmas. They need to balance economic, safety, confidentiality, legal and practice management concerns with ethical principles and professional standards, which dictate responsibilities to respond compassionately and effectively both to individual animals and to society as a whole. Furthermore, with increasing public, legislative and legal attention given to animal welfare issues, failure to fulfil these duties places the profession at risk of adverse criticism and litigation (Robertson, 2010).

To help resolve these issues, the AVMA published a *Practical Guidance for the Effective Response by Veterinarians to Suspected Animal Cruelty, Abuse and Neglect* (Arkow *et al.*, 2011). The objective of this 56-page publication is to help practitioners and their staff to develop practice-specific policies, protocols and procedures for client education and, when warranted, referrals to community agencies, when presenting factors raise an index of suspicion of animal maltreatment.

The *Guidance*, developed by Link and veterinary officials in the USA and UK, includes:

- common scenarios and likelihood of seeing cruelty, abuse and neglect in practice;
- criteria for an index of suspected animal maltreatment;
- diagnostic indicators suggesting possible abuse, including client disclosure, client profile, client behaviour, types of injuries, the animal's behaviour and patient histories;
- risk assessment and reporting decision tree to help clarify the most appropriate response;
- client questionnaire to assess risks for animal maltreatment;
- sample veterinary hospital protocols for suspected abuse and neglect;
- strategies to resolve conflicts between legal, professional and public definitions of cruelty;
- national veterinary association policy statements on reporting suspected abuse;
- state-by-state digest of reporting obligations, liabilities and immunities for reporting abuse;
- digest of state laws covering confidentiality of veterinary records;
- directory of animal shelter resources;
- directory of state anti-cruelty laws;
- sample animal cruelty reporting laws;
- factors in the assessment of dangerousness in perpetrators of animal cruelty; and
- resources and links.

Veterinarians are advised to prepare their practice in advance with policies and protocols. These steps include:

- Identifying whether reporting of abuse is permitted or mandated in the jurisdiction.
- Determining which humane, animal control/services or law enforcement agency should receive reports. The veterinarian is not required to prove a case of alleged cruelty: these agencies will investigate the complaint and take appropriate action, which may or may not include prosecution.

- Establishing an internal decision-making process when a staff member is concerned for an animal's welfare.
- Becoming familiar with telltale diagnostic indicators of abuse, cruelty and neglect.
- Learning procedures for record-keeping, collection and preservation of evidence.

The *Guidance* is available as a free download (http://www.nationallinkcoalition.org/resources).

Responses: Organizational and Institutional Systems

To meet professionals' need for legal authority to report suspected abuse, laws have been enacted that either mandate or permit reports while granting veterinarians absolute or limited civil and criminal immunity for doing so in good faith. Animal welfare acts in some countries, such as Denmark, and in several US states and Canadian provinces, require practitioners to make such reports. Where such laws do not exist, policies and codes of conduct encouraging veterinarians to report abuse have been adopted by national organizations, including the American Animal Hospital Association (AAHA), the American Veterinary Medical Association (AVMA), the Canadian Veterinary Medical Association (CVMA), the Royal College of Veterinary Surgeons (RCVS) and the Veterinary Council of New Zealand (VCNZ) (Arkow *et al.*, 2011).

The AVMA (2012b) policy illustrates the rapidly evolving need for consistent systemic response to this contentious issue. The policy, adopted in 1995 and amended in 2000 and 2009, was further updated in 2012 to require practitioners who observe animal abuse or neglect, as defined by local, state or federal laws, to report such cases promptly to appropriate authorities. Previously, there was no guidance as to when reports must be made. The policy states that veterinarians should attempt to resolve improper animal husbandry that does not meet legal definitions of abuse or neglect through educational approaches with the client: it clarifies that incidents which do meet the legal threshold must be reported.

The rationale underlying the policy is that animal abuse or neglect consistent in type and severity with that covered by cruelty laws should always be reported to an appropriate authority, regardless of whether reporting is mandated by law. This policy is consistent with AVMA's Principles of Veterinary Medical Ethics and Model Veterinary Practice Act.

The 2012 update enables the veterinarian to transcend a traditional animals-only purview into a broader arena consistent with the One Health concept. The policy notes that 'prompt disclosure of abuse is necessary to protect the health and welfare of animals and people. … Prompt reporting of such incidents can be critical to protection of both animals and people (specifically in situations with co-existing domestic violence).' Reporting is for the benefit of the animals, but there are often implications for people, as well (DeHaven, 2012).

AVMA policy parallels other national directives. CVMA declares that veterinarians have a 'moral obligation' to report suspected animal abuse. CVMA recognizes animal abuse as not just an animal welfare issue, but also an important social issue affecting families and communities due to the link between animal abuse and human violence. Reporting can help veterinarians contribute to creating safe and humane communities. 'Veterinarians may be able to play an important role in breaking the cycle of family violence by reporting suspected animal abuse' (Canadian Veterinary Medical Association, 2005).

The VCNZ's Code of Professional Conduct for Veterinarians (2012) declares that veterinarians must not ignore circumstances where they have reasonable grounds to suspect non-compliance with requirements of the Animal Welfare Act and Codes of Welfare. They must act immediately to remedy situations where they have cause to suspect unreasonable or unnecessary pain or distress or possible breaches of animal welfare legislation. If the animal's caregiver is a client, the veterinarian should discuss the situation and develop an action plan to relieve the concerns. If these cannot be discussed with the caregiver, or if the action plan's improvements are not achieved, or if the case involves severe cruelty or neglect, the matter must be reported to an animal welfare inspector. Disclosure of personal information is allowed when there are valid and justifiable reasons for so doing. Because the VCNZ accepts the research linking animal abuse with human violence, veterinarians are encouraged to consider whether people within the home might also be at risk: if so, practitioners should use their best judgement to determine whether police or child, youth and family authorities should be informed. This is wholly consistent with One Health approaches.

The Guide to Professional Conduct for Veterinarians in the UK includes a section on animal abuse, child abuse and domestic violence. Veterinarians are described as one of a number of professionals who may see and hear things in the course of their practice, which arouse suspicion of animal abuse, child abuse and domestic violence, and which are often linked. The Guide encourages veterinarians to include NAI in the differential diagnosis. If the examination of the animal leads to a suspicion of abuse, the veterinarian should first attempt to discuss her or his concerns with the client. Where this would not be appropriate or where the client's reaction increases rather than allays concerns, the veterinarian should contact relevant authorities. Circumstances that are sufficiently serious justify breaching the usual obligations of client confidentiality (Royal College of Veterinarians, 2003).

Conclusion

Animal cruelty is a crime in most, if not all, nations. Increased awareness of animal welfare and the impact of animal abuse on human well-being (Ascione and Arkow, 1999) has led to more aggressive prosecution of animal cruelty cases with increased penalties for offenders. By reporting suspected animal abuse to authorities, veterinarians are taking the first step to resolve unhealthy and dangerous situations and make their communities safer for all.

Since the earliest days of animal protection, veterinarians have worked closely with animal welfare investigators and law enforcement authorities to aid animal victims of human abuse and neglect. The recent addition of veterinary forensics to the animal welfare armamentarium offers veterinarians additional opportunities for the prevention of animal maltreatment.

Animal cruelty cases are being treated with more respect than at any time in the past. Increased public concern for animals, a proliferation of human–animal studies and animal law courses in universities, inclusion of the human–animal bond in veterinary curricula, animal-assisted therapy programmes, and stronger empirical evidence for the links between animal abuse and human violence are generating a renaissance of interest in animal well-being as an indicator and predictor of human health.

This increased attention is helping professionals to do their jobs better, to accord greater protections for animals, and to fulfil the veterinary oath to use their skills for the betterment of society. Veterinarians are ideally placed as sentinels to identify and treat abuse, and where this is severe or cannot be dealt with effectively to report it to appropriate authorities. Practitioners must become an essential part of the public health teams necessary to break the cycle of violence, which often extends from animals to human members of the family and community. In so doing, proactivity by veterinarians has the potential to save human and animal lives and reduce suffering within a One Health approach that unites human and veterinary health in a common concern for the vulnerable, victimized and at risk.

References

Allen, M., Gallagher, B. and Jones, B. (2006) Domestic violence and the abuse of pets: researching the link and its implications in Ireland. *Practice* 18(3), 167–181.

American Humane Association (2003) Non-accidental injury in dogs and cats in Colorado: Final report to Animal Assistance Fund, American Humane, Englewood, Colorado.

American Veterinary Medical Association (2012a) *US Pet Ownership and Demographics Sourcebook*. AVMA, Schaumburg, Illinois.

American Veterinary Medical Association (2012b) Resolution #1 – 2012 Regular Winter Session: Policy on Animal Abuse and Animal Neglect. AVMA, Schaumburg, Illinois. Available at: http://www.avma.org/issues/policy/animal_welfare/abuse.asp (accessed 14 May 2012).

Arkow, P. (1992) The correlations between cruelty to animals and child abuse and the implications for veterinary medicine. *Canadian Veterinary Journal* 33, 518–521.

Arkow, P. (1994) Child abuse, animal abuse, and the veterinarian. *Journal of the American Veterinary Medical Association* 204(7), 1004–1007.

Arkow, P. (2003) *Breaking the Cycles of Violence: A Guide to Multi-Disciplinary Interventions.* A Handbook for Child Protection, Domestic Violence and Animal Protection Agencies. Latham Foundation, Alameda, California.

Arkow, P. and Munro, H. (2008) The veterinary profession's roles in recognizing and preventing family violence: The experiences of the human medicine field and the development of diagnostic indicators of non-accidental injury. In: Ascione, F.R. (ed.) *The International Handbook of Animal Abuse and Cruelty: Theory, Research and Application.* Purdue University Press, West Lafayette, Indiana, pp. 31–58.

Arkow, P., Boyden, P. and Patterson-Kane, E. (2011) *Practical Guidance for the Effective Response by Veterinarians to Suspected Animal Cruelty, Abuse and Neglect.* American Veterinary Medical Association, Schaumburg, Illinois.

Ascione, F.R. (2001) Animal abuse and youth violence. *Juvenile Justice Bulletin,* U.S. Department of Justice, Office of Juvenile Justice and Delinquency Prevention, September, pp. 1–15.

Ascione, F.R. (2007) Emerging research on animal abuse as a risk factor for intimate partner violence. In: Kendall-Tackett, K. and Giacomoni, S. (eds) *Intimate Partner Violence.* Civic Research Institute, Kingston, New Jersey, pp. 3-1–3-17.

Ascione, F.R. (2009) Animal welfare issues related to elder adult abuse and neglect. Presentation at *Cruelty/Crime Connection: Breaking the Chain Conference,* 8 October, Edmonton, Alberta, Canada.

Ascione, F.R. and Arkow, P. (eds) (1999) *Child Abuse, Domestic Violence and Animal Abuse: Linking the Circles of Compassion for Prevention and Intervention.* Purdue University Press, West Lafayette, Indiana.

Becker, F. and French, L. (2004) Making the links: child abuse, animal cruelty, and domestic violence. *Child Abuse Review* 13, 399–414.

Benetato, M.A., Reisman, R. and McCobb, E. (2011) The veterinarian's role in animal cruelty cases. *Journal of the American Veterinary Medical Association* 238(1), 31–34.

Boat, B.W. and Knight, J.C. (2000) Experiences and needs of Adult Protective Services case managers when assisting clients who have companion animals. *Journal of Elder Abuse and Neglect* 12(3/4), 145–155.

Burns, K. (2012) Spreading the one-health concept. *Journal of the American Veterinary Medical Association* 240(2), 112–142.

Canadian Veterinary Medical Association (2005) *Animal Abuse: What Veterinarians Can Do.* Ottawa, Ontario, Canada.

Cooke-Daniels, L. (1999) The connection between animals and elder abuse. *Victimization of the Elderly and Disabled* 2(3), 37–47.

Cooper, J.E. and Cooper, M.E. (2007) *Introduction to Veterinary and Comparative Forensic Medicine.* Wiley-Blackwell, Ames, Iowa.

Crook, A. (2000) The CVMA animal abuse position – how we got here. *Canadian Veterinary Journal* 41, 631–633.

DeGue, S. and DiLillo, D. (2009) Is animal cruelty a 'red flag' for family violence? Investigating co-occurring violence toward children, partners, and pets. *Journal of Interpersonal Violence* 24(6), 1036–1056.

DeHaven, R. (2012) Animal abuse resources for veterinarians. Available at: http://www.avma.org/issues/animal_welfare/abuse/default.asp (accessed 31 January 2012).

DeViney, E., Dickert, J. and Lockwood, R. (1983) The care of pets within child abusing families. *International Journal for the Study of Animal Problems* 4, 321–329.

Doherty, D. and Hornosty, J. (2007) *Exploring the Links: Firearms, Family Violence and Animal Abuse in Rural Communities.* University of New Brunswick Family Violence on the Farm and in Rural Communities Project, Fredericton, New Brunswick, Canada.

Donley, L., Patronek, G.J. and Luke, C. (1999) Animal abuse in Massachusetts: a summary of case reports at the MSPCA and attitudes of Massachusetts veterinarians. *Journal of Applied Animal Welfare Science* 2(1), 59–73.

Enders-Slegers, M.-J. and Janssen, M. (2009) *Cirkel van Geweld: Verbanden Tussen Dierenmishandeling en Huiselijk Geweld.* Stichting DierZijn, Amsterdam, the Netherlands.

Fawcett, N., Gullone, E. and Johnson, J. (2002) Domestic violence and animal abuse: encouraging collaborative relations between animal welfare and human welfare agencies in Australia. *InPsych: The Bulletin of the Australian Psychological Society* 24(2), 36–38.

Felthous, A.R. and Kellert, S.R. (1987) Childhood cruelty and later aggression against people: a review. *American Journal of Psychiatry* 144, 710–717.

Fielding, W.J. (2010) Domestic violence and dog care in New Providence, The Bahamas. *Society and Animals* 18(2), 183–203.

Goodman, P.E. (2006) The relationship between intimate partner violence and other forms of family and societal violence. *Emergency Medicine Clinics of North America – Emergency Medicine and the Public's Health* 24(4), 889–903.

Gullone, E., Johnson, J. and Volant, A. (2004) The link between animal abuse and family violence: a Victoria-wide study. *Australian Veterinary Association, Welfare Conference*, Canberra.

Hildreth, C.J. (2011) Elder abuse. *Journal of the American Medical Association* 306(5), 568.

Hoarding of Animals Research Consortium (2002) Health implications of animal hoarding. *Health and Social Work* 27, 125–136.

Jordan, C.E., Nietzel, M., Walker, R. and Logan, T.K. (2004) *Intimate Partner Violence: Clinical Training Guide for Mental Health Professionals.* Springer Publishing, New York.

Kellert, S.R. and Felthous, A.R. (1985) Childhood cruelty toward animals among criminals and noncriminals. *Human Relations* 38, 1113–1129.

Kempe, C.H., Silverman, F.N., Steele, B.F., Droegenmuller, W. and Silver, H.K. (1962) The battered-child syndrome. *Journal of the American Medical Association* 181, 17–24.

Kessler, D.B. and Hyden, P. (1991) Physical, sexual and emotional abuse of children. *Clinical Symposia* 43(1).

Koop, C.E. and Lundberg, G.D. (1992) Violence in America: a public health emergency: time to bite the bullet back. *Journal of the American Medical Association* 267(22), 3075–3076.

Kovacs, S.J., Adams, C.L. and Carioto, L. (2004) Attitudes, opinions and experiences of veterinary practitioners regarding animal maltreatment: a survey of Southwestern Ontario and the Atlantic Provinces. Presentation at *10th International Conference on Human-Animal Interactions*, International Association of Human-Animal Interaction Organizations, Glasgow, Scotland, 7 –9 October.

Kuehn, B.M. (2002) Animal hoarding: a public health problem veterinarians can take a lead role in solving. *Journal of the American Veterinary Medical Association* 221(8), 1087–1089.

Landau, R. (1999) The veterinarian's role in recognizing and reporting abuse. In: Ascione, F.R. and Arkow, P. (eds) *Child Abuse, Domestic Violence, and Animal Abuse: Linking the Circles of Compassion for Prevention and Intervention.* Purdue University Press, West Lafayette, Indiana, pp. 241–249.

Lembke, L. (1999) Animal abuse and family violence in a rural environment. In: Ascione, F.R. and Arkow, P. (eds) *Child Abuse, Domestic Violence and Animal Abuse: Linking the Circles of Compassion for Prevention and Intervention.* Purdue University Press, West Lafayette, Indiana, pp. 228–240.

Leonard, E.A. (2004) Veterinary forensics. In: Miller, L. and Zawistowski, S. (eds) *Shelter Medicine for Veterinarians and Staff.* Blackwell Publishing, Ames, Iowa, pp. 489–498.

Lockwood, R. (2002) Making the connection between animal cruelty and abuse and neglect of vulnerable adults. *The Latham Letter* 23(1), 10–11.

Maruyama, M. and Ascione, F.R. (2008) Animal abuse: an evolving issue in Japanese society. In: Ascione, F.R. (ed.) *International Handbook of Animal Abuse and Cruelty: Theory, Research, and Application.* Purdue University Press, West Lafayette, Indiana, pp. 269–304.

McCulloch, M.J. (1976, June). Contributions to mental health. In: Anderson, R.K., Fenderson, D.A., Schuman, L.M., Long, E., Byrne, J.P. and Strauman, S. (eds) *A Description of the Responsibilities of Veterinarians as They Relate Directly to Human Health.* University of Minnesota School of Public Health, Minneapolis, Minnesota, pp. 9-1–9-20.

McIntosh, S. (2001) Exploring the links between animal abuse and domestic violence: Calgary research results. *The Latham Letter* 22(4), 14–16.

Merck, M. (2007) *Veterinary Forensics: Animal Cruelty Investigations.* Blackwell Publishing, Ames, Iowa.

Merz-Perez, L. and Heide, K.M. (2004) *Animal Cruelty: Pathway to Violence Against People.* AltaMira Press, Walnut Creek, California.

Miller, K.S. and Knutson, J.F. (1997) Reports of severe physical punishment and exposure to animal cruelty by inmates convicted of felonies and by university students. *Child Abuse and Neglect* 21(1), 59–82.

Munro, H.M.C. (1996) Battered pets. *Irish Veterinary Journal* 49, 712–713.

Munro, H.M.C. and Thrusfield, M.V. (2001a) Battered pets: features that raise suspicion of non-accidental injury. *Journal of Small Animal Practice* 42, 218–226.

Munro, H.M.C. and Thrusfield, M.V. (2001b) Battered pets: non-accidental physical injuries found in dogs and cats. *Journal of Small Animal Practice* 42, 279–290.

Munro, H.M.C. and Thrusfield, M.V. (2001c) Battered pets: sexual abuse. *Journal of Small Animal Practice* 42, 333–337.
Munro, H.M.C. and Thrusfield, M.V. (2001d) Battered pets: Munchausen syndrome by proxy. *Journal of Small Animal Practice* 42, 385–389.
Munro, H.M.C. and Thrusfield, M.V. (2002) The Battered-Pet Syndrome. *Veterinary Times* 32(13), 26–28.
Munro, R. and Munro, H.M.C. (2008) *Animal Abuse and Unlawful Killing: Forensic Veterinary Pathology.* Elsevier/Saunders, Philadelphia, Pennsylvania.
National Center on Elder Abuse (2005) *15 Questions and Answers About Elder Abuse.* National Center on Elder Abuse, Washington, DC.
National League of Cities (2011) *National Municipal Policy and Resolutions 2012.* NLC, Washington, DC.
National Link Coalition (2012) *The Link Between Violence to People and Violence to Animals.* National Link Coalition, Stratford, New Jersey.
Novello, A.C., Shosky, J. and Froehlke, R. (1992) From the Surgeon General, US Public Health Service: A medical response to violence. *Journal of the American Medical Association* 267(22), 3007.
Patronek, G.J. (2004) Animal cruelty, abuse and neglect. In: Miller, L. and Zawistowski, S. (eds) *Shelter Medicine for Veterinarians and Staff.* Blackwell Publishing, Ames, Iowa, pp. 427–452.
Randour, M.L. (2011, June) *What Every Clinician Should Know About the Link Between Pet Abuse and Family Violence.* American Psychological Association, Continuing Education in Psychology Education Directorate, Washington, DC.
Reisman, R. (2004) Medical evaluation and documentation of abuse in the live animal. In: Miller, L. and Zawistowski, S. (eds) *Shelter Medicine for Veterinarians and Staff.* Blackwell Publishing, Ames, Iowa, pp. 453–488.
Robertson, I.A. (2010) Legally protecting and compelling veterinarians in issues of animal abuse and domestic violence. *New Zealand Veterinary Journal* 58(3), 114–120.
Royal College of Veterinarians (2003) *Guide to Professional Conduct for Veterinarians: Animal Abuse, Child Abuse, Domestic Violence.* RCVS, London.
Salber, P.R. and Taliaferro, E. (1995) *Physician's Guide to Domestic Violence: How to Ask the Right Questions and Recognize Abuse.* Volcano Press, Volcano, California.
Schornstein, S.L. (1997) *Domestic Violence and Health Care: What Every Professional Needs to Know.* Sage Publications, Thousand Oaks, California.
Sharpe, M.S. (1999) A survey of veterinarians and a proposal for intervention. In: Ascione, F.R. and Arkow, P. (eds) *Child Abuse, Domestic Violence, and Animal Abuse: Linking the Circles of Compassion for Prevention and Intervention.* Purdue University Press, West Lafayette, Indiana, pp. 250–256.
Simmons, C.A. and Lehmann, P. (2007) Exploring the link between pet abuse and controlling behaviors in violent relationships. *Journal of Interpersonal Violence* 22(9), 1211–1222.
Sinclair, L., Merck, M. and Lockwood, R. (2006) *Forensic Investigation of Animal Cruelty: A Guide for Veterinary and Law Enforcement Professionals.* Humane Society of the US, Washington, DC.
Tiplady, C.M., Walsh, D.B. and Phillips, C.J.C. (2012) Intimate partner violence and companion animal welfare. *Australian Veterinary Journal* 90(1–2), 48–53.
Veterinary Council of New Zealand (2012) *Code of Professional Conduct: Animal Welfare.* Wellington, New Zealand.
Walton-Moss, B.J., Manganello, J., Frye, U. and Campbell, J.C. (2005) Risk factors for interpersonal violence and associated injury among urban women. *Journal of Community Health* 30(5), 377–389.

11 Human/Animal Abuse

Catherine Tiplady, Deborah Walsh and Moo Baulch

Veterinarians are in an ideal position to identify suspected cases of human/animal abuse. Their role and responsibilities in recognizing and reporting animal abuse, domestic violence, child abuse and elder abuse as part of 'One Health' was discussed further by Phil Arkow in Chapter 10.

This chapter discusses the literature surrounding human/animal abuse and collaborates with interpersonal violence practitioners (Deborah Walsh and Moo Baulch) to provide practical guidance on what we can do when confronted with cases of human/animal abuse in veterinary practice.

Animal Abuse and Domestic Violence

> A family pet is often the antithesis of the violence experience – hence in the middle of the chaos the pet can create salvation, serenity, normality.
>
> (Solowiej, 2011, p. 22)

Domestic violence (also known as intimate partner violence) involves any behaviour that causes damage to another person (physical, sexual, emotional or financial), causes someone to live in fear, damages property or threatens to damage a person, pets or property (McDonald, 1998; Walsh, 2004). Domestic violence is all about power and control – by exerting power over somebody it is possible to control them through fear, intimidation and/or threats. A range of tactics (including abuse, threats, stalking, threats of harm toward loved ones) form what is known as 'coercive control' – threats and abuse of pets is part of this. Being told that your much-loved dog or cat will be strangled if you ever leave your partner is a strong deterrent to seeking help or leaving. Unfortunately, many victims of violence delay leaving a violent relationship due to fears their partner will harm the pet (Flynn, 2000). Many feel a strong bond with their animals and do not want to be separated from their pet in order to access emergency accommodation services (Tiplady *et al.*, 2012). Guidelines for domestic violence refuges wishing to provide on-site pet care are provided by Allie Phillips in Chapter 12.

Who are the victims of domestic violence?

Although both women and men of any sexual orientation can experience domestic violence (see section in this chapter by Moo Baulch), women are much more likely than men to be the victim of multiple incidents of abuse, and of sexual violence (Walby and Allen, 2004). Men are more likely to have been physically assaulted by a stranger, whereas women are more often assaulted by a current or previous partner (ABS, 2005). Regardless of the person's gender, all victims of violence experience negative consequences of their exposure and how this is managed will determine the long-term outcome.

Domestic violence is seen in all socio-economic groups around the world but despite our knowledge about the occurrence, most cases remain well hidden (Heise *et al.*, 1999). Less than one-fifth of victims reporting an injury from intimate partner violence sought medical treatment following the injury (US Department of Justice, 2006) and only approximately one-quarter of all physical assaults, one-fifth of all rapes and half of all stalking incidents perpetrated against females by intimate partners are ever reported to the police (Tjaden and Thoennes, 2000). This indicates that domestic violence reporting is only the tip of the iceberg.

Estimates of the prevalence of domestic violence vary between country and setting. European research has found that one in four women experience domestic violence over their lifetimes (Council of Europe, 2002), one in three women in Australia (Mouzos and Makkai, 2004), and in provincial settings in Bangladesh, Ethiopia, Peru and the United Republic of Tanzania 71% of ever-partnered women reported physical and/or sexual violence by a partner (WHO, 2005).

Overwhelmingly, the prevalence data worldwide reveal: that gender is an indicator for being a victim of domestic violence; that socio-economic group is not a protective factor; and that it is a pervasive and chronic social problem confronting people everywhere.

Why are pets harmed during domestic violence?

Threats and abuse of animals is a method used by some perpetrators of intimate partner violence to gain coercive control over their partner (Adams, 1994; Abrahams, 2007). Physically abusing animals can have the same psychological impact on a woman in a violent relationship as physically abusing her (Ganley, 1985), clearly indicating the strong emotional bond human victims may have for their animal. A survey of abused women in a domestic violence shelter found that respondents were more likely to state their pet was a 'very important' source of emotional support if the pet had also experienced abuse (Flynn, 2000).

Companion animals are often regarded as members of the family (McDonald, 1998; Cohen, 2002), but perpetrators of domestic violence are more likely to view animals as property or 'possessions' (Eisikovits and Buchbinder, 2000) and many are willing to hurt animals in order to maintain control over their victim.

Adams (1995) expands on the theme of power and control to list nine reasons why male perpetrators of domestic violence may harm animals, proposing that through animal abuse, men:

1. Demonstrate their power.
2. Teach submission.
3. Isolate the woman from a network of support and relationship.
4. Express rage at self-determined action by women and children.
5. Perpetuate the context of terror.
6. Launch a pre-emptive strike against a woman leaving.
7. Punish and terrorize by stalking and executing an animal.
8. Force the woman to be involved in the animal abuse.
9. Confirm their power.

How are animals affected by living with domestic violence?

Clearly, living with violence is a source of stress to animals, as indicated by the behavioural changes (e.g. running away, aggression toward the perpetrator, proximity seeking to the victimized partner) reported to occur during domestic violent events (Tiplady *et al.*, 2012). Often, these behavioural changes can persist for years after the abusive partner has left the home (Tiplady *et al.*, 2012). These changes are generally fear related and include being frightened of men, hiding and cowering.

Disturbingly, it has been found that in multi-animal homes, animal abuse is not a random event – there is often an individual, 'target' pet, which receives the most severe abuse and this is more likely to be a dog owned or cared for by the woman (Tiplady *et al.*, 2012). The range of abuse experienced by animals living with domestic violence has been found to include:

- *Physical abuse* such as kicking, beating, throwing, hanging, poisoning, decapitation (Tiplady *et al.*, 2012); punching, hitting, choking, drowning, shooting, stabbing (Carlisle-Frank and Flanagan, 2006); shaking, igniting (Ascione, 1998).
- *Deliberate neglect*, such as starving a dog to death (Tiplady *et al.*, 2012).
- *Sexual abuse*, e.g. partners forcing women to engage in sexual abuse activities with animals or watch animal abuse pornography (Roguski, 2012).
- Verbal abuse and threats (Tiplady *et al.*, 2012).

Living with violence can cause emotional injuries as well as physical injuries – even just witnessing domestic violence has been found to have serious adverse effects on the well-being of both animals (Flynn, 2000) and children (Fantuzzo *et al.*, 1991; Zuckerman *et al.*, 1995). A New Zealand study found that abuse of animals can continue after the violent relationship has ended (Roguski, 2012). This included abusers threatening or actually harming or killing pets left in their care, and harming and killing pets belonging to any of the woman's friends and relatives who helped her and the children escape the violence (Roguski, 2012).

Animal abuse by other people

Research has found that those perpetrating the violence against companion animals are not always the perpetrator of the domestic violence. Within a family experiencing domestic violence, the abusive partner is not always the only one who is harming the animals – animal abuse can also occur with the abused partner (or a child in the house) as perpetrator. Motivations for animal harm by a victimized woman can be quite different to that of a male perpetrator. A victimized partner may be coerced into performing sexually abusive acts with an animal (Walker, 1979), may take out their anger on pets (Walker, 1984) or may kill their pets to prevent them from suffering further at the hands of their abusive partner. One victim of domestic violence chose to drown her much-loved kittens rather than let her husband 'take pot shots at them' with his rifle (Hunter, 2006, p. 188). Welfare of pets may assume less importance by the time a woman leaves a violent relationship due to maintaining safety for herself and her children (Roguski, 2012). Abused women have also been forced to assist their abuser in perpetrating animal cruelty. One horrific case of domestic violence involved a man making his girlfriend hold a puppy while he bored an electric drill into its head (Hicks, 2012). Police reportedly later found 29 dog carcases on the property, illegal guns, tools covered in blood and hair, and what appeared to be the pelt of a beagle and dogs' eyes in a jar (Hicks, 2012). This case is a good example of how various professionals can form an effective team to help human and animal victims of violence. Forensic investigators, animal control officers, lawyers and police were all involved and financial support for the prosecution was pledged by the Animal Legal Defense Fund (Hicks, 2012).

Children, Domestic Violence and Animal Abuse

Domestic violence and child abuse coexist in some families (Saunders, 2003), and children living with domestic violence may show higher levels of animal cruelty (Currie, 2006) than those not living among domestic violence. Domestic violence has been suggested as potentially being one of the risk factors for childhood animal cruelty and subsequent adult violence (Duncan and Miller, 2002). Some studies suggest a progression from abuse of animals during childhood and/or adolescence to violence toward humans during adulthood (Kellert and Felthous, 1985; Flynn, 1999; Muscari, 2004), highlighting the need for early intervention. Veterinarians who encounter animals abused by children should speak to the parents and suggest the family meet with a professional counsellor who is experienced in this issue. Assessment and treatment guides for counsellors working with animal abusers are found in the *AniCare Child* handbook for children up to 17 years of age (Randour *et al.*, 2005) and the *AniCare Model of Treatment for Animal Abuse* for those over 17 years of age (Jory and Randour, 1999). As of 2010, 27 states in the USA authorize judges to order counselling for people convicted of animal abuse (ASI, n.d.), such as in the case where a man stuck needles in hotdogs and left them out for animals to eat, resulting in the death of his neighbour's dog (Irwin, 2012).

Workshops and online courses are available to instruct people in using AniCare for animal abusers (ASI, n.d.).

There are many humane education programmes undertaken by welfare and veterinary organizations around the world to encourage children to care for animals. One of these, 'CARE', was created for children who have lived with domestic violence and is described in Chapter 13.

Children who live with domestic violence are more likely to have displayed animal cruelty (17%) than those who do not live with domestic violence (7%), as reported by their mothers in a case-control study of 47 women with a history of domestic violence and 45 women with no such history (Currie, 2006).

Children may be coerced into harming animals within abusive homes and may be forced to alternate between the roles of abuser and victim in order to survive. In one such case, an animal protection agency investigated a case that involved a father teaching his 18-month-old son to beat an 8-week-old puppy with a chain, telling the child 'Now you beat the dog with the chain or I'll beat you with it' (Loar and Colman, 2004, p. 12). It has been suggested that homophobia is driving much of the 'hypermasculine aggression' seen in men who encourage their sons to abuse animals and not cry or cower 'like a woman' (Loar and Colman, 2004, p. 12). Homophobia and animal abuse may be linked. In the USA, an arson attack on a barn of horses (owned by a gay man) was believed to be motivated by homophobia – eight horses died in the fire, including a pregnant mare and a foal, and homophobic graffiti were sprayed on to the barn walls (Ninemsn, 2011).

Assisting those who are living with domestic violence and animal abuse

For those working in domestic violence services and refuges, it is vital to enquire about animal ownership and animal abuse on your intake forms and know options for safe pet accommodation in your area. Housing abused adults, children and pets together during their rehabilitation is now possible, with the assistance of excellent programmes such as the Sheltering Animals and Families Together (SAF-T) programme (see Allie Phillips' Chapter 12 for guidelines).

For those who are experiencing domestic violence and have animals there are services to help you, your children and pets find safe accommodation. Nobody should have to remain in a violent relationship because they are afraid their animals will be harmed.

The following guidelines have been adapted from a Humane Society of the United States publication (HSUS, 2004):

If you are able to safely prepare before you and your pets leave domestic violence:

- Establish ownership of the animal (have your details as the owner on receipts for veterinary treatment, microchip forms, registration and vaccination certificates).
- Having the animal's vaccinations up to date will assist greatly in helping find foster care or boarding for the animal (and ensures that risk of contracting infectious disease is reduced).
- Assemble vaccination certificates and medical records and store them in a safe place where your abuser will not find them.
- Investigate options for temporary pet accommodation (such as boarding kennels and catteries, boarding with a friend/relative) and make contact with your local domestic violence service and/or veterinarian to discuss pet accommodation options.
- Make sure you have collars, leads and a suitable pet carry-box (a pillow case can be a temporary cat carrier in an emergency).
- Assemble bowls, brushes, toys and favourite bedding.
- Create new identification tags with the telephone number of a friend or veterinarian on them – remember to replace old tags with the new ones when you leave.
- Have any necessary medication the animal requires.
- Write information about the animal's preferred foods and feeding schedule, medical conditions and medication routine, likes and dislikes and any behavioural issues on a piece of paper to be given to the temporary carer.

For those who have to leave without their pet:

- Ask the police to escort you home to collect your pets in safety.
- Leave sufficient water, food, clean litter and bedding for your pet until you can return (Maryland's People's Law Library, 2010).

An additional suggestion is to consider desexing your pet. If this cannot be done before leaving, this may be able to be provided during foster care by a humane society or domestic violence pet fostering service at a reduced fee. Desexing has a range of health and behavioural benefits and eliminates the possibility of unwanted litters at a time when helping people and pets safely relocate with minimum stress is the goal.

What To Do When You Suspect Domestic Violence and When Someone Discloses That They Are Experiencing It

Dr Deborah Walsh, a social work practitioner, trauma counsellor and clinical supervisor in the area of domestic and family violence

You suspect a client is experiencing domestic violence

There will come a time in your practice that you suspect that an owner might be a victim of domestic violence and you consider that you would like to approach the issue to see if you can help. There are a couple of things you need to know. First, trust your sense that there may be something going on even if the person denies that anything is going on at home. Many victims of violence have stated that while they did not disclose when asked, they appreciated the fact that someone cared enough to inquire (Stratigos, 2000). There have been a number of studies conducted in human healthcare settings, with particular emphasis on pregnancy and antenatal care, where it has now been well established that women victims of violence want to be asked and will disclose when they feel they can trust the service provider that the information will be confidential and that the victim will be in control of how the information will be handled (Rodriguez *et al.*, 2001; Renker and Tonkin, 2006). It is clear that victims want to be asked when a service provider suspects there is violence and, in order to help service providers with the delicate task of asking, Alpert (1995) developed a helpful tool that a number of healthcare providers have now implemented.

The system is referred to as the RADAR (Alpert, 1995; Massachusetts Medical Society, 1999; Institute for Safer Families, 2002). When implementing this system into a practice, workers are encouraged to 'use the RADAR when you suspect or detect domestic violence in your population' (ibid). RADAR is an acronym for a domestic violence intervention, which stands for the following:

R = Remember to ask

Always interview someone who you may suspect to be a victim of violence alone. Victims of violence will disclose if they trust the professional who is asking.

A = Ask directly

The worker needs to ask simple, direct questions in a non-judgemental way. For an example, 'I have noticed that you and the animal have injuries – is there anyone at home doing this to you? I am concerned about you and the animal. Is everything alright at home?'

If the owner answers 'yes' to the first question, then your responses will be important.

Encourage the owner to talk about it.

Listen non-judgementally (never, ever criticize the perpetrator[1] – focus on the victim and their experiences) and gather enough information to be able to provide the person with the referrals they may need.

Validate the experience. For example, it can be very reassuring to say that there are a lot of people in the same situation, which is why there is a range of services available to help them. Remember that the victim is never to blame for the violence perpetrated on them.

If the owner says that there is nothing going on at home and you still feel that there is

[1] Criticism of the perpetrator is experienced by victims of violence as a criticism of their choice of partner and is likely to alienate them.

something not quite right, it will be important to respect what the owner says and leave the issue alone. You can reassure the person that if ever they wanted to talk to you in the future, the door would always be open.

D = Document findings

If you observe clinical injuries not consistent with the story provided, it is important that your observation is noted along with any other findings in the case file. So if you were to ask directly and the owner stated that everything was fine at home, then you record this in the file. If you ask questions directly and the owner discloses that they are experiencing violence, then your record will be very important. Your notes will need to be specific about what was disclosed and what you did about that. For example, what services did you refer the owner on to and was any follow-up required? If you observed physical injuries on the owner and the animal, it may be important to supplement the written record by a body map with the injuries noted. Any documents you have may be required in a later court process, so they will need to be accurate and up to date.

A = Assess safety

Assessing the safety of the owner after a disclosure is critical. Asking simply whether they are safe to go home later is an important question and will determine the referral pathway. Do not attempt to provide printed domestic violence information without checking with the victim whether it is safe for them to take the information home by asking the questions: 'Does your partner go through your things? Is it safe for you to take this information with you?' Women victims of domestic violence are at the greatest risk of being murdered if the violent partner finds out she has disclosed to a professional or separates (Family Violence Professional Education Taskforce, 1994, p. 102; Women's Coalition Against Family Violence, 1994, p. 65; Mouzos and Makkai, 2004).

If the owner is not safe to go home, then a referral to a 24-hour crisis domestic violence accommodation service is often the only option if family and friends are not appropriate.

R = Respond, review and refer

Respond empathically without blame or judgement. Review what you have been told and discuss the available options with the owner and refer on. There are many domestic violence services that are very well qualified to undertake the work required to support the owner who experiences domestic violence. You may be the first person in this owner's experience who took the time to care. If it is the owner's decision to stay with the partner and do nothing about the violence, then respecting that decision is critically important. For many victims of violence, having someone who has heard their story empathically can have a profound impact on them and may be a catalyst for thinking about options in the future. We will often never know the long-term impact of what we do or say. Leaving the door open can be a vital step in the pathway to safety in the future.

Working with domestic violence can be challenging and may bring up a range of issues that can impact on you as a professional and as a person generally. It can be very helpful to have access to debriefing with a colleague who has similar view points as yourself. Remember the oxygen mask.

Having a resource folder that is updated annually with domestic violence services and how and when they operate will be an important addition to your practice. In addition, access continuing education and training provided for professionals in your area on how to work with domestic violence issues, and having ongoing conversations with other professionals will be helpful as you expand your knowledge about the issue. Document and share any successes you have had by publishing case studies so others can learn from your practice.

Domestic violence is a crime and is everyone's business, so if you see it in your practice it is important to act in ways that do not silence victims and that help keep the issue a secret.

Domestic Violence, Pets and LGBTIQ Families

Moo Baulch

It is a truth universally acknowledged that pets play a significant role in many LGBTIQ (lesbian, gay, bisexual, transgender, intersex and 'queer') families. Consumer indexes indicate that our rates of pet ownership tend to be higher and that we spend more disposable income on them; a study from the USA found that 71% of GLBT people have a pet, in comparison with 63% of heterosexual adults (Harris Interactive/Witeck Combs, 2007). You only have to visit an LGBTIQ community event such as Mardi Gras Fair Day to see evidence of the love (and the money) that we lavish on our non-human dependents.

The concept of 'family' in the LGBTIQ world can differ from the traditional nuclear family model; as we come out and form relationships we often tend to adopt new family members along the way. We share the most intimate ups and downs of our lives with our LGBTIQ friends who become our 'chosen family'. Inevitably, our pets are an important part of these families.

The 2006 Private Lives research examined the health of 5500 LGBTIQ Australians and noted that many respondents nominated their pets as among the three best things in their life (Pitts *et al.*, 2006). For people living with HIV and other chronic illnesses, pets can be more than just a comfort – they provide support, pleasure and have been linked to a healthier, more motivated lifestyle (Siegel *et al.*, 1999; *Fenuxe Magazine*, 2010). Extraordinary long-term relationships are formed between LGBTIQ people and their pets, whether we have human partners and biological offspring or not.

The majority of LGBTIQ relationships are healthy, loving and respectful, but as is the case in the broader population, some are abusive and controlling. People who experience domestic or family violence (DV) in their relationship are often isolated from support networks and reluctant to seek help. This is further compounded in abusive LGBTIQ relationships when people are afraid that they might be 'outed' or that DV services will not believe or help them because they do not fit into a gendered model of a woman being battered by their male partner. Some may be afraid to leave even when the violence is severe, because they have been convinced by their abuser that no one else will want them. Others (particularly those in their first relationships) may believe that this is a 'normal' dynamic in LGBTIQ relationships. Even those who break the cycle of abuse may be reluctant to talk about the existence of DV for fear of giving all LGBTIQ relationships a bad name. Transgender and intersex people are often exposed to such extreme levels of socially sanctioned prejudice and violence in daily life that they may struggle to identify the DV as abusive.

Despite these unique dynamics, in terms of the impact of DV there are also significant commonalities with the broader population. Family pets can be secondary victims of the abuse. They can be used as pawns in the cycle of manipulative control: 'If you leave me, you will never see the dog again' or 'If you don't do as I say then Fluffy gets it'.

To date there is little Australian research exploring the abuse of pets in LGBTIQ relationships, although explicit inclusion in programmes such as the RSPCA's Safe Beds for Pets initiative acknowledges the role of pets in our families and the fact that we may need someone to look after them when we leave abusive relationships (Another Closet, n.d.). Despite a lack of dedicated research, we know that:

- Roughly one in three gay and lesbian people experience some sort of abuse in the context of a relationship. For transgender and intersex people it is significantly higher (Pitts *et al.*, 2006).
- LGBTIQ people are far more likely to ask a friend, work colleague or other informal supports for help than go to the police, a DV service or other formal support services (Farrell and Cerise, 2006).
- In a 1992 US study, 38% of women with pets and in abusive lesbian relationships reported maltreatment of the pets by their partners (Renzetti, 1992).

Vets and clinical staff can play a vital role in the informal DV screening process. By asking the right questions and being prepared to refer clients on to specialist services, you might save a life (human or animal).

So what can you do? Here are some ideas to get you started:

- If something seems wrong and you suspect that there is DV occurring, do not be afraid to ask if your client is okay. It is always better to be wrong than to wonder (with hindsight) whether you should have said something.

- Make your clinic a LGBTIQ-friendly space by displaying posters, having LGBTIQ press in your reception, and listing LGBTIQ people as a client group on your website – remember that clients may feel more comfortable talking to you than the police or a DV service (for more tips, download 'Is your service LGBTIQ friendly?' from http://www.acon.org.au/anti-violence/resources/GLBTIQDV-toolkit).
- Train your staff to understand DV and the diversity of clients. Challenge homophobic or heterosexist comments in your workplace and speak openly about your support of LGBTIQ people.
- Connect with your local LGBTIQ community and networks, work with them and participate in community events such as Mardi Gras or Pride Fair Day (it is also great for business!).
- Use the language your client uses – if a woman talks about her partner as her wife, do the same. If someone talks about their partner who appears 'female' but uses male pronouns, you should also.
- Ask yourself, 'If I were LGBTIQ would I feel comfortable to be open about my life/sexuality/sex/gender at this service?'

For more information contact your local LGBTIQ organization and ask them for help

Another Closet is a New South Wales-based site with information for LGBTIQ people experiencing abuse and links to resources for service providers (http://www.anothercloset.com.au/).

There is a range of organizations that can help you connect with your local LGBTIQ communities and assist you to understand better the needs of LGBTIQ people and families.

Abuse of elderly and/or people with a disability

It is not surprising that perpetrators of violence toward animals would also harm elderly or disabled people. The elderly and disabled are vulnerable members of the community and may be unable to defend themselves against physical, sexual, emotional, verbal and financial abuse. Abusers may be family members of the elderly person, their carers or members of the public.

What to do when you suspect a child is being harmed where there is animal abuse
Deborah Walsh

In the majority of countries there are laws protecting children, with supportive legislation around mandatory child abuse and neglect notification requirements. In many instances people are able to anonymously provide information to a telephone helpline about the suspected abuse of children or, if preferred, a person can choose to reveal their details. In some countries there is legal protection available that protects the identity of the person who notified the child protection agency.

It is important that professionals establish the protocols and requirements in their own country and state that govern this area, as there are so many variations across countries. Keeping this information up to date is an important part of delivering services to the community.

What to do when you suspect an elderly person is being harmed where there is animal abuse occurring
Deborah Walsh

Recognition of elder abuse is relatively new, and protection is spasmodic and in some cases fragmented. There are a few areas in the USA that mandate professionals to notify if they suspect or detect elder abuse. However, other countries such as Australia have strongly opposed this, arguing that mandating professionals has the potential to send elder abuse underground, with the Elder Abuse Prevention Unit (2006) arguing that there is no convincing evidence that mandatory reporting creates better outcomes for older people.

If this is a concern in a veterinary practice, it would be advisable for the staff to find out the resources available for this very vulnerable group and establish what your own reporting requirements might be in your state or territory.

Continued

What to do when you suspect a person with a disability is being harmed where there is animal abuse occurring
Deborah Walsh

In this situation, if the person is an adult and the person caring for them is the perpetrator then there are variations between countries and states about the requirements if professionals suspect or detect domestic violence in this population group. Similarly to the information provided for elder abuse victims, establish the protocols and resources available in your country and state.

When owners or family members have a reduced capacity to care safely for animals
Deborah Walsh

There is a great deal of information on the benefits of companion animals for a whole range of circumstances; however, when owners or families have a reduced capacity to care adequately or safely for these animals then someone needs to act. Sadly, there are those in our community with a disability by birth or acquired by accident where the capacity to adequately care for an animal is compromised. In addition, there are those who face debilitating mental health issues who may also have reduced capacity to care safely and adequately for animals. In these instances, if a plan for supervision cannot guarantee that the animal can be cared for then a recommendation may need to come from the veterinarian to state clearly that an animal may need to be cared for by an alternative person or be rehoused. In some instances arrangements for visitation may be possible until safe and adequate care can be guaranteed, but in others a directive may need to be made that clearly states that the person should not have responsibility for an animal.

These types of situations in professional practice can be very stressful for all concerned, and place the veterinarian in a very challenging and confronting position. This is an example of practice where the veterinarian is likely to need to draw on some peer support and apply the 'oxygen mask' (Walsh, 1998 and see section on self care, Chapter 14). Discussing these situations with someone who understands the issues involved can reduce the long-term impact on the individual veterinarian and alleviate the immediate concerns that many have around whether or not they did the right thing. In cases such as these, the health and well-being of the animal is the primary concern.

References

Abrahams, H. (2007) *Supporting Women After Domestic Violence: loss, trauma and recovery*. Jessica Kingsley Publishers, London.

ABS (2005) Personal Safety Australia (Reissue). Australian Bureau of Statistics. Available at: http://www.abs.gov.au/ausstats/abs@.nsf/mf/4906.0 (accessed 29 March 2012).

Adams, C.J. (1994) Bringing peace home: a feminist philosophical perspective on the abuse of women, children and pet animals. *Hypatia* 9, 63–84.

Adams, C.J. (1995) Woman-battering and harm to animals. In: Adams, C.J. and Donovan, J. (eds) *Animals and Women: Feminist theoretical explorations*. Duke University Press, Durham, North Carolina, pp. 55–84.

Alpert, E. (1995) Violence in intimate relationships and the practicing internist: new disease or new agenda. *Annals of Internal Medicine* 123(10), 774–781.

Another Closet (n.d.) Domestic violence in gay and lesbian relationships – pets. Available at: http://www.anothercloset.com.au/pets/ (accessed 3 June 2012).

Ascione, F.R. (1998) Battered women's reports of their partners' and their children's cruelty to animals. *Journal of Emotional Abuse* 1(1), 119–133.

ASI (n.d.) The AniCare approach: Interrupting the cycle of violence. Animals and Society Institute brochure. Available at: http://www.animalsandsociety.org/files/AniCare%20Approach%20Brochure.pdf (accessed 22 April 2012).

Carlisle-Frank, P. and Flanagan, T. (2006) *Silent Victims: Recognizing and Stopping Abuse of the Family Pet*. University Press of America, Lanham, Maryland.

Cohen, S. (2002) Can pets function as family members? *Western Journal of Nursing Research* 24, 621–628.

Council of Europe (2002) *Recommendation of the Committee of Ministers to member States on the protection of women against violence adopted on 30 April 2002 and Explanatory Memorandum*. Council of Europe. Strasbourg, France.

Currie, C.L. (2006) Animal cruelty by children exposed to domestic violence. *Child Abuse & Neglect* 30(4), 425–435.

Duncan, A. and Miller, C. (2002) The impact of an abusive family context on childhood animal cruelty and adult violence. *Aggression and Violent Behaviour* 7, 365–383.

Eisikovits, Z. and Buchbinder, E. (2000) *Locked in a Violent Embrace: understanding & intervening in domestic violence*. Sage Publications, Thousand Oaks, California.

Elder Abuse Prevention Unit (2006) *Position Statement on Mandatory Reporting of Elder Abuse*. Elder Abuse Prevention Unit, Brisbane, Australia.

Family Violence Professional Education Taskforce (1994) *Family Violence: Everybody's Business Somebody's Life*. Federation Press, Annandale, New South Wales, Australia.

Fantuzzo, J., DePaola, L. and Lambert, L. (1991) Effects of interparental violence on the psychological adjustment and competencies of young children. *Journal of Consulting and Clinical Psychology* 59, 258–265.

Farrell, J. and Cerise, S. (2006) *Fair's Fair – a snapshot of violence and abuse in Sydney LGBT relationships*. ACON and the Same Sex Domestic Violence Interagency Working Group, Brookvale, Sydney, Australia.

Fenuxe Magazine (2010) A gay's best friend. 12 August. Available at: http://www.fenuxe.com/2010/08/12/a-gays-best-friend/ (accessed 3 June 2012).

Flynn, C.P. (1999) Animal abuse in childhood and later support for interpersonal violence in families. *Society and Animals* 7(2), 161–172.

Flynn, C.P. (2000) Women's best friend: pet abuse and the role of companion animals in the lives of battered women. *Violence Against Women* 6(2), 162–177.

Ganley, A.L. (1985) *Court-mandated Counselling for Men Who Batter: A Three-day Workshop for Mental Health Professionals*. Centre for Women Policy Studies, Washington, DC.

Harris Interactive/Witeck Combs (2007) GLBT Adults more likely to own a pet than heterosexuals. Available at: http://www.witeckcombs.com/news/releases/20071217_pets.pdf (accessed 3 June 2012).

Heise, L., Ellsberg, M. and Gottemoeller, M. (1999) *Ending Violence Against Women*. Population Reports, Series L, No. 11. Johns Hopkins University School of Public Health, Population Information Program, Baltimore, Maryland.

Hicks, I. (2012) Guilty in dog torture case. The Intelligencer/Wheeling News-Register April 5. Available at: http://theintelligencer.net/page/content.detail/id/568137/Guilty-In-Dog-Torture-Case.html (accessed 11 April 2012).

HSUS (2004) *Starting a Safe Havens for Animals™ program*. Humane Society of the United States, Washington, DC.

Hunter, R. (2006) *Point Last Seen*. Debut Publishing, Sunshine Coast, Australia.

Institute for Safer Families (2002) *RADAR Pocket card*. Institute for Safer Families, Philadelphia, Pennsylvania.

Irwin, T. (2012) Mich. Man gets 30 days for neighbour's dog's death. *Toledo Blade*, 30 March. Available at: http://www.toledoblade.com/Courts/2012/03/30/Mich-man-gets-30-days-for-neighbor-dog-s-death.html (accessed 22 April 2012).

Jory, B. and Randour, M. (1999) *The AniCare Model of Treatment for Animal Abuse*. Psychologists for the Ethical Treatment of Animals, Maryland.

Kellert, S.R. and Felthous, A.R. (1985) Childhood cruelty toward animals among criminals and noncriminals. *Human Relations* 38, 1113–1129.

Loar, L. and Colman, L. (2004) *Teaching Empathy: animal-assisted therapy programs for children and families exposed to violence*. A Latham Foundation Publication, Alameda, California.

Maryland's People's Law Library (2010) Domestic violence/companion animals. Maryland State Law Library. Available at: http://www.peoples-law.org/node/642 (accessed 9 April 2012).

Massachusetts Medical Society (1999) *RADAR Training for Health and Medical Professionals*. Massachusetts Medical Society, Massachusetts.

McDonald, H. (1998) What's in a name? Definitions and domestic violence. Discussion paper no. 1. Domestic Violence and Incest Resource Centre, Melbourne, Australia.

Mouzos, J. and Makkai, T. (2004) Women's experiences of male violence: findings from the Australian component of the International Violence against Women Survey. Australian Institute of Criminology, *Research and Public Policy Series no. 56*. Canberra, Australia.

Muscari, M. (2004) Juvenile animal abuse: Practice and policy implications for PNPs. *Journal of Pediatric Health Care* 18, 15–21.

Ninemsn (2011) Eight horses killed in gay-hate barn fire. 28 April. Available at: http://news.ninemsn.com.au/world/8241954/eight-horses-killed-in-gay-hate-barn-fire (accessed 28 April 2011).

Pitts, M., Smith, A., Mitchell, A. and Patel, S. (2006) *Private Lives: A Report on the Health and Well-being of GLBTI Australians*. Australian Research Centre in Sex, Health and Society, La Trobe University, Melbourne, Australia.

Randour, M., Krinsk, S. and Wolf, J.L. (2005) *AniCare Child – an assessment and treatment approach for childhood animal abuse*. Psychologists for the Ethical Treatment of Animals, Maryland.

Renker, P.R. and Tonkin, P. (2006) Women's views of prenatal violence screening: Acceptability and confidentiality issues. *Obstetrics and Gynecology* 107, 348–354.

Renzetti, C. (1992) *Violent Betrayal: Partner Abuse in Lesbian Relationships*. Sage Publications, London.

Rodriguez, M., Sheldon, W., Bauer, H. and Perez-Stable, E. (2001) The factors associated with disclosures of intimate partner abuse to clinicians. *Journal of Family Practice* 50, 338–344.

Roguski, M. (2012) *Pets as Pawns: The Co-existence of Animal Cruelty and Family Violence*. Royal New Zealand Society for the Prevention of Cruelty to Animals and The National Collective of Independent Women's Refuges, Auckland, New Zealand.

Saunders, B.E. (2003) Understanding children exposed to violence: toward an integration of overlapping fields. *Journal of Interpersonal Violence* 18, 356–376.

Siegel, J.M., Angulo, F.J., Detels, R., Wesch, J. and Mullen, A. (1999) AIDS diagnosis and depression in the Multicenter AIDS Cohort Study: the ameliorating impact of pet ownership. *AIDS Care* 11(2), 157–170.

Solowiej, A. (2011) We made it home: the betrayed, traumatised look in their eyes is finally gone. The relationship between domestic and family violence and pet maltreatment: do we need more pet friendly options for women and children experiencing homelessness? Parity 24(4), 22–23.

Stratigos, S. (2000) Domestic violence screening and pregnancy. *Proceedings of The Way Forward: Children, Young People and Domestic violence*. Partnerships Against Domestic Violence, Melbourne, 26–27 April, pp. 45–50.

Tiplady, C.M., Walsh, D.B. and Phillips, C.J.C. (2012) Intimate partner violence and companion animal welfare. *Australian Veterinary Journal* 90(1–2), 48–53.

Tjaden, P. and Thoennes, N. (2000) *Extent, Nature and Consequences of Intimate Partner Violence: Findings from the National Violence Against Women Survey*. National Institute of Justice and the Centers of Disease Control and Prevention, Rockville, Maryland.

US Department of Justice (2006) *Intimate Partner Violence in the United States*. Bureau of Justice Statistics, Northwest, Washington, DC.

Walby, S. and Allen, J. (2004) *Domestic Violence, Sexual Assault and Stalking: Findings from the British Crime Survey*. Home Office Research, Development and Statistics Directorate, London.

Walker, L.E. (1979) *The Battered Woman*. Harper and Row, New York.

Walker, L.E. (1984) *The Battered Woman Syndrome*. Springer Publishing, New York.

Walsh, D.B. (1998) *Introduction to Working with Domestic Violence Training*. Deborah Walsh Domestic Violence Training Services, Melbourne, Australia.

Walsh, D.B. (2004) Silent suffering: the extent, level and nature of violence against women during pregnancy. A study of 400 Australian women. PhD thesis, University of Melbourne, Victoria, Australia.

Women's Coalition Against Family Violence (1994) *Blood on Whose Hands? The killing of women and children in domestic homicide*. Arena Printing, Fitzroy, Melbourne, Australia.

World Health Organization (2005) WHO multi-country study on women's health and domestic violence against women: Summary report of initial results on prevalence, health outcomes and women's responses. Available at: http://www.who.int/gender/violence/who_multicountry_study/ (accessed 12 April 2009).

Zuckerman, B., Augustyn, M., Groves, B. and Parker, S. (1995) Silent victims revised: the special case of domestic violence. *Pediatrics* 96, 511–513.

12 Sheltering Animals & Families Together (SAF-T)™: Working Together to Protect Families and Pets from Abuse

Allie Phillips

Introduction

It was March 2011 and Barbara was safely at a family violence shelter in California along with her three children and two dogs (note: Barbara's name and the names of her dogs have been changed to safeguard her privacy). Their path to safety, however, was prompted by a tragedy. Barbara's two sons had been chronically beaten by their father; he would strike Barbara so hard that she would see stars. The battering had gone on for years and became more brutal as her husband progressed to abusing the three family dogs. Barbara recounted how he had sexual intercourse with one of the dogs in front of her; she was paralysed in fear and unable to help the dog. Although he kicked the dogs frequently, one day he went too far. Riley strayed out of the yard and her husband 'lost it'. With her lip quivering in an attempt to hold back the tears and rage, Barbara explained how her husband grabbed one of his guns, took Riley to the back yard, and shot her dead in front of Barbara and the children. When the children wailed out in agony, he slapped the oldest son so hard that he himself began to cry. When her husband took off in their truck, she packed up the kids and the two remaining dogs and headed for safety. Lucky for Barbara, she found her way to one of a small number of US family violence shelters that allow pets on site.

It is stories like Barbara's, along with many years spent as a prosecuting attorney handling domestic violence cases, that prompted me to create Sheltering Animals & Families Together (SAF-T)™, a widespread initiative and with written guidelines to help family violence shelters house pets on site. The idea came to me in the mid-1990s when I was a frontline prosecuting attorney and saw too many victims of domestic violence return to their abusers, in order to protect their pet. At that time, only a couple of American shelters were housing pets of domestic violence. It quickly became clear to me that criminal justice professionals were not addressing animals caught in family violence situations and did not have the tools or resources to help. After one fateful day where my case was dismissed when my victim left the courthouse hand-in-hand with her abuser in order to protect her pets, I learned that shelters were not recognizing that pets need to evacuate abusive homes with their human family members, I took action in hope of showing the simplicity of on-site pet housing to shelters across the USA.

Research Studies

International research studies consistently demonstrate that if someone intentionally harms an animal, they are likely also to harm a person. And within a home environment, animals who are part of the family are also victims of domestic violence. Twelve independent research studies found that between 18 and 48% of women in abusive relationships delayed or refused leaving their abuser out of fear for leaving their pet or livestock behind (Ascione, 2007). A 2007 American study found that women seeking refuge at family violence shelters were nearly 11 times more likely to report that their partner had hurt or killed their pet, and four times more likely to report that their pet had been threatened (Ascione *et al.*, 2007). 'Batterers who also abuse their pets are both more controlling and use more dangerous forms of violence [sexual violence, marital rape, emotional violence and stalking] than batterers who do not' (Simmons and Lehmann, 2007). And with 62–76% of animal abuse in the home occurring in front of children (Faver and Strand, 2003), studies have found a strong link between witnessing animal abuse and subsequently perpetrating animal abuse (DeGue and DiLillo, 2009).

The foundation of SAF-T recognizes the human–animal connection and that some people refuse to be separated from their pets during a time of crisis. SAF-T celebrates that bond and understands that when a family has lost everything, having the family pet within arm's reach can provide immediate comfort and healing when life may seem grim and uncertain.

The Reach of SAF-T

When I started training criminal justice professionals on these guidelines in 2004 and published them in February 2008, there were only four known family violence shelters in the USA allowing pets on site, and there was no common network or online portal listing shelters that allowed pets on site. I was also unaware of any shelters internationally that were housing pets. With approximately 2500 shelters in the USA, this situation was unacceptable. As of early 2013, there are now 70 family shelters in the USA that accommodate pets on site with their families, and another five in progress. Jessie Street Domestic Violence Services in New South Wales is the first-known Australian shelter to house pets on site. Shelters from the UK, Canada and other countries have also expressed interest in implementing SAF-T and the concept is being shared in South America and the Netherlands.

SAF-T Start-Up Manual

In January 2012, an updated edition of the SAF-T Start-Up Manual was launched to demonstrate the simplicity of housing pets on site. SAF-T recommends three housing options. Shelters may implement one option or a combination to help accommodate families with pets.

1. Option One: Pets are housed with their families directly in the rooms. Shelters participating in this option allow the pet to either free-roam in the room or be housed in a crate when the family is not in the room. There is minimal, if any, set-up cost for this option. The SAF-T Start-Up Manual addresses ways to address the concern about pet allergies with other residents, including creating 'pet-friendly rooms' and 'no-pet rooms'. Families prefer this option since they can sleep with their pet, which may help calm the pet and avoid excessive barking or meowing.

2. Option Two: Pets are housed in an indoor kennel. The indoor kennel is a separate room within the shelter. Shelters participating in this option have used office space, a utility room or a basement. Crates are placed in the room to house animals of all sizes. Animals are housed in the crates, but allowed out to interact with their family. The primary cost of set-up is the crates and some pet supplies. Asking your community pet store or partner animal protection organization for donated or low-cost items will help to minimize costs. This option is popular for keeping pets indoors while containing allergens in one location.

3. Option Three: Pets are housed in an outdoor kennel. The kennel may involve renovating an outdoor building, renovating a garage, or erecting a small shed in the backyard. Shelters opting for this model do so because of the concern about pet allergies or limited space inside the shelter. Many shelters have built an outdoor dog run/play area where families can interact with and exercise their pets (primarily dogs). Smaller pets or pets with separation anxiety may not fare well in these outdoor kennels, so it may be important to offer a different option for them. The outdoor kennels are the most expensive to implement since this may involve erecting a building, installing heating/cooling and ventilation systems. Also, be sure to install security features (padlocks or security cameras) to prevent others from accessing the pets.

There are four foundational principles that make SAF-T a success:

1. *Working together:* a family violence shelter will create and sustain a successful SAF-T programme if they incorporate all criminal justice agencies in the process: attorneys, judges and court staff, law enforcement, animal shelters and animal protection officers, veterinarians, social workers (both child and adult) and medical and counselling professionals. You will also want to let your community know that you are helping pets. Doing so will result in donors wishing to provide funding or supplies to help maintain your programme.

2. *Partnering with an animal protection organization:* family violence shelter staff are typically not trained in how to care for and house family pets. Therefore, identifying and partnering with an animal shelter or animal rescue group locally will help with the set-up and maintenance of the programme. The partner animal protection organization can advise about local laws regarding kennel set-up and maintenance, housing pets, as well as being available to house aggressive or stressed pets, pets that are unable to be accommodated at the family violence shelter (e.g. exotic pets, livestock) or pets if the SAF-T facility is full. The partner animal shelter may be able to help with obtaining free or low-cost pet food and other pet-related supplies. This partnership also prevents family pets from being surrendered to an animal shelter due to family violence.

3. *Partnering with a veterinarian:* locating a veterinarian who will provide free or low-cost services to your SAF-T programme is essential. Pets may arrive with fresh or healing injuries from abuse requiring medical attention, or may be in poor health due to an inability to access veterinary care. Most SAF-T shelters have located veterinarians who will provide free on-site services (such as a wellness exam, vaccinations, flea/parasite treatments, grooming) and low-cost services at the veterinary clinic (for treatment of injuries, spaying/neutering). Veterinarians who support SAF-T feel proud to give back to their community and to help a population of pets who are often the silent victims of family violence.

4. *The family cares for their pet:* it is important that the family care for their pet on site, including walking/exercising the dog, playing with the cat, feeding, and spending time to help the pet adjust to their new surroundings. The shelter SAF-T director or other designated staff should be the only other persons having access to the pets. Pets should never free-roam in the shelter and among other residents. Some residents may be fearful of animals, have allergies or may approach an animal improperly thus increasing the likelihood of being bitten or scratched. Because pets may be stressed from being abused or from living in a new environment, this policy avoids the concern about dog bites, cat scratches and other animal-related injuries. Since you will probably need to obtain an insurance rider for housing pets on site, this policy will ease the concerns of the insurance carrier. The goal of SAF-T is for all to be safe.

The guidelines in the SAF-T Start-Up Manual are straightforward: if you keep it simple, you will implement in a short amount of time with limited expenses and garner the support of your community; whereas if you complicate the process with extravagant designs, construction processes and burdensome policies, it will take many months, sometimes years, and excessive expenditures of money before your on-site programme is ready to take its first client. If you are in a heavily populated metropolitan area, you may require a more complicated set-up. However, most shelters are smaller and have succeeded with the simple approach.

The SAF-T Start-Up Manual outlines all of the issues to consider when implementing the programme, including allergies, fear of pets, legal issues, zoning issues, fundraising and even includes sample forms. You can download the manual and other pet safety planning materials at www.animalsandfamilies.org. For those family violence shelters wishing to first help pets with off-site housing (foster care programme or boarding at a veterinary clinic, animal shelter or boarding facility), Dr Frank Ascione's *Safe Havens Guidelines* (Ascione, 2000) provide excellent resources and tools for starting a programme.

How Veterinarians Can Help

As discussed above, veterinarians are a key component to a successful SAF-T programme. The generosity of veterinarians currently assisting SAF-T programmes is allowing more family pets to receive critical and basic care that they have otherwise been denied due to violence in the home. Some veterinarians have even offered to board certain pets that are suffering from ailments or behavioural problems because they have the staff equipped to handle these situations. Supporting a SAF-T programme will not only allow a veterinarian to feel good about helping pets caught in the crossfire of family violence, but will spread throughout the community and bring goodwill to that veterinary practice. In essence, if you give, you will receive.

Conclusion

While those people who love animals may find it difficult to understand why family violence shelters have only recently recognized that pets are part of the family and that pets can be targets of domestic violence, we are now at a tipping point across the globe where a small number of shelters are pushing the movement to make on-site housing of pets mainstream. For people like Barbara who had children and pets to protect, SAF-T saved their lives before another tragedy like Riley could unfold. SAF-T is available as a resource to provide step-by-step guidance on how to allow families to safely escape abusive homes with their pets. To learn more about this programme, please visit http://www.animalsandfamilies.org.

References

Ascione, F.R. (2000) *Safe Havens for Pets: Guidelines for Programs Sheltering Pets for Women Who Are Battered.* Available at: http://www.humananimalconnection.org/PDF/ascione_safe_havens.pdf (accessed 14 May 2012).

Ascione, F.R. (2007) Emerging research on animal abuse as a risk factor for intimate partner violence. In: Kendall-Tackett, K. and Giacomoni, S. (eds) *Intimate Partner Violence.* Civic Research Institute, Kingston, New Jersey, pp. 3.1–3.17.

Ascione, F.R., Weber, C.V., Thompson, T.M., Heath, J., Maruyana, M. and Hayashi, K. (2007) Battered pets and domestic violence: animal abuse reported by women experiencing intimate violence and by non-abused women. *Violence Against Women* 13(4), 354–373.

DeGue, S. and DiLillo, D. (2009) Is animal cruelty a 'red flag' for family violence? Investigating co-occurring violence toward children, partners and pets. *Journal of Interpersonal Violence* 24(6), 1036–1056.

Faver, C.A. and Strand, E B. (2003) Domestic violence and animal cruelty: untangling the web of abuse. *Journal of Social Work Education* 39(2), 237–253.

Simmons, C.A. and Lehmann, P. (2007) Exploring the link between pet abuse and controlling behaviors in violent relationships. *Journal of Interpersonal Violence* 22(9), 1211–1222.

13 CARE Programme (Children and Animals; Respect and Empathy): Pet Therapy for Children from Abusive Homes

Zoe Hinds and Jenna Ooi

History of the CARE Programme

In 2010, after attending a Humane Education Conference in New Zealand, the Education Director at the Animal Welfare League of Queensland (AWLQ) had the idea to use shelter animals to help child victims of domestic violence.

The idea was conceived after hearing a speaker at the conference talk about a programme that was assisting the child victims of the tragic 2009 'Black Saturday' bushfires. These bushfires claimed over 200 lives in rural Victoria (Australia); hundreds of families lost their homes, livelihoods and loved ones in the fires, which were deliberately lit by an arsonist. The events were particularly traumatizing for the children of these communities, being displaced from their homes, families and school communities.

In response to concerns raised by parents and teachers in the aftermath of Black Saturday, about their children having extreme nightmares, not being able to sleep and not being able to function at school, a local educator developed an animal-assisted therapy programme using guinea pigs. The programme eventually proved to have significant, lasting benefits for the children, improving their sleep, lessening the reoccurrence of nightmares and reducing their anxiety and fear levels.

It was deduced that if such a programme was effective for these children, it may also be effective for children suffering trauma and displacement due to domestic violence, and that the AWLQ was in a position to develop such a programme.

The Education Director contacted the local women's refuge, Macleod Accommodation Support Service, and gained the support of the Domestic Violence Child Support Worker who could also see the potential of such a programme. At the 2010 Queensland Council of Social Sevices conference, refuge staff had seen a presentation on the BARK programme (Building Animal Relationships with Kids), a similar collaboration between Malaga RSPCA and the Patricia Giles Centre in Perth. The staff at the Patricia Giles Centre were very helpful and provided programme information to the refuge. The two organizations, AWL and Macleod, began developing the programme plan collaboratively in late 2010, and in early 2011 the first pilot of CARE began.

The CARE programme is based on the premise that young children who become victims of parental abuse and neglect are at greater risk of engaging in antisocial behaviour and continuing the cycle of abuse as they get older. This is because the development of healthy behaviour in children, such as displaying empathy and compassion, comes from the early formation of strong bonds to family, school and community (Crawford and Bodine, 1996). Children who have been exposed to violence or experienced trauma in their lives may have missed opportunities to develop these early bonds and therefore may display limited empathy and respond abnormally to the distress of others (including animals) (Redfeld, 2006).

Early intervention programmes such as CARE, which explicitly teach empathy and respect, may help child victims of domestic violence by promoting the formation of these bonds. The key to the programme's success is using animals to facilitate the learning – children are easily motivated by the idea of working with animals; because of this eagerness, the children are open to instruction and in the best frame of mind for learning new, healthy behaviours. The children have the opportunity to observe empathy, respect and compassion, modelled by their instructors and they in turn are positively rewarded with praise and more time with the animals, for displaying these qualities themselves.

Children seem to understand intuitively that there is a connection between the way the world treats animals and the way it treats children (Loar and Coleman, 2004). As with domestic animals, the lives of children are circumscribed by the families with whom they live. It is because of this dependency on others that children and animals are the two groups in society most susceptible to abuse and neglect (Loar and Coleman, 2004). Animal welfare workers such as those who work at the AWLQ see first-hand the devastating effects of neglect and abuse on the animals in our society; child welfare workers likewise see the same in the children in their care. It makes sense then that an animal welfare organization should team with a social welfare organization to help improve the outcomes for both of these vulnerable groups.

Aim of the Programme

To develop a sense of empathy and respect for animals in child victims of domestic violence with the aim of breaking the cycle of abuse that often occurs with children exposed to family violence.

How the CARE Programme Works

Children are given the opportunity to visit the Animal Welfare League Queensland Rehoming and Education Centre to engage in a series of structured activities. Each session is an hour long and they are carried out over 2 weeks (two sessions per week). The programme aims to provide children with opportunities to develop a sense of empathy, respect, compassion and responsibility by teaching them how to care for and nurture an animal (Figs 13.1 and 13.2).

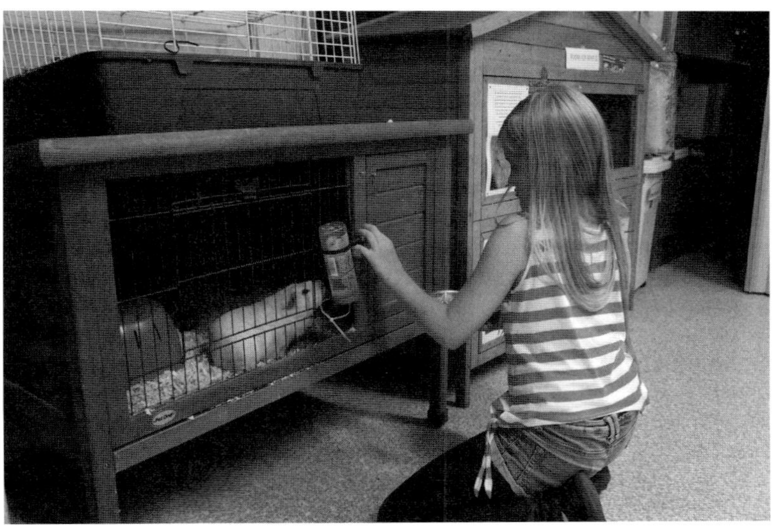

Fig. 13.1. A child taking part in a humane education workshop. Cleaning the guinea pigs' cages is one way the children learn what it means to be responsible for another living creature. The child featured in this photograph is taking part in a humane education workshop that covers similar activities to the CARE Program. Permission to use this photograph was granted by the child's parents. (Photograph courtesy of Zoe Hinds and Jenna Ooi.)

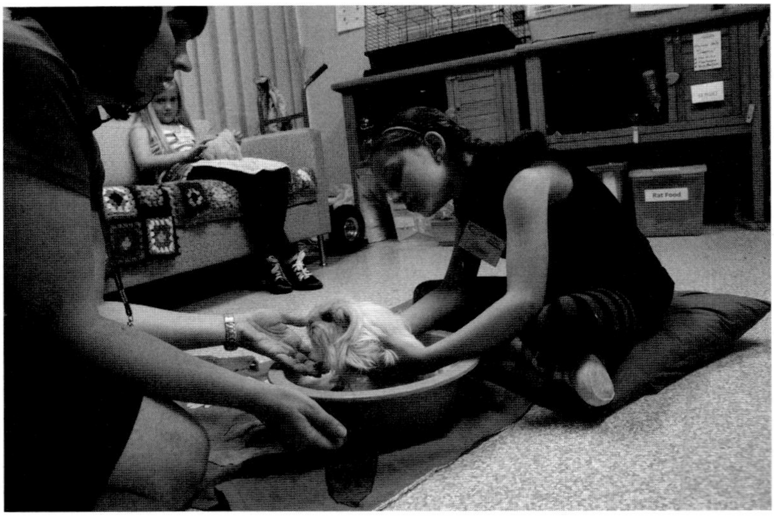

Fig. 13.2. As part of the programme, the children bathe and groom their guinea pigs. Children featured in this photograph are taking part in a humane education workshop that covers similar activities to the CARE Program. Permission to use this photograph was granted by the parents. (Photograph courtesy of Zoe Hinds and Jenna Ooi.)

The children who are selected to participate have all come from domestic violence situations where they may have been direct victims of violence but may also have witnessed the perpetrator abuse other family members, including the family pet. Some of these children may have even begun hurting their peers and/or animals themselves, as a reaction to their situation.

In order to break the cycle of abuse that often occurs with children who have come from violent backgrounds, it is essential they have opportunities to observe and practise empathy and respect – qualities they have not had the opportunity to observe in a household where the perpetrator of violence controls their victims through abuse and fear.

Programme outcomes

At the end of the four-session programme, the children should be able to:

- demonstrate empathetic responses to an animal or person in need;
- understand the concept of responsibility and know what their own responsibilities are in different roles;
- understand how to respect the personal space of another person/animal;
- know how to keep themselves safe and who to turn to when in need; and
- know the meaning of compassion and how to demonstrate compassion towards another person or an animal in need.

Each session was developed with a 'theme' that relates to the qualities of empathy and respect. The session begins with spending quality 'calm' time with a chosen animal; petting, grooming and feeding.

The session then moves into the active learning phase where the children learn something new about caring for and understanding animals – this being related to the 'theme' for that session. This new learning is then related to their own experiences and the lesson shifts from being about care for animals to care for themselves and others.

Each session is then ended with 'family time', where the children's mothers and siblings (if available) are invited into the session to share time with the animals and engage with the programme. It is important that the children's mothers are NOT present throughout the main part of the session, so as to give the children a feeling of autonomy and personal responsibility for their CARE animal.

If there are mothers accompanying their children, a quiet, relaxing space, separate from the learning space should be provided for the mothers to wait while their child participates in the programme.

Implementing the CARE Programme

Implementing the pilot CARE programme required careful thinking and planning. After developing the outline of each session, the AWLQ Education Director and Domestic Violence Child Support Worker also had to consider, among other things, the number of participants, the type of instruction, selection of animals to use and the type of learning space. Below is the session outline, as well as an overview of some of the considerations to do with therapy animal selection and design of the learning space.

Outline of sessions

Table 13.1 is an outline of each session in the CARE programme. While it is important to be organized and have a plan for each session, instructors must ensure that each session is structured 'gently'. The children should be allowed the freedom to explore their feelings about each activity, ask questions and tell stories about their own experiences (if they feel so inclined).

Programme participants and instructors

- The programme is targeted at children aged approximately 5–10 years old.
- No more than six children per programme should be participating at any one time. The small student/AWLQ Education Officer/social worker ratio allows for small group activities and maximum interaction with the AWLQ animals.
- AWLQ Education Officers involved in the CARE programme must be experienced and knowledgeable about the animal-related content within the programme outline.
- Education Officers must also have experience working with and an affinity for young children, in particular children in crisis and/or children at risk. They must hold or be willing to obtain a 'Suitability for Working with Children' Blue Card.
- Each group of participating children must be accompanied in each session by an experienced child social worker, who is familiar with the programme content and is willing to teach the sessions in partnership with the AWLQ Education Officer.
- Education Officers will be employed by the AWLQ and directly answerable to the AWLQ Education Division.

The therapy animals

The animals used for the CARE programme must be carefully considered. The success of the entire programme (i.e. the enjoyment of the children involved) depends entirely on their experience with the therapy animals.

All activities with the animals should allow positive experiences for the children. Even one negative experience (i.e. the animal scratches the child) may negatively impact the child's entire time in the programme. Therefore, animals must not only be selected carefully, but also the children's interactions with the animals must be managed carefully.

Selecting the animals

All animals used in such a programme should be non-threatening and non-challenging for the children. This needs to be thought out carefully, because even a small, fluffy, white dog that bounces around the room could be considered threatening for a small child sitting cross-legged on the floor; particularly a child who is uncomfortable with being touched, a dog that jumps up and licks their face all over would be very challenging and even distressing.

It is for this reason that the AWLQ Education Director chose to use mainly guinea pigs for the CARE programme. This is because: (i) guinea pigs were used with much success in the programme by which CARE was inspired; and (ii) guinea pigs are very benign, predictable

Table 13.1. An outline of sessions from the CARE programme.

Session theme	Description of activities	Activity leader(s)	Resources required
Session 1: Responsibility	• Tour of AWLQ refuge (15 min) ✓ Take children on guided tour, led by an AWLQ Education Officer, of refuge with their mothers and siblings included, so as to gain a context for where they are during the duration of the programme.	Zoe; Rachel	• Education guinea pigs • Guinea pig brushes • Assortment of chopped fruit and veggies for the guinea pigs • Easel with butcher's paper • Permanent marker
	• 'Housekeeping' and rules (5 min) ✓ Discuss briefly with children expectations of their behaviour during their time at the AWLQ – outline the '4 Respects': Respect for our Animals; Respect for our Peers; Respect for our Instructors; Respect for Ourselves. ✓ Point out where the lockers and toilets are. Explain what their mothers will be doing whilst they are engaged in the programme activities. ✓ Outline how each session will run – i.e. they will start with 'guinea pig time', then have a 'sharing session' and then finish with 'family time' each week.	Zoe; Rachel	
	• Meet-and-greet with guinea pigs (20 min) ✓ Introduce each guinea pig in turn and tell them their 'story' of how they came to be at AWLQ. ✓ Explain to children that they will each be allocated a guinea pig that will be their special animal to care for at each session over the course of the programme. Show children how to groom their guinea pig, feed, clean its cage, etc.	Zoe; Rachel	
	• Sharing session: 'Circles of Responsibility' (10 min) ✓ Seat children in a circle around the mat – instructor is seated at front of circle next to the easel. Draw up the easel paper with three circles. ✓ Ask children 'what are responsibilities to our pets?' – write responses in the corresponding circle. Ask children 'what are our responsibilities to our family?' – write responses in the corresponding circle. Ask children 'what are responsibilities to our friends?' – write responses in the corresponding circle.	Jenna	
	• Family time (10 min) ✓ Invite the children's mothers and siblings to come into the classroom and join them while they cuddle their guinea pigs and talk about the things they have been learning about in the sharing session.		

Continued

Table 13.1. Continued.

Session theme	Description of activities	Activity leader(s)	Resources required
Session 2: Respect	• Guinea pig care (20 min) ✓ Instruct children through the process of cleaning the guinea pig cages. Explain that as a pet owner, you are responsible for the life of a living creature. It is your responsibility to ensure they are clean, fed, watered, nurtured and healthy.	Zoe; Rachel	• Education guinea pigs • Guinea pig brushes • Assortment of chopped fruit and veggies for the guinea pigs • Easel with butchers paper • Permanent marker • Book *Hands are Not for Hitting* by Martine Agassi
	• Treating animals and people with respect (20 min) ✓ Allow children to spend some time with their guinea pigs, brushing, feeding and stroking them. ✓ Explain to students that when we are around animals, it is very important to 'respect' them by handling them gently. ✓ Talk about how we treat our friends and families with respect and write some of their ideas on the easel. ✓ Read 'Hands are not for Hitting' as a group.	Zoe; Rachel, Jenna	
	• Family time (10 min) ✓ Invite the children's mothers and siblings to come into the classroom and join them whilst they cuddle their guinea pigs and talk about the things they have been learning about in the sharing session.		
Session 3: Safety	• Guinea pig time and photo (10 min) ✓ Allow children to spend some time with their guinea pigs, brushing, feeding and stroking them. ✓ Take a photo of each of the children with their guinea pig, so it can be designed into a special keepsake card for the next session.	Zoe; Rachel	• Education guinea pigs • Guinea pig brushes • Assortment of chopped fruit and veggies for the guinea pigs
	• Meet-and-greet with a shelter puppy – 'safety paw' (15 min) ✓ Introduce the shelter puppy to the children and tell them its story. Allow them to feed it food treats and give it pats. ✓ Ask children: 'how can we keep pet dogs safe?' On the easel, draw up a dog's paw as shown in (**Resource 4**). Explain the 'safety paw' by discussing each point in turn, saying that together these are all the ways in which we can keep dogs safe.	Zoe; Rachel	• Digital camera • Shelter puppy • Easel • Easel and butcher's paper • Permanent marker
	• Sharing session: 'safety hand' (15 min) ✓ Draw up a 'safety hand'. Ask children: 'if we were in trouble, who could we go to in order to be safe?' Hear the children's answers and write the five key people inside each of the hand's fingers.	Jenna	
	• Family time (10 min) ✓ Invite the children's mothers and siblings to come into the classroom and join them while they cuddle their guinea pigs and talk about the things they have been learning about in the sharing session.		

Continued

Table 13.1. Continued.

Session theme	Description of activities	Activity leader(s)	Resources required
Session 4: Care and Compassion	• Guinea pig time (10 min) ✓ Allow children to spend some time with their guinea pigs, brushing, feeding and stroking them.	Zoe; Rachel	• Education guinea pigs • Guinea pig brushes • Assortment of chopped fruit and veggies for the guinea pigs
	• Feed the farm animals (20 min) ✓ Take children over to the 'farm yard' and give them each a small bucket filled with fresh scraps to feed the poultry and goat. Encourage them to stroke the animals and talk to them about how our animal attendants care for all our animals equally – the chickens, ducks and goats are as important and matter just as much as the dogs and cats.	Zoe; Rachel	• Access to farm animals • Assortment of chopped fruit and veggies for the poultry and goat
	• Sharing session: 'Everyone matters' care and compassion (10 min) ✓ Seat children in a circle around the mat – instructor is seated at front of circle next to the easel. Direct children's attention to the 'Everyone Matters' poster. Ask children: 'What can we see in this poster? What do you think it might mean?' ✓ Lead into a discussion about how the poster is trying to show that all living things in our world matter and they should all be treated with compassion. ✓ Discuss with children the meaning of the word 'compassion'. Ask children: 'How can we be a "hero of compassion"?' Ask children to take some of these ideas and try and do at least one of these things on the list before your next session.	Zoe; Rachel	• Easel with butcher's paper • Permanent marker • Poster 'everyone matters'
	• Family time and presentation of photos and certificates (20 min) ✓ Seat children in the 'sharing time' circle. Present each child in turn with their certificate of completion and their special keepsake card with the picture of their guinea pig. ✓ Celebrate the end of the programme with a small 'party', with some treats for them and their family members. ✓ Present each child with the special AWLQ bag of 'goodies'.	Zoe; Rachel, Jenna	• Education guinea pigs • Guinea pig brushes • Assortment of chopped fruit and veggies for the guinea pigs • Certificates and keepsake cards • Selection of party food • Paper cups and soft drink/juice • AWLQ bag of 'goodies'

and unthreatening animals that, as long as properly socialized, enjoy human handling.

It is important that within the programme, each child feels a certain amount of responsibility and personal connection to one or more of the therapy animals. In order for this to happen the children need lots of contact with the animals and, preferably, there are enough animals so that children do not have to share with another child (i.e. each child has their 'own' animal with which to interact). Using guinea pigs makes this much easier to do, because of their small size and that they are easy for a child to manage handling on their own (unlike a cat or dog).

Guinea pigs are also extremely safe. They are in no way aggressive animals – even when frightened they will very rarely express their fear with a display of aggression. To put it plainly, guinea pigs very rarely will bite a human. This makes them a good choice to use with children, especially those who may not be used to handling animals gently, as a slight mishandling here or there on the child's part will probably not result in the child getting injured. Similarly, a slight mishandling by the child will not result in the guinea pig becoming personally fearful of that child – unlike cats or dogs, who will shy away from a particular child if they feel distrustful. Of course, having said this, the aim is to have the children NOT mishandle the animals; however, it is always good practice to consider the risks and 'worst case scenario'.

Managing the animals

Good management of the animals in any therapy or educational programme that requires children to interact closely with animals comes down to structure and group size. As long as the children's time with the animals is structured with purposeful activities and done in small groups, then both the children and the animals should enjoy the experience.

There should always be at least one adult supervising for every two children. If there is a child in the group who is nervous about handling animals, take it slowly and allocate an adult to supervise just this child – never push the child to handle the animal if they are unsure or do not want to. Let the child decide when and if they are ready.

The learning space

It is important to create a learning environment where the children feel safe, comfortable and inspired.

AWLQ is lucky enough to have a purpose-built Education Centre, with a 'lounge room'-style classroom where the small animals' enclosures are kept. The guinea pig cages are situated around the perimeter of the room, with a three-seater sofa at one end of the room and a large rug in the middle of the floor. When the CARE children visit, large cushions are scattered around the rug and the children can choose to sit either on the sofa or on the cushions. The adults are encouraged to sit on the floor with the children. There are posters with positive messages about responsible animal care on the walls. The idea is to make the space as 'soft' and inviting as possible, with easy access to the therapy animals. The space should also be clean and tidy, with easy access to bathroom and hand-washing facilities.

Evaluating the CARE Programme

Evaluation of the pilot CARE programme was carried out for the following purposes.

1. Evaluating the effectiveness of instruction and how instruction methods may be developed and improved.
2. Evaluating both the cognitive and emotional effect of the experience on the children involved.
3. Evaluating the structure of the programme and the resources used and how these aspects may be improved in the future.

Evaluation on point 2 was carried out mostly using anecdotal feedback from the Child Welfare Social Workers and the parents of the children involved. The AWLQ Education Director also developed a 'reflection diary' for each child to fill in after each session, in hope that this may gain some insight into how the child was feeling about the experience. In practice, it was difficult to get the children to complete these diaries, as it may have been too close to a 'homework' task, which did not seem to motivate them. In the end, verbal feedback from the children (during and after the sessions) and written feedback from the parents/social workers was the most effective form of feedback.

Evaluation on points 1 and 3 was carried out on completion of the pilot programme in consultation with the social worker who originally developed the programme with the AWLQ Education Director. The main issues to resolve concerned the duration of the programme (as in weeks) and the difficulty in retaining the same group of children over a lengthy period in order to complete the programme in its entirety.

Originally the programme was developed to have six 1-hour sessions, over 6 weeks. This allowed for more content and allowed the children to develop a deeper connection with their instructors and therapy animals; however, due to the transient nature of the children's living circumstances (all children engaged in the programme were living in temporary crisis accommodation), it was difficult for the children's mothers to commit to a regular appointment 6 weeks into the future (as the family may not have known where they would be living in 6 weeks' time).

It was decided that in order to increase the likelihood of retaining the same children over the course of the programme, the programme should be condensed to four sessions that could be completed in 2 weeks (two 1-hour sessions per week).

Benefits of the CARE Programme

The most effective way to demonstrate the benefits that this programme can have for a child, is to let one of the child welfare social workers describe her experience with the CARE programme:

> I wish to convey a very special thank you to Zoe and Jenna (co facilitators) and Laurel (volunteer) for organising an exceptional C.A.R.E. program for children that have experience trauma and abuse in their short lives.
>
> The C.A.R.E program provided an opportunity for children to discover and explore fascinating facts about animal behaviour, their habitat and appropriate care.
>
> I believe the small interactive groups allowed children to feel safe, and confident enough to participate in hands on activities and group discussions.
>
> All of the children that attended the program expressed how much fun they had when we sat in a circle on a mat on the floor surrounded by bright coloured cushions nursing, brushing and feeding our favourite guinea pigs. They also mentioned how much they enjoyed gathering food from the veggie and herb garden, and sharing their fruit for afternoon tea with their guinea pigs.
>
> It was a poignant moment for me as I had not witnessed these children so calm, relaxed and engaged in an activity before.
>
> Animals are often attachment objects for children – touch, proximity and mind and body interaction with animals has been found to contribute to stress reduction and trauma recovery in adults and children.
>
> I have witnessed first-hand the change that can and did occur within seconds of an animal entering a room.
>
> A quiet withdrawn (7 year old) girl engaged immediately when Leroy the dog was led into the room.
>
> A young (4 year old) boy had not spoken a single word while staying at the refuge until he attended the C.A.R.E program. He only said one word while interacting with a variety of animals, e.g. guinea pigs, rats, mice, kittens, dogs, goat, pig and cats, but that one word was the beginning of his healing and recovery process.
>
> By the end of the six week program I had observed the positive effects of 'Contact Comfort', a tactile process whereby unconditional attachment bonds form between the animals and children inducing relaxation and a reduction in stress.
>
> The children that attended the C.A.R.E. program appeared to be less anxious, more confident and had a greater perception of happiness after their visits to the animal shelter.
>
> (Sonia Lebby, Support Worker)

References

Crawford, D. and Bodine, R. (1996) *Conflict Resolution Education: A Guide to Implementing Programs in Schools, Youth-Serving Organizations, and Community and Juvenile Justice Settings.* US Department of Justice and US Department of Education, Washington, DC.

Loar, L. and Colman, L. (2004) *Teaching Empathy: animal-assisted therapy programs for children and families exposed to violence.* A Latham Foundation Publication, Alameda, California.

Redfeld, L. (2006) Report to lotteries commission of Western Australia on the links between family violence and pet abuse. Patricia Giles Centre, Perth, Western Australia.

14 Mental Health Issues of Working with Animal Abuse

Catherine Tiplady and Deborah Walsh

Introduction

While working with abused animals is very important work providing a range of rewards, it can also be distressing, particularly when there are other vulnerable victims involved. Becoming distressed when confronted with animals that have been deliberately harmed is a normal reaction – understanding our reactions and knowing what we can do can limit the detrimental effects of these events on our lives. Being healthy and well supported can give us the benefit of being able to support ourselves, our colleagues and clients and continue our work with animals.

This chapter collaborates with Dr Deborah Walsh, a social work practitioner, trauma counsellor and clinical supervisor in the area of domestic and family violence. Deborah will provide a range of information and guidance to help professionals think about establishing information for when difficult situations arise in practice and the prioritizing of self-care as part of occupational health and safety maintenance.

Mental Health Issues and Stress

Most people who enter animal care work and veterinary science do so with a genuine desire to save animals' lives and relieve suffering, and can be unprepared for cases of animal abuse. Unfortunately, veterinary schools do little to train students in this area, despite there being a high likelihood of being confronted with cases of animal abuse during their career (Green and Gullone, 2005). Not surprisingly, working with abused animals is distressing to many veterinarians (Tiplady *et al.*, 2012, unpublished results).

Both mental and physical health can be affected if stress levels are chronic and enduring – one in three veterinarians have reported poor psychological health, particularly in women, those who are younger and those who have recently graduated (Fritschi *et al.*, 2009). Increasing hours spent at work appeared to correlate with an increase in distress and anxiety. Veterinarians also have one of the highest rates of suicide of any profession. Among UK veterinarians, the chance of death being due to suicide is approximately four times greater than in the general population and about twice that of other healthcare professionals (Bartram and Baldwin, 2010).

One of the duties that can cause veterinarians a lot of distress is being required to euthanize animals.

Dealing with euthanasia

The stress of caring for animals as well as having to euthanize them has been referred to as the 'caring–killing paradox' (Arluke, 1994). 'Moral stress' (Rollin, 2006) such as this arises when people are required to do things they have difficulty justifying on moral grounds. Performing euthanasia of abused animals is more distressing to many veterinarians than euthanasia of animals suffering chronic disease such as renal failure or cancer (Tiplady *et al.*, 2012, unpublished results), as abused animals are otherwise healthy but their 'injury' has been caused by unacceptable behaviour in humans. Should veterinarians become distressed around issues of injustice generally it is likely that facing issues such as this may cause distress, particularly if attempts to treat or rehome the animal have not been successful.

People who euthanize animals as a regular part of their jobs have been found to suffer a wide range of distressing reactions, including grief, anger and depression (White, 1998) and may experience traumatic symptoms of nightmares, recurrent thoughts and feelings (intrusion) and avoidance of emotions and ideas associated with the euthanasia of animals (avoidance) (Rohlf and Bennett, 2005). Active participation in traumatic events may result in 'perpetration-induced traumatic stress' or PITS (MacNair, 2002). This stress has also been identified in war veterans (MacNair, 2002) and police officers (Loo, 1986) who have shot or killed people as part of their duties.

A survey of over 300 animal shelter staff in America enquired about what could be done to assist them in dealing with euthanasia-related stress (Rogelberg *et al.*, 2007). Responses included: support from management, providing counselling to employees, job rotation, skills-based training, time off and more breaks during work, stress and coping seminars and morale-boosting initiatives. This research raises some serious concerns about occupational health and safety issues for shelter staff that need attention. Practical guidelines for performing euthanasia humanely are outlined in Chapter 19.

Considering ways to improve the mental and physical health of students and staff is essential for the health and future of the veterinary profession – for example, arranging workshops in coping with stress and grief and providing access to counsellors for their staff and students. Some associations for veterinarians and veterinary nurses and technicians offer telephone or face-to-face counselling for their members and immediate family who are seeking assistance with work or personal issues. For veterinary practices and shelters, a visit from a counsellor could be arranged on a regular basis, to hold workshops in issues such as grief, coping with stress and caring for yourself.

What is the Well-being of Veterinary Staff?

A trauma counsellor who originally trained and worked as a veterinary nurse undertook research into the psychological and physical well-being of veterinary nurses, veterinarians and clinic staff (Overfield, 2010). Her survey of over 500 respondents found:

- 90% stated their reasons for working with animals were 'a love of animals' and 'to care for animals'.
- 83% feel worn out because of their work.
- 80% never detach, or find it difficult to detach, from their work at the end of the day.
- 70% struggle to fall asleep or lose sleep, over their patients in the practice.
- Handling difficult clients and insufficient time were top stressors in 64% of cases.
- Nearly 1 in 3 (29%) found seeing injured and ill animals to be a top stressor.
- 85% were often too exhausted to do anything else after their shifts.

People who choose to work with abused animals are often extremely compassionate people driven by a strong desire to prevent animal suffering. These people may initially be full of enthusiasm to help animals but later become stressed and disenchanted with the way some members of society treat animals. Encouraging people to contribute to education campaigns and other community education initiatives may relieve the frustration and helplessness that these issues can generate as the energy can be channelled into prevention of cruelty.

What Can Happen to Those Who Work with Animal Abuse

While some will turn distress around and use this energy to become advocates for abused animals, others will find the situation too overwhelming and may develop unhealthy coping mechanisms (i.e. alcohol dependence). Others may develop mental health issues and a small population may walk away from the profession completely. One of the first steps toward self-care is to identify the range of reactions that may confront workers and recognize them so they can be addressed before becoming entrenched behaviour.

Four phases that employees working in the animal welfare field may experience have been identified (Smith and Fakkema, 2009).

1. *Ready to change the world.* In this initial phase, people feel energized and enthusiastic to the cause of helping animals. Total obsession with animal work may overtake friendships and cause isolation. Simple solutions may be assigned to complex problems – for example, the belief that every animal should be desexed and no animal euthanized.
2. *Depression.* The energy and enthusiasm of phase one are replaced by a realization that animals are still being abused and neglected. There are feelings of exhaustion and sadness as there seems to be no end to the euthanasia and nobody seems to understand. Families are ignored, work is not discussed and dreams are filled with horror. At this stage some turn to unhealthy behaviours such as living on junk food, drugs and alcohol to try and take away the feelings of hopelessness.
3. *Anger.* The depression of phase two turns outward and hopelessness turns to rage. There is hatred toward any person who has not devoted their life to animals and even thoughts that people who abuse animals should be 'euthanized'. Disagreement and hatred of co-workers may be seen. Even the animals we work with seem distant and unreal.
4. *Realization.* Although some people may not reach this phase or may alternate between phases, phase four is where people come to terms with the inherent stress and sadness of animal work. There is a realization that, although all problems have not been solved, a difference has been made to the lives of dozens, hundreds or thousands of animals. People who abuse and neglect animals are acknowledged as a minority and no longer hated. Weekends and holidays are used for relaxing and isolation, alcohol, drugs and food are not used to hide feelings of anger, depression and sadness. The recognition of the potential to help animals and change the world one step at a time is seen.

One way of avoiding long-term negative consequences of facing difficult situations is to reach out for help and support (see section on 'Finding the Oxygen Mask' below). A range of negative reactions to ongoing distress has been identified and a number of these will be outlined below. Definitions will be provided along with ways of managing this in your professional life.

Burnout

'Burnout' is the emotional and physical exhaustion in a person who experiences excessive pressure and not enough satisfaction (Figley and Roop, 2006).

Symptoms include (Figley and Roop, 2006):

- poor motivation and a lack of desire to advance yourself at work;
- dread of going to work – feeling overworked, unappreciated, demoralized and unenthusiastic;
- sense of alienation – avoiding socializing or talking to colleagues;
- aggression – easily annoyed and impatient with the perceived incompetence of others; and
- health problems – including headaches, backaches, insomnia, depression and increased alcohol consumption.

Compassion fatigue

Compassion and empathy are great assets for veterinarians and animal carers; however, continually trying to alleviate the suffering of others can result in feeling traumatized and exhausted. This puts people at a greater than usual risk of developing compassion fatigue.

Compassion fatigue is a form of post-traumatic stress disorder (PTSD), a condition that includes reliving a stressful event, avoiding reminders of the event and experiencing physical distress when remembering the event (Figley and Roop, 2006).

Symptoms of compassion fatigue include the following (Durrance, 2007):

- loss of interest in work;
- emotional numbness;
- withdrawal from previously enjoyable activities;
- indifference to and withdrawal from relationships;
- sleeping and eating difficulties;
- episodes of high anxiety;
- feeling drained and overwhelmed;
- feeling unable to recover from a patient's death;
- feeling trapped by responsibilities and victimized by your job; and
- experiencing acute emotional pain.

Factors contributing to compassion fatigue include (Figley and Roop, 2006):

- prolonged exposure to suffering without a sufficient break or holiday;
- traumatic memories – unresolved distress when remembering a traumatic event; and
- other life demands, such as stress in personal relationships.

The Professional Quality Of Life (ProQOL) scale: compassion satisfaction and compassion fatigue (Hudnall Stamm, 2009) is a scale that can be of assistance in identifying our risk of compassion fatigue and burnout (Appendix 4).

To understand how we can avoid compassion fatigue we need to understand how to care for ourselves. Dr Deborah Walsh describes methods of minimizing the risk of compassion fatigue and burnout.

Caring For Yourself – 'Finding the Oxygen Mask'

Deborah Walsh

Working in a profession where caring is central to your role can be very rewarding, but if workers are not vigilant it can also have a dark side. The dark side is burnout and/or compassion fatigue, which can sneak up on the unsuspecting worker if they do not look after themselves. Being overwhelmed by the demands of others can be draining and can deplete a person's ordinary coping resources. However, the best way to beat burnout and/or compassion fatigue is to avoid it in the first place. Maslach (2003, p. 240), a world-renowned specialist on burnout, states:

> If all knowledge and advice about how to beat burnout could be summed up in one word, that word would be balance. Balance between giving and getting, balance between stress and calm, balance between work and home.

To achieve an even balance may be challenging at times, but it is critical if workers are to avoid burnout and compassion fatigue. Many women, in particular, succumb to the notion of self-sacrifice or the martyr syndrome and give, give and give; this is a clear pathway toward burnout. Remember balance – care out needs care in. Self-care should not be considered selfish – it is survival.

A good analogy that can be applied to self-care is what Walsh (1998) refers to as the 'oxygen mask'. In training health and welfare workers to work in the area of domestic violence she emphasizes self-care as critical to worker survival. Walsh (1998) cites the instructions flight attendants give to their passengers during the inflight emergency procedure briefing. The flight attendants are careful to remind passengers that when the oxygen masks fall they should fit their own mask first before attempting to help others. This, Walsh (1998) says, is sage advice for us all for if we replenish ourselves regularly by self-care we will be able to continue the care of others (in this case – animals) and reduce the risk of burnout and compassion fatigue.

Walsh (1998) likens burnout to a well of water and describes caring as giving out the water a bucket at a time and, if the water is not replenished, then it dries up. If water is not forthcoming then we risk the bottom of the well becoming brittle and cracked, not allowing any water to be held in the well without major repair work. The best way to avoid major repair work is by investing time and energy in self-care.

While cumulative exposure to the demands of work can sneak up on a worker, the other important issue to be aware of is the 'critical incident'. The definition of a critical incident should be left to the individual to define for themselves, as each individual will have different thresholds and if an incident has an impact on the person's ability to cope then that is critical to them. Should a worker experience a traumatic event or a critical incident at work, it is very important to have some critical incident stress management (CISM) plan in place (Harms, 2007). This can be as simple as taking the time to listen to a co-worker who is distressed about dealing with a case that is particularly difficult and checking they are alright. Or it could be an occupational health and safety issue of ensuring staff are rotated on work duties so they do not spend too long on particularly distressing tasks such as euthanizing animals. Taking time to care for yourself and colleagues contributes to the work culture and longevity of caring workplaces. Each workplace is unique and has differing needs, so any support plan needs to be developed by staff members in consultation with management so that the plan is useful to everyone.

There is a range of private psychological service providers who specialize in working with critical incident stress management, and it will be important to build connections with at least two of these service providers so that the workplace can include how to contact these services in the event that a critical incident occurs that is outside the expertise of the existing staff. The level of seriousness that might trigger the activation of a CISM plan will need to be determined by the individual workplace in consultation with management.

A list of these service providers and their availability will be a critical part of the CISM plan. Access to a list of private providers who have this expertise can be made by contacting your region's psychological society branch. It would be a wise professional move to develop a CISM plan prior to any incident occurring, so that this is well and truly in place with all staff knowing how to access the plan should it ever be required. A proactive approach to management issues provides clarity around processes and protocols and safety for staff.

A CISM plan needs to be easy to follow and accessible in the event of an emergency or a critical incident occurring. It is well documented that most of our higher functioning cognition and skills become depleted during and immediately after a critical incident, so a simple, clear, step-by-step process of what to do and who to contact and in what order should be how this plan is developed (Figley, 2002). In order to develop such a plan, all parties in the organization must agree to a set of steps, with all decisions made prior to an event that requires one or more staff to activate the plan. Doing a search to see if others have already developed such a plan and using this as a basis to begin your own can save time. If not, then developing a plan and publishing it can help promote your practice and increase your publications.

Self-care in the caring professions is critical for a worker's survival, and being proactively engaged in self-care is one way of ensuring that burnout and compassion fatigue can be reduced.

Tips for Animal Advocates to Avoid and Recover from Burnout

Tips for animal advocates to avoid and recover from burnout have been given the following mnemonic of ACTIVE (Hawthorne, 2008):

> **A**llow yourself to be human and have a break;
> **C**reate a file of your achievements to remind yourself of the positive changes you have helped bring about;
> **T**alk to other animal advocates and if necessary, a therapist; share your concerns and fears;
> **I**gnore upsetting images and reports of animal cruelty until you feel stronger;
> **V**isit an animal sanctuary and spend time with the animals you are working to help;
> **E**xercise regularly, consult a doctor and consider walking, yoga and meditation.

Yoga and meditation sessions need not be lengthy to be beneficial, making this an option worth considering for busy veterinarians and animal workers.

Research has found that even 15 minutes of seated yoga or meditation practice reduced perceived stress among office workers and improved several physiological and psychological markers of stress (Melville *et al.*, 2012).

A 'pocket card' that briefly lists strategies to improve your resiliency and minimize compassion fatigue is available for free at www.proqol.org/Helper_Pocket_Card.html.

Grief

Grief is commonly encountered in veterinary practices and shelters due to the frequent exposure to death and euthanasia of animals. How people are affected by grief and for how long varies between individuals. Dr Deborah Walsh provides guidance on coping with, and assisting others with, grief.

Coping with Grief
Deborah Walsh

> Grief takes time and everyone grieves in their own way and in their own time.
>
> (Ashfield, 2010, p. 286)

Grief has been described as the emotional reaction to loss, which can include a wide range of emotions ranging from sadness through to despair (Raphael, 1987). Essentially the process of grief is the business of dealing with all the emotions associated with coming to terms with the loss of something or someone. The depth of feeling associated with this process will directly relate to the level of attachment someone has to what or who is gone. So the message here is that people will experience a range of emotions when faced with loss, and these emotions are part of a grieving process that is not only associated with death and dying. These feelings are natural and normal and, when they are experienced, humans do better if they have good supports around them.

People will experience grief-type responses in a range of circumstances when loss has occurred. As an example, if someone loses a job they may experience a range of emotional responses that include shock, numbness, disbelief, sadness, anger, helplessness and sometimes despair, and over time when the person comes to terms with the loss the feelings abate. When dealing with a death of a loved one the emotional response will include all those same feelings, but the degree to which the pain and suffering will be experienced will directly relate to how attached they were to that person. In some situations when a life partner dies the intense pain may ease but may never actually go completely, and this is normal and natural.

During the intense experience of grief the comfort and consolation from others is important. While people are not always comfortable being around sadness and acute grieving, it is an important part of being human and contributing to the support of others is a valuable part of being a community.

Veterinarians work with sick and dying animals as part of their occupation and, while most will find this distressing, this is normal. Individuals will have a range of ways to deal with these emotions. A very common way people deal with this issue is to talk with someone else that understands, does not judge and can provide support. This helps the person to begin to process what has happened and to make sense of their feelings associated with it. The listener often will not really have to do much except listen, which is a vital skill in this situation.

Another area where veterinarians will face grief issues is when a companion animal dies and the owner begins to grieve the loss of that companion. Providing the immediate support is critical, and allowing time for the information to filter through the layers of numbness and disbelief is important. Sometimes the person will need to see the animal and say goodbye while others will not want to do that. To respect differences is also important. It would always be important for the veterinarian to feel confident that the person was in a position to drive safely prior to the person getting in a vehicle and driving home. Ashfield (2010, pp. 285–286) provides some suggestions that are valuable to consider when supporting someone who is distressed. They include:

- Try to be a good listener and show by body language, eye contact and attentiveness that you are interested.
- Allow the person to express emotions such as guilt, blame, anger and regret.
- Respect the person and do not try to take over.
- Avoid giving advice or using clichés.
- Avoid making any promises to support if you are unable to commit to them.

There is a range of very good resources available online, and one of these is the Australian Centre for Grief and Bereavement. The site has a range of online resources that are very helpful for people who want to understand grief and obtain some suggestions about how to help (http://www.grief.org.au/). The site also has information available for professionals who are supporting people experiencing grief, which provides valuable resources for those in that situation.

While grief and bereavement are painful experiences they are an inevitable part of life, love and the journey we undertake while on this earth. The only true way to survive it is to go through it and, if we have support during this process, it will make it a little easier.

Working with Perpetrators of Animal Abuse

It is likely that veterinarians and animal carers will come into contact with abusive people at some point. In certain situations, violent people may assault or threaten veterinary clinic staff. Many people who abuse animals will also abuse people – this can also make you vulnerable to threats and verbal and physical abuse. Some cruelty inspectors, such as those in the Massachusetts SPCA, have bullet-proof vests, guns and cans of mace available to them (Arluke, 2004). For the majority of people working with animals however, this equipment is not available, or even desirable.

In this section, Dr Deborah Walsh provides guidance for those of us who may have to work with potentially violent people.

Personal Safety Issues When Working with Abusive People

Deborah Walsh

Many of those who use violence in the home do not use violence in any other setting (Bancroft, 2002). In addition, given the statistical prevalence of domestic violence in our communities it is likely that each of us knows someone who is a perpetrator because perpetrators of domestic violence are indistinguishable from their peers – they can hold good jobs or not, can have a high degree of education or not and do all the things the average person does except when these people go home another picture of who they are emerges (Family Violence Professional Education Taskforce, 1994; Bancroft, 2002). Many perpetrators will go to extreme lengths to develop friendly and helpful social behaviour, but this is often a mask to hide the truth. However, it is important to understand that violence is an instrument used to establish power and control over intimate partners and family members and, unless an outsider poses a threat to this power and control, it is not likely that violence will be used outside the family. There are exceptions to this, but in the main family violence is confined to the home and those within it.

Veterinarians working in isolated areas, doing house calls and working late at night need to consider their own personal safety. While the information above may defuse certain anxieties about those who use domestic violence in the home, personal safety should be a priority. If there is prior knowledge that a person or people in the household are known to be aggressive, then putting a safety plan in place is wise. However, it is also good practice to have policies and plans in place for general day-to-day working if you do work in an isolated area, do house calls and/or work late at night.

General safety precautions for house calls can include the following:

- Always have a mobile phone fully charged and functioning.
- Ensure that there is more than enough fuel in the vehicle for your return trip.
- Have a safety checking system at the office where someone else knows where you are going and what time you are expected back. Some services have a staff location/movement board where all staff record their whereabouts and, if they are leaving the premises, they are required to provide details on the board (this board or book should never be visible to the public) and verbally to one other individual who then becomes the contact person (in some services this role can fall to the administration person). The person leaving the office to attend a house call would then be required to contact when they have arrived safely at the destination and to estimate the time needed at the location, and then again when leaving with an estimated time of arrival back at the office or home. If times vary a check-in is needed to adjust the time. If the person does not phone at the nominated time then the contact person would phone to check whether everything was alright. Check-in phone calls are important as they remind personnel of the responsibility they have for safety procedures. There needs to be an agreed plan in place for what the contact person needs to do in a step-by-step procedure if no contact can be made or the person has not arrived back at their destination at the nominated time.

- If there is any information about situations where veterinarians are going to visit, then this needs to feature in any staff safety plan and plans adjusted accordingly. For instance, if the farmer you are visiting has a history of aggression then plan to take someone else with you. This is particularly important as the presence of two people may act as a deterrent; or should you need to lay a police complaint, then the presence of someone else can be helpful as a witness.
- Develop your house call policy and procedure with the view that it should be reviewed from time to time in order to ensure it is relevant and able to be implemented by all it was designed to assist.

General safety precautions for working late at night:

- Once the time passes the usual working hours it is good policy to ensure that once office administration staff leave for the day, all external doors should be locked and all phones diverted to message.
- After-hours policy should include a process for people to let the staff inside know they have someone waiting outside. As an example, an after-hours doorbell that can be activated and deactivated from inside the building so it is used only when needed (an outside bell that was active all of the time could be problematic, with anyone being able to use it).
- Ensure that there is a visible way of identifying anyone who is outside the door, for example a surveillance camera or a peephole.
- Some services are able to have a policy where no one person is permitted in the building alone after hours. This is expensive for private practices, so other precautions can be implemented such as letting someone know that you are working alone and have a phone check-in procedure in place.

Personal safety is an occupational health and safety issue and should be everyone's business. Developing policy and procedures into which all staff have had input can highlight the importance of staff safety. It cannot prevent external threats, but when something happens everyone will know what to do.

Positive Aspects to Working with Animal Abuse

Despite the difficulties of working with animal abuse, there are rewards.

You are not only helping that individual animal, you are providing a service to society, inspiring others to protect those who are defenceless. You have invested a great deal of time and money in your education and, to ensure you maximize the long-term benefits of this, you need to invest in the ongoing emotional and psychological work that keeps you healthy. By caring for yourself you will be best equipped to continue to care for animals for years to come. The following case study uses the example of rescue of shot waterbirds to illustrate some of the stressors to which animal carers and veterinarians may be exposed during their animal abuse work.

Case Study

The emotional impact of working with animal abuse can be considerable. One area of animal work that is particularly challenging is rescuing, treating and rehabilitating animals that have been hunted and maimed as 'sport'.

Veterinarians and animal carers who oppose the hunting of animals for sport may volunteer to rescue and treat these injured animals and are motivated by compassion and a desire to prevent animal suffering. Ironically, by caring for vulnerable animals, these volunteers may themselves become the targets of abuse and threats from hunters.

Being confronted with such human aggression and animal suffering is extremely distressing, particularly when it is allowed by authorities. Dr Howard Ralph is an experienced wildlife veterinarian who works from a mobile veterinary clinic to treat waterbirds shot during the legal hunting season in Australia. Dr Ralph has written the following case study to provide in detail the experiences and emotions of a veterinarian working at the front line of animal abuse in extremely challenging conditions. Reading this account illustrates the profound psychological impact animal cruelty has on those who work to prevent it and, as such, is ideally situated within the mental health chapter.

Waterbird Massacre Also Known as Duck Shooting: a personal account of a veterinarian's experiences of treating waterbirds injured during legal duck shooting
Dr Howard Ralph BVSc (Hons1), MBBS (Hons), MVS (Wildlife Medicine), JCCA Accred. (Anaesth), Dip TESL, A/Dip Fine Arts, Cert Ed NSW

Well before first light the conflagration began. In excess of an estimated 3000 shooters began their assault on the waterbirds of Lake Cowal, New South Wales, Australia. An untold number of birds and other species were subject to the annual massacre sanctioned by the authority responsible for national parks and wildlife. Many birds other than the so called 'legal species' were shot. They included herons, pelicans, freckled ducks, grebes and darters. The shooting toll also included a fish, a tortoise, a snake, two humans (rescuers) and a dog.

Shooters had the support of the authorities and the police were there in force, many of them spending time with the shooters and National Parks rangers, issuing infringement notices to the rescuers for a range of spurious transgressions and keeping rescuers under constant surveillance.

It was notable that the authorities were absent at night when the shooters were most active, tormenting and harassing the rescuers.

As the shooting began in the morning darkness, the world erupted into a cacophony of gunshots such that all conversation was precluded. The alternative was to stand beside the lake and shout in despair for the helpless victims of the unleashed trauma. That made no difference of course, but encouraged the rescuers to wade into the lake, determined to brave the shooters with their brutality and threats of abuse, shooting, kidnap and rape. The rescue of crippled wildlife that had failed to fly from their roost early enough or had returned later in the day in time for the afternoon massacre, continued all day and into the night.

A small contingent of rescuers arrived at the lake the previous evening to find the camping area littered with hostile shooters. Our appearance incited a not unexpected reaction of abuse, threats and beer can missiles. Eventually we sourced an area equidistant from shooters enclaves and set up a camp in the manner of the wild west covered wagons. That proved to be a fortuitous decision as the ensuing evening provided the shooters with ready entertainment such as further abuse, beer can and other missile launching, motorcycle circling and bright spot lighting of rescuers. After such a harrowing nocturnal experience, the appearance of a convoy of friendly car headlights in the early morning darkness was cause for celebration. The battalion of rescuers that had camped away from the lake arrived and immediately set to work preparing for the difficult day ahead.

The shooting that began in the dark continued during the morning until the heat of the day intervened and the shooting became sporadic for a few hours. The rescues continued with new injured wildlife presenting regularly to the veterinary facility. The birds were generally quiet and dazed but distressed. Some were severely injured with body parts such as wings, legs and parts of their heads and body missing. Some could not be saved and were humanely euthanized. Others required emergency resuscitation and pain management. After their suffering was relieved they joined their colleagues in the recovery area that was quiet, warm and undisturbed.

The contact between shooters and rescuers was expectedly strained. Rescuers were trained to not respond to threats and abuse but to observe from a safe distance and to rescue shot, but still living, birds. They were trained to handle the birds in such a manner as to calm them and reduce stress and pain. Injured birds were then transported to the veterinary hospital facility as soon as possible. The barrage of insults and abuse discharged from the shooters at the rescuers was distressing but did not deter the main focus of waterbird rescue. Female rescuers were the main targets for threats of various types. Shooters sometimes demonstrated overt cruelty to the birds presumably to upset the watching rescuers. The child of one shooter was encouraged to perform such public cruelty and then taunt the rescuers. The heat of the day prompted a temporary reprieve for the wildlife as many shooters returned to the sanctity of their camps.

Meanwhile the triple conjoint of authorities and shooters embarked on a noisy lunch that combined eating, drinking and tormenting whenever possible. We were so busy with the injured birds that the heckling and abuse was irrelevant.

Later in the day the killing and trauma resumed, as shooters, large guns, boats and decoys headed for areas on the lake that were thought to be hidden from unwanted attention by rescuers. As the waterbirds returned to the 'sanctuary', in the afternoon, the shooting began again in earnest.

This carnage was repeated the next day, Sunday, after which many of the shooters packed and left. Presumably they had to return to their jobs during the week. The impact of such cruelty and suffering

continued

was profound. Some of the rescuers were significantly traumatized. For those who had not attended the massacre previously, many could not understand how and why such blatant cruelty could be condoned in a so-called civilized society. Others were emotionally and physically exhausted from the constant activity and abuse.

As a result of the shooting there were many rescued birds that then required veterinary attention including resuscitation, wound and fracture repair, treatment of stress and myopathy and rehabilitation. Later complications for not only the rescued birds but also for those remaining at the 'sanctuary', were myopathy, lead poisoning, starvation, botulism and amyloidosis, non-fatal injury allowing predation, drowning, septicaemia and other causes of eventual miserable death. Many bags of dead and dismembered bodies, of so called protected species, such as freckled ducks, were retrieved from beneath, and tied to, reed beds. They were secreted away by shooters to avoid detection and perhaps to be collected at a later time when convenient.

Survivors of the carnage were transported to a veterinary facility for further assessment, reparative and definitive surgery and rehabilitation. The commonest treatable injuries were compound fractures of wings and/or legs. Most of these required internal fixation with bone pins, under general anaesthesia, and supportive splinting, anti-infective therapy and pain management. After recovery they were released into a safer area and their progress monitored.

Attendance at the massacre leaves a lasting impression of outrage and sadness for the victims, disgust for the fact that such an event can even occur and contempt for the trio of protagonists that strutted around with large guns or protected and encouraged each other. It is notable that rescuers were targeted to be subject to infringement notices purporting to be breaches (spurious or otherwise) of the law, while dangerous and threatening behaviour including gunshot wounds, throwing of potentially injurious missiles, drinking associated with shooting, verbal abuse and intentional animal cruelty, by shooters and their colleagues, were generally ignored or tolerated by 'authorities'.

Rescuers who experienced the horror and barbarity shall not forget. Some find difficulty in facing such terrible carnage again. Others become determined to try to stop the slaughter and as a general position to try to prevent similar assaults on other species. We all are traumatized to some degree but shall never accept that such horror and cruelty is acceptable. Never!

References

Arluke, A. (1994) Managing emotions in an animal shelter. In: Manning, A. and Serpell, J. (eds) *Animals and Human Society.* Routledge, New York, pp. 145–165.

Arluke, A. (2004) *Brute Force.* Purdue University Press, West Lafayette, Indiana.

Ashfield, J. (2010) *Taking Care of Yourself and Your Family – a resource book for good mental health.* Peacock Publications, Norwood, South Australia.

Bancroft, L. (2002) *Why Does He Do That? Inside the minds of angry and controlling men.* Berkley Books, New York.

Bartram, D.J. and Baldwin, D.S. (2010) Veterinarians and suicide: a structured review of possible influences on increased risk. *Veterinary Record* 166, 388–397.

Durrance, D. (2007) Recognize symptoms of compassion fatigue: are you a wounded caregiver? *DVM* 38, 1. Available at: http://veterinarynews.dvm360.com/dvm/article/articleDetail.jsp?id=398288 (accessed 4 June 2012).

Family Violence Professional Education Taskforce (1994) *Family Violence: Everybody's business somebody's life.* Federation Press, Annandale, New South Wales, Australia.

Figley, C.R. (ed.)(2002) *Treating Compassion Fatigue.* Routledge, New York.

Figley, C.R. and Roop, R.G. (2006) *Compassion Fatigue in the Animal-Care Community.* Humane Society Press, Washington, DC.

Fritschi, L., Morrison, D., Shirangi, A. and Day, L. (2009) Psychological well-being of Australian veterinarians. *Australian Veterinary Journal* 87(3), 76–81.

Green, P.C. and Gullone, E. (2005) Knowledge and attitudes of Australian veterinarians to animal abuse and human interpersonal violence. *Australian Veterinary Journal* 83(10), 619–625.

Harms, L. (2007) *Working with People: communication skills for reflective practice.* Oxford University Press, Melbourne, Australia.

Hawthorne, M. (2008) *Striking at the Roots – a practical guide to animal activism.* O-Books, Ropley, UK.
Hudnall Stamm, B. (2009) The ProQOL (Professional quality of life scale: Compassion satisfaction and compassion fatigue). Pocatello, Idaho. Available at: http://www.proqol.org (accessed 6 May 2011).
Loo, R. (1986) Post-shooting stress reactions among police officers. *Journal of Human Stress* 12, 27–31.
MacNair, R.M. (2002) *Perpetration-induced Traumatic Stress.* Praeger Publishers, London.
Maslach, C. (2003) *Burnout: the cost of caring.* Malor Books, Cambridge, Massachusetts.
Melville, G.W., Chang, D., Colagiuri, B., Marshall, P.W. and Cheema, B.S. (2012) Fifteen minutes of chair-based yoga postures or guided meditation performed in the office can elicit a relaxation response. *Evidence-Based Complementary and Alternative Medicine* 2012, 1–9.
Overfield, R. (2010) Compassion fatigue part two: survey results of stress, fatigue and wellness in veterinary nurses and animal care workers. *The Australian Veterinary Nurses' Journal* 16, 6.
Raphael, B. (1987) *The Anatomy of Bereavement: a handbook for the caring professions.* Hutchinson Education, London.
Rogelberg, S.G., DiGiacomo, N., Reeve, C.L., Spitzmüller, C., Clark, O.L., Teeter, L., Walker, A.G., Carter, N.T. and Starling, P.G. (2007) What shelters can do about euthanasia-related stress: an examination of recommendations from those on the front line. *Journal of Applied Animal Welfare Science* 20(4), 331–347.
Rohlf, V. and Bennett, P. (2005) Perpetration-induced traumatic stress in persons who euthanize nonhuman animals in surgeries, animal shelters, and laboratories. *Society and Animals* 13(3), 201–219.
Rollin, B.E. (2006) *An Introduction to Veterinary Medical Ethics: theory and cases.* Blackwell Publishing, Oxford, UK.
Smith, P. and Fakkema, D. (2009) Four phases of career evolution. In: *To Weep for a Stranger: Compassion Fatigue in Caregiving.* Createspace, Mt View, California, pp. 106–111.
Walsh, D.B. (1998) *Introduction to Working With Domestic Violence Training.* Deborah Walsh Domestic Violence Training Services, Melbourne, Australia.
White, D. (1998) It's a dog's life – animal shelter workers share the psychological impact of having to euthanize animals as part of their daily routine. *Psychology Today*, November–December, 10.

Part IV

Animal Abuse: the Animal Side – Helping the Animals Involved

Behavioural issues in animals from abusive pasts are often encountered by veterinarians and shelter workers.

Knowledge of how and why these behavioural changes manifest will best enable us to consider ways we can assist those animals during their rehabilitation. This part of the book describes the behavioural consequences of animal abuse and its remedies, outlining the ways animals may behave when they have had an abusive past. This section also covers the reporting of suspected animal abuse cases, outlining the information required by animal cruelty investigators. Veterinarians who report animal abuse may be required to attend a court trial as an expert witness, yet typically, little attention is paid to legal matters during veterinary training. The role of the veterinary and legal team in prosecuting animal cruelty and neglect is described here.

Practical advice for treating animal abuse and neglect cases are provided in this section, using case studies and photographs from around the world. Some abused animals, however, will not be candidates for treatment and rehabilitation. For these animals, humane methods of euthanasia are described, with the intention of minimizing stress for both animals and their carers.

15 Behavioural Consequences of Animal Abuse and its Remedies

Cam Day and Cassandra Day

Behavioural Consequences of Abuse in Dogs

Case studies

Tex, an 18-month-old Kelpie, was adopted into a family of three. He is very anxious around unknown people, and as a result is showing aggression with a fight/flight response. He came from a farm in North Queensland, where he missed out on vital socialization experiences in his critical period, and the previous owner was a scholar of the traditional, 'push–pull' and dominance methods of interacting with dogs.

Pixie and Caramelo, two 4-year old female Chihuahuas, were rescued by the RSPCA from a 'puppy mill'. They were eventually sent to a foster home for rehabilitation. They presented with high levels of fear of humans, aggression if they thought they were cornered, fear of loud noises and a malady of health problems.

Belle and Lizzie are two adult dogs, a Cocker Spaniel and a Beagle respectively, who were rescued from a 'puppy mill' by the RSPCA. Belle has been blind since birth and there is inter-dog aggression between the two dogs. Belle especially is anxious when discovering new things and new people.

The behavioural consequences of abuse in dogs are many and varied, with both owners and animal professionals unaware of the correct methods of handling these dogs. Improper handling can cause more damage than intended for both human and dog, so due care must be taken when interacting with the animals. It is important to understand the behaviour of a formerly abused dog, so that the correct remedies and methods can be used.

Dogs who have been abused in the past may present as very fearful with higher rates of house-soiling and compulsions and generally have 'significantly lower rates of aggression, trainability, chasing small animals, excitability, and energy' (McMillan *et al.*, 2011). In this case, this is referring to adult dogs that were used as breeding stock in 'puppy mills'.

These observations in regard to abused dog behaviour are corroborated by animal foster parents from the RSPCA: 'Pixie and Caramelo would not relax in the same room as us; they would find another room together. It took about 10 months to get these dogs to relax around us enough so that they could be rehomed' (N. Graham, personal communication, 2012).

Indeed, this has been observed in the clinic, where Tex, a blonde Kelpie, aged 18 months, has shown immense fear and distrust of humans other than his current owner. Tex presented in the clinic with aggression towards strangers (people) and high levels of anxiety and fear. The aggression was a result of his anxiety in being in the presence of strangers and, despite the anxiety, was posing a serious risk to visitors and other unknown people. This risk was evident to the clinicians throughout the course of the therapies, and much care was needed to ensure everyone's safety.

Munro and Thrusfield (2001) have noted that, for dogs abused in the home, the behaviour of the owner is important to observe as well as that of the dog, and that the owner's behaviour may be a stronger indication of animal abuse rather than the dog's behaviour. These owner characteristics identified include 'phrases such as "implausible and aggressive", "obvious discomfort and embarrassment", "uneasy", "reluctant to give history", "lack of concern", "angry on questioning" and "not reacting as expected to news (of a stab wound)"' (Munro and Thrusfield, 2001, p. 224). The authors also used these phrases to describe the behaviour of the abused animal: '"fear of owner", "dull demeanour", "became very timid with humans", "depressed", [and] "psychological damage"' (Munro and Thrusfield, 2001, p. 224).

Anxieties and Other Mood Disorders of Pets

Cam Day

Do pets have moods?

You would only have to own a pet for 5 minutes to know the answer to that is 'yes', but to what extent do the moods of pets reflect the moods of people?

Do pets suffer from panic attacks? Do pets ever develop post-traumatic stress disorder and do pets experience generalized anxiety disorders or suffer from compulsions?

Let's take a trip through the mood disorders of humans and determine if there are pet correlates.

What is the difference between fear and anxiety?

Fear and anxiety are confusing terms and they are often used synonymously.

You have heard about the flight–fight response and know, for instance, that a gazelle noting a lion racing through the bush towards it will flee in a desperate attempt to save its life.

Is this gazelle anxious or fearful?

This is a fearful response. The gazelle's autonomic nervous system kicks in and the gazelle does 'what comes naturally' to escape from the lion. The gazelle does not have to learn this response – it is an innate, hard-wired, self-protective mechanism.

However, a gazelle that has survived the experience of a lion's charge will then be more vigilant.

When hearing the rustling of bushes nearby it will be on guard and start running, even though the rustling of bushes may have been caused by an innocuous animal such as a nesting bird.

So the gazelle is 'predicting the doom' of a lion's chase – the gazelle is anxious.

But the anxiety was born from a fear-induced response, which is an innate life-saving response common in most species – including us humans.

So, anxiety is most easily remembered as the 'prediction of a doom-full event, location, object or situation'.

For instance, you may be anxious when needing to enter your backyard shed when the last time you entered it, a huntsman spider scurried across the wall in front of you. You are predicting the doom of entering the shed and you are expecting to see the same spider when in reality it is very likely no spider will be present.

Your dog may be anxious when walking past a house on a street where previously an aggressive dog has lunged at him or her through the gate of that house, even though that dog may not be present every time the house is passed.

Your cat may be anxious when you approach him or her because in the past you have placed a flea control preparation on its neck even though you only apply a flea control preparation to your cat once per month.

While anxiety is a normal and useful reaction to perceived dangers, an anxiety disorder is when the anxiety is abnormal or inappropriate.

You pet may have an anxiety disorder if its anxiety occurs in the absence of an appropriate stimulus or where the reaction is out of proportion to the stimulus it is experiencing. Metaphorically we talk about dogs barking when a butterfly sneezes in the distance – an abnormally high reaction to a normal, everyday stimulus.

Types of anxiety disorder

Acute stress disorder (acute anxiety disorder)

Acute stress disorder is a result of a person or animal experiencing a traumatic event that, in humans at least, involves threatened or actual serious injury or death (of another person).

If you have an acute anxiety disorder you may experience intense fear and helplessness at such times. Various symptoms occur in humans, including dissociative symptoms such as numbing, detachment, a reduction in awareness of the surroundings and derealization or depersonalization. Some people mentally re-experience the trauma and avoid stimuli that could be associated with it. Significant anxiety occurs, including irritability, poor concentration, difficulty sleeping, and restlessness.

Not many of these symptoms equate to the behaviours we see in pets, but some do.

In humans, the symptoms must be present for a *minimum of 2 days and a maximum of 4 weeks* of the traumatic event for a diagnosis to be made.

Do pets experience this in the same way?

I think they do.

Pets often experience threatened or actual serious injury. The commonest we see is *inter-dog aggression* and *inter-cat aggression.*

If your dog was attacked by another in a dog park your dog could perceive that as a serious, life-threatening event – and yes, it could cause death.

As a consequence, if your dog showed reluctance to enter that dog park on your next visit, it is 'avoiding that stimulus' and showing 'significant anxiety'.

If your cat was out one night in your garden and was attacked by the neighbourhood 'thug cat' with all the associated caterwauling and commotion then this is threatened or actual serious injury, although death when one cat attacks another is rarely an immediate consequence.

To fit the human model, for a pet to suffer an acute anxiety disorder the errant mood must be present after 2 days and up to 4 weeks.

Certainly this occurs with pets.

Pets can develop a 'doom-full prediction' of an event or location and get over it within a month, especially if the trauma is not repeated. In such cases the anxiety heals almost as if it evaporates but *pour some 'liquid of emotion' on to the pet by allowing it to re-experience the same trauma and the anxiety can be prolonged for a lot longer.*

One big difference between humans and pets is that, unlike humans, pets cannot easily control their own moods.

This means that when a pet gets an anxiety disorder, the anxiety often feeds off itself and through self-reinforcement worsens – often rapidly.

For this reason, pets with anxieties need rapid treatment or an acute anxiety disorder can develop into a generalized anxiety disorder or a post-traumatic stress disorder

One big difference with pets is that, when compared with humans, *pets have a lot more difficulty in 'self-healing' their emotions,* so to heal their own acute anxiety disorder is hard for them. So, your pet will recover much more quickly if you render it assistance.

With us humans, if an anxiety disorder extends beyond 1 month then it can develop into either a generalized anxiety disorder or a post-traumatic stress disorder. With pets, we do not formally know if the 1 month marker is relevant – but in my experiences, it seems to be. Our goal is always to create remedies as quickly as possible to stop the disorder growing into a more severe one, which could be much more difficult to eradicate.

Generalized anxiety disorder

In humans, generalized anxiety disorder (GAD) is characterized by excessive, exaggerated anxiety and worry about life's everyday normal events.

While it is normal for people to worry about life's general challenges, humans with GAD worry excessively with no obvious reasons for their worry.

People with symptoms of GAD tend to always expect disaster and are unable to stop worrying about common everyday events such as money matters, health, family issues, work or school.

Most of us would know someone that fits that description.

GAD develops over a period of time with humans and may not be noticed until it is significant enough to cause problems with functioning. Unlike acute anxiety disorder, it is usually not associated with a clearly defined traumatic event.

In humans, GAD is evidenced by general feelings of anxiety such as mild heart palpitations, dizziness and excessive worry. Mostly the anxiety needs to be present for more than 6 months for this condition to be diagnosed.

So does this occur with pets?

It is easy to argue that *wild animals are genetically programmed to have a GAD*. Prey animals such as sheep, cattle and our gazelle mentioned earlier are always 'on guard', worrying in their own way about being attacked by a predator.

But our most common pets, cats and dogs, are predators, not prey animals.

In our clinics we see behaviours that if they are not GAD, they are very close.

So, we see *pets that are over-reactive to the normal challenges of everyday life*. We see dogs that bark excessively when a 'butterfly sneezes in the distance'.

We see cats that are always on guard, running and hiding at the slightest stimulus. These pets certainly have an anxiety to everyday life events, which is characterized by excessive reactions.

With pets, we can often see an initiating cause of their GAD.

Dogs with noise fears would be the commonest example. While we see the dog develops an anxiety when he or she can detect an approaching storm, we also see the anxiety becomes generalized to life's normal events.

Dogs with a fear of storms react to approaching darkness of dusk because it looks like the darkness of a storm. They react to the flicking of a fluorescent light because it looks like and sounds like a lightning flash and they react to trees swaying in a stiff breeze because the trees do the same thing in a storm.

Simple phobias

A phobia is an *extreme anxiety or fear of a specific object or situation* that is often disruptive to everyday functioning. Common phobias in people include fear of heights, the dark, water, enclosed spaces and animals (such as dogs) or bugs such as spiders.

People with a phobia often avoid the situation that creates their phobia. For example, a person may resign from a job because they need to work in a high-rise building or to use an elevator to access their office.

Pets certainly show phobias.

For example, with dogs an anxiety of a 'specific object' that is 'disruptive to everyday functioning' would certainly include the common problem that many owners experience when trying to get their dog go into the garden if their dog was *fearful of the garden*.

Why would a dog be fearful of the garden? Wet grass is the commonest scenario for small dogs and can certainly disrupt everyday functioning for dogs and their owners, even to the stage of causing house-soiling.

My own dog has a fear of the garden because she was *attacked by a carpet python* on her first night outside when she was 4 months old.

With dogs we talk commonly about separation anxiety. *This malady could more correctly be called a separation phobia* because it is an anxiety that severely disrupts everyday life and is associated with the specific situation where the dogs' owners leave each morning and are then absent for several hours.

Panic disorder

In humans, a panic disorder is characterized by *sudden attacks of intense fear or anxiety, usually associated with numerous physical symptoms* such as heart palpitations, rapid breathing or shortness of breath, blurred vision, dizziness and racing thoughts.

Often these symptoms are thought to be a heart attack by the individual, and many cases are diagnosed in hospital emergency rooms.

In humans the causes can be quite subtle, but in some cases are caused by a previous adverse event.

We definitely see panic disorders in pets. *A common condition is noise anxieties*. While a pet can show a GAD to, for instance, thunder and may be anxious as a storm approaches, the *pet proceeds to a panic disorder* when the thunderstorm arrives.

At this time an affected dog does show the human signs of '*intense fear or anxiety*', and that occurs along with the physical symptoms of hyperventilation, hyperactivity, a need to escape from the stimulus and sometimes the need to hide from the stimulus. Dogs that are affected cause significant damage to themselves and their owner's property when consumed by their panic disorder. Dogs with panic disorders created by noise phobias often rip their claws from their feet in scraping at fences to escape or the back door to 'inscape'. They regularly break their teeth (and sometimes their jaws) and cause themselves other harm.

Many owners consider their dog might 'have a heart attack' at the height of its panic disorder, albeit this does not occur with pets.

Panic disorders also occur with cats. The most common cause would be a house-confined cat's reaction to another cat wandering through its visually owned territory when the house-cat looks out of a window and sees the trespasser outside.

At such times cats show intense fear and anxiety, with hissing, spitting and yowling and they will often transfer their aggression to an in-contact cat or to their owner.

Post-traumatic stress disorder

Post-traumatic stress disorder (PTSD) is the ugly relative of an acute stress disorder.

Whereas an acute stress disorder is short term (less than 1 month), *PTSD is long term – in humans longer than 1 month.*

It follows a traumatic event where that event causes *intense fear and/or helplessness.*

Typically the symptoms develop shortly after the event, but may take years. Symptoms need to exist for at least 1 month to confirm a diagnosis (Cantor, 2009).

In humans symptoms include re-experiencing the trauma through nightmares, obsessive thoughts and flashbacks (sufferers feel as if they are actually in the traumatic situation again).

Affected people show an avoidance component where situations, people or objects that remind him or her about the traumatic event are avoided. For instance, a person suffering PTSD after a serious car accident might avoid driving or being a passenger in a car.

Finally, there is increased anxiety in general, possibly with a heightened startle response where the person may be very jumpy and may be easily startled by noises.

Yes, traumatic events causing fear or helplessness are very commonly experienced by pets.

Animal abuse (human to animal) would be a typical cause. Aggressive attacks by another animal of the same species (dog to dog or cat to cat aggression) or by a different species (dog to cat, cat to dog, livestock to dog, snake to cat, snake to dog aggression and so forth) are also very common causes.

Following such harmful experiences, many pets then show behavioural change, which certainly lasts longer than a month and can be lifelong.

Pets experiencing traumas that cause long-term behaviour change often show avoidance of the situation, object, person or animal, as do humans.

For instance, a cat that is abused by a person may distrust all people and hide when people are near. A dog when attacked by another in a dog park may be reluctant to enter the dog park.

Just like humans, we also see pets that are very reactive to noises in their environment and show a startle response. Dogs experiencing thunder is a common example, but some dogs show reactive barking when hearing other dogs near their territory (i.e. their house and garden) because they are anxious that the barking dog means they may be attacked again. So these pets are exhibiting all the signs of PTSD.

What we do not know is whether pets re-experience the trauma through nightmares, flashbacks or obsessive thoughts. Certainly pets dream, and perhaps some are re-experiencing a trauma.

Obsessions and compulsions

Obsessions in humans are described as persistent ideas, thoughts, images or impulses that are experienced by the sufferer as anxiety provoking or distressing. The sufferer has difficulty switching his or her train of thought on to another topic (Anxiety Treatment Australia, n.d.).

We do not know if pets have persistent ideas or thoughts that are akin to this because they are unable to tell us.

But compulsions are the next step. Compulsions are observable, or covert, repetitive behaviours or mental acts that are performed to prevent or reduce the anxiety and distress of obsessions.

We certainly see repetitive behaviours with pets, which are senseless and purposeless and often self-damaging.

Typical examples with dogs include:

- pacing, circling, spinning and tail-chasing;
- fly snapping (of imaginary flies);
- some forms of barking;
- self-chewing and self-harm; and
- food-related compulsions and the licking or ingestion of non-food objects such as rocks, pebbles and the droppings of other animals.

Fixing mood disorders (deflation) and training for rehabilitation

Mood disorders such as PTSD and acute stress disorder may be eliminated in a number of ways. Some mood disorders can 'deflate' on their own, while others may need a helping hand – this all depends on the severity of the mood disorder and whether or not the disorder has been able to infiltrate the animal's well-being more than once.

Training, medications and pheromones

Synthetic pheromones (available as a spray, plug-in diffuser or impregnated collar) and/or medications may be advisable in some cases; however, consulting with a veterinary behavioural specialist and trainer is strongly recommended. Positive reinforcement-based training is a humane way of training and works to reward animals for desired behaviours rather than punishing unwanted behaviours. Groups such as the Delta Professional Dog Training Society provide training for those wishing to become accredited trainers or seek advice for animal behaviour issues.

References

Anxiety Treatment Australia (n.d.) Anxiety Treatment Australia. Available at: http://www.anxietyaustralia.com.au/index.shtml (accessed 13 July 2012).

Cantor, C. (2009) Post-traumatic stress disorder: evolutionary perspectives. *Australian and New Zealand Journal of Psychiatry* 43(11), 1038–1048.

McMillan, F.D., Duffy, D.L. and Serpell, J.A. (2011) Mental health of dogs formerly used as 'breeding stock' in commercial breeding establishments. *Applied Animal Behaviour Science* 135(1–2), 86–94.

Munro, H.M.C. and Thrusfield, M.V. (2001) 'Battered pets': features that raise suspicion of non-accidental injury. *Journal of Small Animal Practice* 42, 218–226.

16 Reporting Suspected Animal Abuse

Catherine Tiplady

Whether or not you live in a jurisdiction that mandates you to report suspected animal abuse, it is unacceptable to do nothing about animal suffering. In some cases, owners can be educated on how to provide the correct care for their animals but this may not always be feasible or desirable. If in doubt about what to do, contact your veterinary association for advice. This chapter discusses procedures involved with making a cruelty complaint and how this complaint may be investigated.

To Whom Do I Report My Concerns?

This varies depending on where you are practising as a vet and the type and number of animals involved. To find out the best place to lodge your concern about an animal's welfare contact your local veterinary association, humane society, government animal welfare department or society for the prevention of cruelty to animals. The police service may also be able to assist.

Can I Be Anonymous?

Although you can remain anonymous, it is strongly recommended that you provide your name and contact details. This will enable the investigator to contact you if they need additional details and can strengthen any case against the alleged perpetrator. Due to the large number of false complaints received it is very important inspectors can verify complaints – as this cannot happen in anonymous complaints the inspector may not act on these unless they believe there is a strong enough case to do so (A. Buchanan, personal communication, 28 March 2012).

What Happens Next?

Your concerns may be handed to a complaints coordinator who will assess the urgency of the issue and prioritize, or 'triage' according to whether it is a life-threatening matter, a major or minor incident. From there, an inspector will deal with cases.

What Do Animal Cruelty Inspectors Do?

The inspectors' primary role is (RSPCA Qld, n.d.):

- To investigate complaints of animal cruelty and neglect.
- To provide guidance and education to animal owners.
- To initiate prosecutions for offences.

- To attend to sick and injured stray animals or those that have been abandoned.
- To carry out regular inspections of places where animals are kept for sale, breeding, boarding, transportation, slaughter, farming and entertainment.

What If I Suspect a Human Is Being Harmed as Well?

This issue is covered further in Chapter 11.

Reporting Animal Cruelty

Reporting suspected animal abuse may be done:

- in person, at a Humane Society, RSPCA, SPCA or similar;
- via the telephone to a cruelty complaints number run by the above organizations;
- in writing and sent in the post or via fax or e-mail; or
- using an online cruelty complaint form.

Whichever way you report animal abuse it is essential to provide as many details about the case as possible. When you suspect co-occurrence of abuse of humans, such as elder abuse, child abuse or domestic violence, it is advisable to make this known in your complaint so that the relevant team can be ready. People working with animal abuse need to protect their own safety, so if the alleged offender is known or suspected to be violent, verbally abusive or has weapons it is vital they are informed. This should be requested as standard questions whenever a complaint is registered.

What Do I Have To Tell Them?

An online cruelty form will typically request the following information, some of which is required for the complaint to be processed. An example form from the RSPCA South Australia website (2011) provides a good basis for the information required and includes the following.

Details of animal cruelty (= required information)*

- Description of the alleged cruelty.*
- Number of animals involved.
- Type, size and colour of the animal/s.
- Estimated body condition of the animal/s (an explanation of the body condition score made available).
- When the complainant last saw the animal/s.*
- Whether the complainant personally witnessed the alleged cruelty* or, if not, how they became aware of the alleged cruelty.

Location

- Address.
- Whether the incident occurred in a car, at a commercial property, at a residential property or other location.*
- Closest cross-roads or landmarks.

Animal Owner/Offender Details

- Name of owner/alleged offender.
- Address of owner/alleged offender.*
- Telephone numbers of owner/alleged offender.

Details of complainant

- Name.*
- Address.*
- Telephone number.*
- E-mail address.

Body Condition Scoring

Body condition scoring scales involve assessing the animal visually and by palpating areas of the body, such as the ribs and lumbar processes. The scoring systems vary between countries and depending on the species of animal. In the USA, the ASPCA use a five-point scale to cover underweight animals from 1 (ideal) to 5 (emaciated) (ASPCA, 2001). In the UK, the PDSA use a five-point scale ranging from 1 (very thin), to 3 (ideal) and 5 (obese) (PDSA, 2008). In Australia, a nine-point condition scale is commonly used to cover condition from 1 (emaciated) to 4–5 (ideal) and 9 (grossly obese) (Nestlé Purina, n.d.). Body condition scoring results may vary, depending on who is examining the animal, so if in doubt ask an experienced colleague to check your results. Whichever method you use, be consistent and record what the score is out of. Recording '5' alone is insufficient, writing 'bcs 5/9, ideal' is better.

In hoarding cases, the HOMES Scale (Health, Obstacles, Mental Health, Endangerment, Structure and Safety) allows rapid assessment of the different issues associated with hoarding (Bratiotis, 2009). The Tufts Animal Care and Condition Scales (TACC, 1997) were specifically developed for assessing dog welfare, body condition and physical health as well as environmental conditions, sanitation and physical care such as grooming and nails.

Note: Abused animals may exhibit any body condition from emaciated to grossly obese.

Questions to Ask when Clients Report Suspected Animal Abuse

People reporting animal abuse may be emotionally distressed; however, for the sake of the animals it is essential that they provide as much relevant information as possible. The following points serve as a guide. Other services, such as the police, may need to be informed in some instances, for example to gain access to a property or vehicle. If possible, take the complainant's contact details and name early in the complaint in case the phone call is cut off and in case inspectors need to contact them later should further information be required. It is essential to record details of where and how the animal is kept and any details of the owner of the animal, such as name, car numberplate, telephone number and description of the suspected offender. At this stage any suspected offender should be referred to as a 'Person of Interest'.

Abandonment

- Have the owners moved away or are they on holiday?
- When was the owner or a carer last seen with the animals?
- Do you have contact details for the owner/carer?
- What is the address of where the animal is?
- If abandoned at a house or business, do you have details of the landlord, owner or rental agency?
- Is the animal abandoned in a garden? At a business premises? In a house? In a vehicle? (If in a vehicle – is it in the sun? How long has the animal been there? Does it have water? Are the windows down or is the air conditioning on?)
- What condition is the animal in?
- Does the animal appear distressed or injured?
- Have the animals been left with water and/or food?
- Is the animal a guard dog or a possibly dangerous animal?
- Is the animal caged, tethered or chained?
- Is the animal a juvenile, adult or elderly?
- Does the animal have any shelter available?

Animal's environment

Assessing an animal's environment is important in animal abuse cases and this should be photographed as evidence. The dog in Figure 16.1 appears thin with visibly protruding dorsal vertebral processes. There appears to be no shelter and no access to food or water. Examining the amount and condition of faeces around this

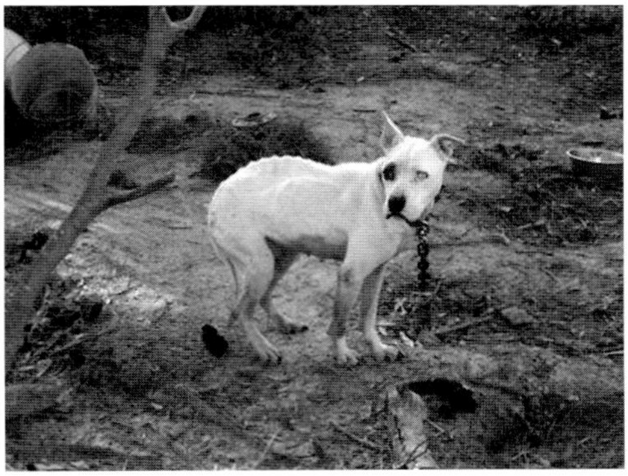

Fig. 16.1. Providing photographic evidence of an animal's environment is important in animal abuse cases. This dog is in poor condition and is chained without shelter. (Photograph courtesy of ASPCA.)

animal will help indicate how long it was tethered. Chained or tethered dogs have an inability to flee from adverse stimuli and may become highly territorial and anxious when someone invades their limited space (Carlisle-Frank and Flanagan, 2006). A tethered dog is more likely to bite (Gershman *et al.*, 1994), so exercise caution when approaching.

Baiting/Poisoning

- Describe the incident.
- What type of animal was involved?
- If a domestic animal, who is the owner?
- If a wild/pest animal, was a licensed pest exterminator used?
- Type of poison used (if known).
- Is a sample of the poison available?
- Has a veterinarian examined the animal and tested for poisoning?
- Were any threats made toward you or the animal prior to the suspected poisoning?

Cruelty

- What is the nature of the suspected cruelty?
- What type of animal was involved?
- How many animals were involved?
- Who is the owner of the animal?
- Is the animal injured?
- What are the animal's injuries?
- Has the animal been treated by a veterinarian?
- If a domestic animal, is the owner aware of the suspected cruelty?
- Where is the animal kept?

Fighting (e.g. dog fighting, cock fighting)

- Describe the incident.
- How many animals were involved?
- What types of animals were involved?
- Where did the fight take place?
- Were the events organized?
- How often are the fights held?
- Who are the organizers?

Neglect/failure to treat illness or injuries

- Describe the neglect (note that some cases of suspected 'neglect' may not qualify as such under law).
- What condition is the animal in?
- What is the nature of any illness or injuries?
- Who is the owner and what are their details?

What Happens Once a Complaint is Received

Once details of the alleged animal abuse have been received, complaints are 'triaged' or prioritized into the order of urgency and passed on to the animal cruelty inspectors or similar staff. A life-threatening emergency (e.g. a horse that was shot and lying injured and bleeding on a road) will probably receive priority over a thin but constantly tethered dog that has access to shelter and water. Depending on the organization, certain types of owned/domestic animals may receive priority over a wild animal.

Once the inspector has been informed of the complaint the following procedures may happen, as outlined by Annabel Buchanan, Chief Inspector (Prosecutions) at RSPCA Queensland (A. Buchanan, personal communication, 28 March 2012):

Assess the animal welfare incident

- What are the broad concerns or issues for the animal's welfare?
- Does the situation require a response under the relevant legislation, and if so, how urgent is the situation?

Find a fit for the incident under the relevant legislation

- What offences could arise under the relevant legislation?
- Examination of key terms under the legislation.

Preparing the response

- What other information might be useful?
- What must I do before exercising any power under the relevant legislation?
- What are my possible powers of entry going to be?
- What other powers might I need to exercise under the relevant legislation?
- Contact complainant for verification and further information.
- Contact other relevant witnesses if applicable.
- Contact the owner of the animals if applicable.
- Assemble equipment needed and assess the need for an expert witness.
- Workplace Health and Safety issues – risk analysis in regard to potential aggression.

Responding to the incident

- Address the immediate welfare needs of the animal.
- Assess grounds for the exercise of further powers under the relevant legislation.
- In light of observations and information obtained on site, reassess the seriousness of the incident and the possible offences.
- To successfully resolve most incidents, the best process is by educating the person responsible for the care of the animal.
- In certain circumstances, the inspector will conduct further investigations including field interviews, photographs.

References

ASPCA (2001) Body condition assessment. In: Merck, M.D. (ed.) (2007) *Veterinary Forensics: Animal Cruelty Investigations.* Blackwell Publishing, Oxford, UK, Appendix 6, p. 273.

Bratiotis, C. (2009) HOMES multi-disciplinary hoarding risk assessment. Available at: http://vet.tufts.edu/hoarding/pubs/HOMES_SCALE.pdf (accessed 23 April 2012).

Carlisle-Frank, P. and Flanagan, T. (2006) *Silent Victims – recognizing and stopping abuse of the family pet.* University Press of America, Maryland.

Gershman, K., Sacks, J. and Wright, J. (1994) Which dogs bite: a case-control study of risk factors. *Pediatrics* 93(6), 913–917.

Nestlé Purina (n.d.) Body condition system. Available at: http://www.purinaveterinarydiets.com/resources/Files/dog_chart.pdf (accessed 1 March 2012).

PDSA (2008) People's Dispensary for Sick Animals: Healthy shape poster. Available at: http://www.pdsa.org.uk (accessed 1 March 2012).

RSPCA Qld (n.d.) Inspectorate. Available at: http://www.rspca.org.au/what-we-do/inspectorate.html (accessed 28 March 2012).

RSPCA South Australia (2011) Reporting cruelty form. Available at: http://www.rspcasa.asn.au/how-to-help/report-cruelty (accessed 28 May 2011).

TACC (1997) Tufts Animal Care and Condition Scale. In: Merck, M.D. (ed.) (2007) *Veterinary Forensics: Animal Cruelty Investigations.* Blackwell Publishing Ltd, Oxford, UK, Appendix 21, pp. 291–292.

17 Prosecuting Animal Cruelty and Neglect Matters

Michael Byrne and Tracy-Lynne Geysen

This chapter is partly adapted from papers presented by Michael Byrne QC at the Queensland Law Society and Law Council of Australia Occupational and Health Seminar on 29 November 2007 (Brisbane) and the Central Queensland Law Association Conference 2008 (Rockhampton).

This paper will traverse five areas in which the particular duties of prosecutors of animal cruelty and neglect matters will be examined.

These are:

1. Prosecuting generally.
2. Presenting the prosecution case.
3. Cross-examination.
4. Sentencing process.
5. Prosecuting animal cruelty and neglect matters.

Prosecuting Generally

Some time ago the High Court of Australia had the opportunity to examine the role of the prosecutor (Libke v The Queen, 2007).

In the course of the judgement, his Honour Hayne J adopted the formulation:

> (The role of a prosecutor is) not to obtain a conviction, it is to lay before a jury what the Crown considers to be credible evidence relevant to what is alleged to be a crime. Counsel have a duty to see that all available legal proof of the facts is presented: it should be done firmly and pressed to its legitimate strength but it must also be done fairly. The role of prosecutor excludes any notion of winning or losing; his function is a matter of public duty than which in civil life there can be none charged with greater personal responsibility. It is to be efficiently performed *with an ingrained sense of the dignity, the seriousness and the justness of judicial proceedings* [italics added].
>
> (Libke v The Queen, 2007, point 71).

Justice Hayne then summarized that role in this sentence:

> A central, even the central, element in that role is ensuring that the (prosecution) case is presented with fairness to the (defendant).

While this statement may be at odds with other commentators both curially and extracurially, for example: (i) 'prosecuting counsel represents the State' (Deane, 1983); or (ii) 'the role of the prosecutor is described as representing the public interest' (Willis, 1996), it has to be said however that both the State and the 'public interest'[1] are major stakeholders in the justice system. And any justice system that does not give paramount importance to the protection of persons (real or corporate or animals) accused of breaching the law is not a justice system.

Briefly, it is necessary to discuss the distinction between 'public interest' and 'public opinion'.

[1] Care should be taken to properly distinguish between 'public interest' and 'public opinion'.

The media refer to the 'shock/horror' of actually releasing prisoners who have served the full prison sentence imposed by courts. It may well be a correct perception of public opinion that the comfort of the majority is more important than the liberty of an individual. Public interest, however, is better served by adherence to the rule of law.

Back then, to the general duty of a prosecutor. And to expand upon what has been described as the 'central' element of fairness, this does not, in any sense, mean that a prosecutor is to be simply passive. He or she may be robust and be expected and required to conduct the prosecution conscientiously and firmly (Libke v The Queen, 2007, point 35).

In so acting, the prosecutor is expected by courts and the community to endeavour to establish the whole truth in accordance with the procedures and rules of evidence applicable to the contest (Whitehorn v The Queen, 1983).

Presenting the Prosecution Case

The touchstone in this area is that a prosecutor must offer all evidence relevant to the prosecution case.

This should be done objectively in the sense that a prosecutor should not align himself or herself to the prosecution case. There should be no resort to prejudice or emotion.

To give an example, in most of the animal cruelty or neglect matters that come before the courts, an animal has suffered serious injury or neglect or has been killed.

Prosecutors in such cases should be careful not to create the impression (either to the animal's owner or generally) that they are acting for the animal or in any way presenting a case on the animal's behalf. Prosecutors are required to act objectively and not pursue a conviction. Rather, and as part of an advocate's duty to the court, a prosecutor is required to inform the court of authorities or statutory provisions relevant to the case, even when those matters are adverse to the prosecution case.

Cross-examination

It is necessary to emphasize that in conducting a cross-examination of a witness, a prosecutor does have duties and responsibilities.

A clear expression of those is contained in the following quotation:

> (A prosecutor must) conduct him/herself with restraint and with due regard to the rights and dignity of (defendants). A cross-examination must naturally be as full and effective as possible, but it is unbecoming in a legal representative – especially in a prosecutor – to subject a witness and particularly a (defendant) who is a witness, to a harassing and badgering cross-examination.
>
> (S v Booi, 1964).

In addition, so far as cross-examination is concerned, a prosecutor must put the relevant points forward to fully test the witness. It is neither attractive nor helpful to an advocate's case to descend into an argument with the witness nor to be seen by the tribunal of fact to be a bully.

Sentencing Process

As referred to above, a prosecutor need not be passive. An earlier view of the duty of a prosecutor in sentencing was expressed by a commentator, albeit some 60 years ago:

> In the matter of sentence (a prosecutor) will exercise no grain of pressure towards severity and will leave his opponent to say what he may in the matter of mitigation.
>
> (Humphries, 1955)

Today, in Queensland, courts expect the prosecutor to 'assist' them in a number of regards.

These include:

1. Clearly stating the maximum penalty and, if necessary, how one arrives at it.
2. Set out the factual basis of the offence in a structured way.
3. To acknowledge mitigating factors such as cooperation in an investigation and an early plea of guilty.
4. In an appropriate case to point to aggravating aspects that may bring into play sentencing principles such as deterrence and denunciation.
5. To assist the court in avoiding appellable error, usually by reference to comparable cases.
6. To bring to the attention of the sentencer not only previous convictions of a defendant, but to properly explain the facts and circumstances of

such previous convictions, as well as pointing out the, then, maximum penalty.

The above is a summary of the duties of prosecutors in different phases of a court hearing.

By way of overview, a Justice of the High Court once expressed the overall position as:

> (The) function (of the prosecutor) is ultimately to assist in the attainment of justice between the (prosecution) and the (defendant). In this respect the (prosecutor) may have added responsibilities in comparison with other counsel but it does not mean that his is a detached or disinterested role in the trial process
> (Whitehorn v The Queen, 1983, point 17)

Prosecuting Animal Matters

BLEATS

BLEATS (Brisbane Lawyers Educating and Advocating for Tougher Sentences) started in October 2007 and currently comprises a panel of more than 300 lawyers (about 150 barristers including three Queens Counsel, six Senior Counsel and about 150 solicitors) as well as 150 support staff (including psychologists, psychiatrists, administrative staff and university students).

BLEATS conducts legal work on a pro bono basis for the RSPCA and prosecutes animal cruelty and neglect matters by enforcing the maximum penalties and sentences under the current legislation, the Animal Care and Protection Act 2001 (Qld) ('the Act').

The role of the BLEATS prosecutor is to assist the magistrate or judge in handing down an appropriate sentence in accordance with the law, which reflects all the mitigating and aggravating factors of the case. It is the prosecutor's job to supply the court with the facts and circumstances of the case (for example, injuries suffered and veterinarian reports) and the offender's criminal history.

In most circumstances a prosecutor will provide the court with a schedule of other animal cruelty or neglect cases and the penalties that were handed down in those cases. If there is a precedent reflective of an appropriate sentence, then it is certainly appropriate to provide this as a reference to the court.

The Animal Care and Protection Act 2001 (Qld)

The RSPCA pursues defendants charged by the RSPCA under the relevant sections of the Animal Care and Protection Act 2001 (Qld).

Historically and currently, a gap exists between the maximum penalties found in the Act (2 years' imprisonment or $100,000 penalty), which reflects society's high moral regard for animals and the realities of enforcement.

Appropriate sentences

The maximum penalties in the Act are not necessarily reserved for the worst case possible, but are an indication of what parliament and the people consider is a reasonable penalty for cases that fall into the worst category of such offences (R v Tait and Bartley, 1979).

Some of the relevant aggravating factors may include:

- The defendant acted with intent or malice.
- Where there is a severe degree of harm, multiple animals suffered and/or the suffering was for a long duration.
- Failure to heed RSPCA warnings or advice.
- No mitigation of pain (especially where it was reasonable, or not impractical for the harm to be mitigated or avoided).
- The defendant acted with extreme violence, weapons, committed multiple or prolonged attacks and/or attacked the animal's head.

Some of the relevant mitigating factors may include:

- The defendant entered guilty plea early in proceedings.
- The defendant usually has good character (look at job, family, societal status, volunteer work, friends, usual behaviour is inconsistent with the conviction).
- Age of the offender.
- Mental capacity.
- The defendant was not directly involved in the offence and was not primarily responsible for the harm suffered.

It may be appropriate where there is a single offence with no intent, and little harm inflicted on the animal that the offender receive a penalty to deter them from committing the offence again.

If the offence was so serious that the animal or animals suffered significant harm and the defendant acted with intent and malice, the sentence should be one that: (i) deters the offender from acting in such a way again; (ii) protects the community from more harmful acts; and (iii) acts to deter other persons from committing such behaviour. In such circumstances an appropriate sentence would be a longer term of imprisonment.

A BLEATS prosecutor should consider the principles they are trying to invoke in advocating for certain sentences and may consider sentences that achieve, for example, protection, deterrence, retribution, denunciation, rehabilitation, reparation and/or restoration. Regard should also be had to consideration that animals are sentient beings and are vulnerable and dependant on owners/humans.

A fine or good behaviour bond is the least severe and most common sentence applied to offenders found guilty of animal cruelty or neglect offences.

Community service or work orders are more severe orders and not as common as fines.

Sentencing range in other jurisdictions

Finally, as a prosecutor, regard may be had to penalties and sentences in other jurisdictions.

For example, the UK is currently reviewing the animal cruelty system in place to prosecute offenders. The new system will enable the courts to have greater guidance in handing down sentences and it is expected this will give rise to higher precedents in sentencing for courts to use in later cases. The new system will implement a range into the legislation, giving appropriate minimum standard orders in each range. The least serious cases of cruelty (for example, an impulsive act, short-term neglect, where there is little or no injury to the animal) the sentence is a community service or substantial fine. Where the defendant has committed a more serious act of cruelty (for example, ill treatment or medium-term neglect) the order is to be a longer-term community service, fine, or small-term jail sentence. In the worst cases of animal cruelty (for example, where the defendant has killed, tortured or committed prolonged neglect, or where there were multiple animals affected, or multiple malicious attacks, causing significant pain and suffering) there is a minimum standard order of substantial term imprisonment.

Conclusion

The basic principles of prosecuting and advocacy apply in animal cruelty and neglect cases in much the same way that they do in cases where the victim is human.

The principal difference is that in animal cases the victim cannot communicate to the court what it has suffered and the circumstances of that abuse.

Hence the prosecution team's role is to be able to act as interpreter for the harmed creature through the use of aids such as expert veterinary opinion, photographs, analysis of infections and the exclusion of persons and causes other than the defendant(s) as the perpetrator(s).

Society and our own law makers are on an upward learning curve as to the seriousness and hence need for deterrence in relation to animal cruelty and neglect.

As lawyers, our task is to foster such learning and expose animal cruelty and neglect in the courts to the best of our abilities.

References

Deane (1983) cited in: Libke v The Queen (2007) High Court of Australia, case number 30, point 34. 20 June. Available at: http://www.austlii.edu.au/au/cases/cth/HCA/2007/30.html (accessed 20 June 2012).

Humphries, C. (1955) The duties and responsibilities of prosecuting counsel. *Criminal Law Review (UK)* 739, 747–748.

Libke v The Queen (2007) High Court of Australia, case number 30. 20 June. Available at: http://www.austlii.edu.au/au/cases/cth/HCA/2007/30.html (accessed 20 June 2012).

R v Tait and Bartley (1979) 24 *Australian Law Reports* 473, 484–485.

S v Booi (1964) cited in Libke v The Queen (2007) High Court of Australia, case number 30, point 122. 20 June. Available at: http://www.austlii.edu.au/au/cases/cth/HCA/2007/30.html (accessed 20 June 2012).

Whitehorn v The Queen (1983) Commonwealth Law Reports. Available at: http://www.austlii.edu.au/au/cases/cth/HCA/1983/42.html (accessed 20 June 2012).

Willis, J. (1996) Some aspects of the prosecutor's role at sentencing. *Journal of Judicial Administration* 6(1), 38–55.

18 Animal Abuse Case Studies and Treatment

Catherine Tiplady

This chapter will discuss how to recognize, treat and rehabilitate abused animals, with guidelines on maximizing their quality of life. Some injury types listed will include a brief first aid advice section while others will include case studies and/or rehabilitation guidelines.

According to Munro (1999), animal abuse should be considered when:

- the owner's account of the accident does not fit with the injury observed;
- the owner refuses to comment on how the injury occurred;
- the owner shows lack of concern for the animal's injuries;
- the owner delayed seeking veterinary treatment;
- behavioural signs in the animal may be noted – e.g. fear of the owner; and/or
- multiple injuries/fractures at various stages of healing that do not fit the history provided.

It is difficult to know if an animal has been abused or neglected just by looking at it.

All the photographs in Fig. 18.1 show dogs in very poor condition, yet without further investigation we are unable to assume which, if any, were victims of abuse/neglect.

Types of Abuse Seen By Veterinarians

Surveys of veterinarians in several countries (the UK, Republic of Ireland and Australia) have found that the following types of injuries are being seen by veterinarians in practice, raising suspicion of animal abuse (Table 18.1).

Other types of abuse/neglect that veterinarians may encounter include:

- failure to treat wounds/injuries/illnesses;
- animal fight wounds from organized fighting;
- harness wounds;
- ingrown collars;
- malnutrition and starvation; and
- matted hair/overgrown claws/horns/hooves.

This section will now cover treatment for animals presenting with some of the commonly seen physical injuries resulting from abuse or neglect.

The aim in trauma cases is to deal first with potentially life-threatening problems (e.g. control haemorrhage and shock), keep the patient as comfortable and stable as possible and avoid further complications such as contamination of wounds.

All animals must be evaluated for pain and given suitable analgesia if and when required. See Appendix for Glasgow Pain Scoring chart.

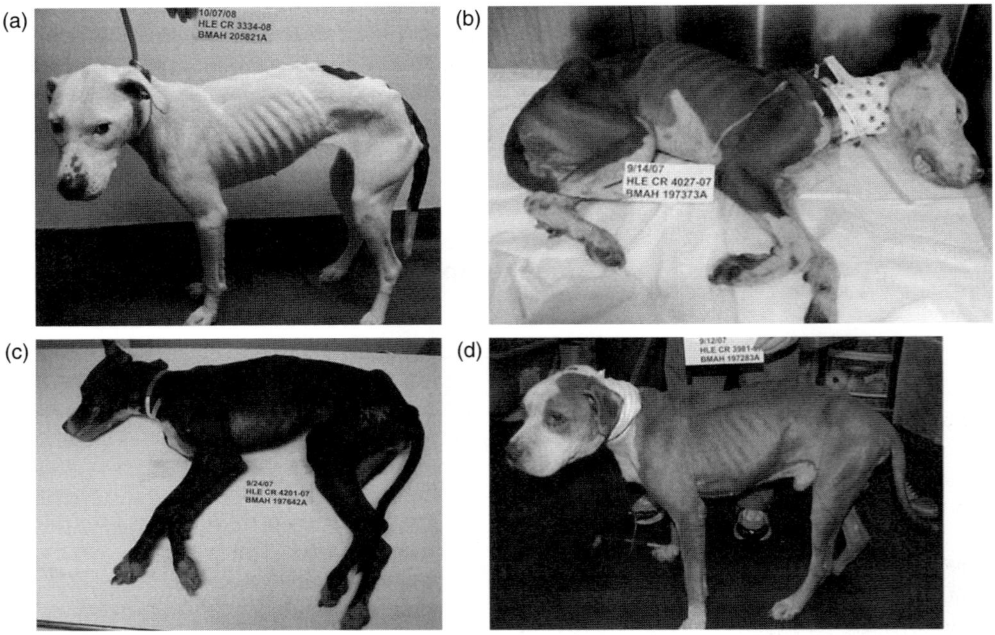

Fig. 18.1. (a) Dog with exocrine pancreatic insufficiency; (b) dog with intestinal lymphosarcoma; (c) 8-month-old puppy with parvovirus; and (d) a dog with chronic hookworm parasitism with secondary inflammatory bowel disease. Of the four dogs, the last was the only case that was prosecuted. (Photographs courtesy of ASPCA.)

Table 18.1. Clinical signs raising suspicion of animal abuse, as reported by veterinarians. Data from: Munro and Thrusfield (2001a–d); Green and Gullone (2005); McGuinness *et al.* (2005).

Bruising
Fractures
Repetitive injuries
Burns and scalds
Ocular injuries
Internal thoracic and abdominal injuries
Administration of drugs/poisons
Drowning
Asphyxiation
Sexual abuse
Munchausen syndrome by proxy
Gunshot/pellet wound
Laceration/stab wound
Broken/missing teeth
Concussion

In abuse cases, adequate records will assist investigation and prosecution but should not take up time that could be used saving the animal's life.

An initial physical examination in an emergency situation should focus on the major body systems (Jasani, 2011):

- cardiovascular – heart rate, sounds and rhythm; pulse quality and rate; mucous membrane colour and capillary refill time;
- respiratory – respiratory rate, respiratory effort and respiratory pattern and noise; and
- central nervous system – mentation, ability to stand and ambulate.

A more thorough physical examination can be performed once the animal's condition is stabilized.

In trauma cases, the initial investigative plan (following a complete physical examination) should include (Pead and Langley-Hobbs, 2007):

- conscious thoracic and abdominal radiographs;
- an electrocardiogram (ECG); and
- evaluation of blood packed cell volume (PCV) and total solids.

Broken bones

Broken bones include: skull or jaw fracture, spinal/tail injuries, fractures of limbs, pelvis and ribs or any combination of these. Fractures may be accidental or resulting from a range of abuse such as being kicked, struck, hit with an object, hit against a wall or thrown (Fig. 18.2). Presence of multiple fractures in various stages of healing suggests the possibility of repetitive abuse (Munro, 1999; Merck, 2007).

Examination of the animal

The animal may be in pain, be limping, vocalizing and have crepitus, swelling or distortion around the fracture site. Radiographs will confirm the presence of fracture/s and can be used as evidence in cruelty investigations (Fig. 18.3). Other problems that need to be checked for include neurological deficits, ruptured bladder, diaphragmatic hernia and pneumothorax.

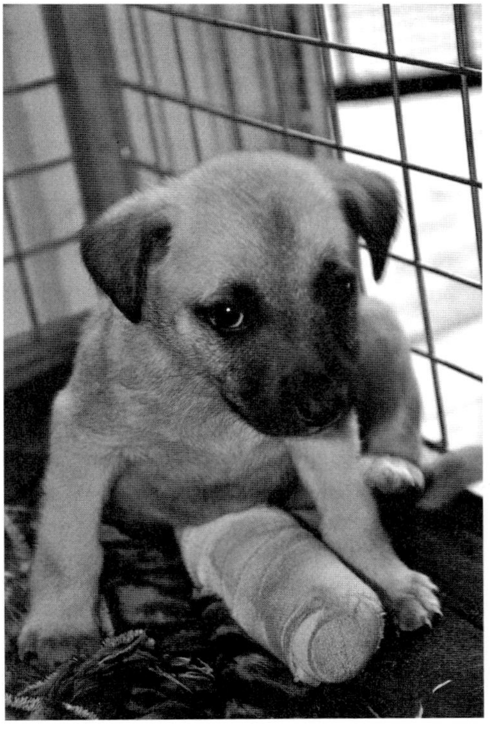

Fig. 18.2. This young male puppy was 'thrown around' by some children and his right hind leg was broken. He was admitted to Mdzananda Animal Clinic in South Africa. He is recovering well in hospital with a splint on his leg and cage rest. Young animals, which are otherwise healthy, often heal broken bones very well when given the correct care. (Photograph courtesy of IFAW.)

Treatment

Treatment of fractures depends largely on the severity and type of fracture, the bone/s involved and whether it is an open or closed fracture.

First aid

Principles of emergency treatment for fractures are (Pead and Langley-Hobbs, 2007):

- Limit swelling.
- Prevent further compromise of blood supply.
- Limit further soft tissue damage.
- Increase patient comfort and minimize patient movement.

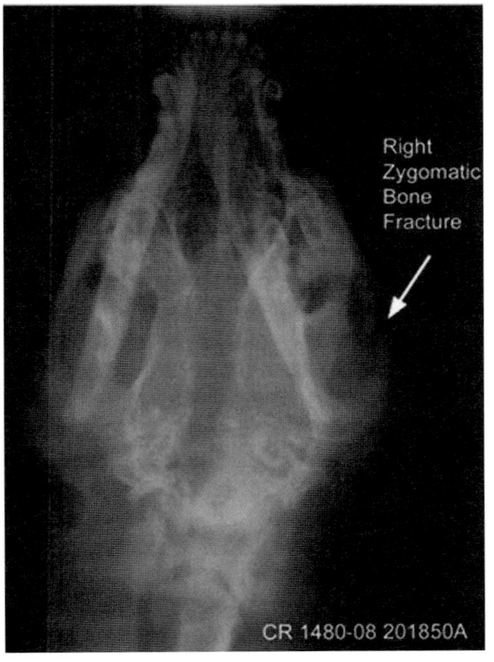

Fig. 18.3. Radiographs (X-rays) of the entire animal (if possible) are vital pieces of evidence in suspected animal cruelty cases, as well as being essential for diagnosis and treatment of fractures and other issues such as pneumothorax. This radiograph shows a fracture to the zygomatic arch in the skull of a dog. (Photograph courtesy of ASPCA.)

- Provide analgesia.
- Treat wounds over the fracture site.

The need to be vigilant in your examination is seen in the following example.

A dog that had experienced facial trauma and fracture of the zygomatic arch 7 days previously was found to have bradycardia with first-degree atrioventricular (AV) block and prolonged uncorrected QT interval when assessed with a 6-lead electrocardiogram (ECG) (Ghaffari *et al.*, 2009). These ECG signs were completely resolved after administration of atropine, supporting the authors' hypothesis that the ECG changes were related to stimulation of parasympathetic fibres in the periosteum of the damaged zygomatic bone (Ghaffari *et al.*, 2009).

Burns

Burns (Fig. 18.4) can occur from heat, sunburn, fire, boiling liquids, friction, chemicals, electricity and radiation.

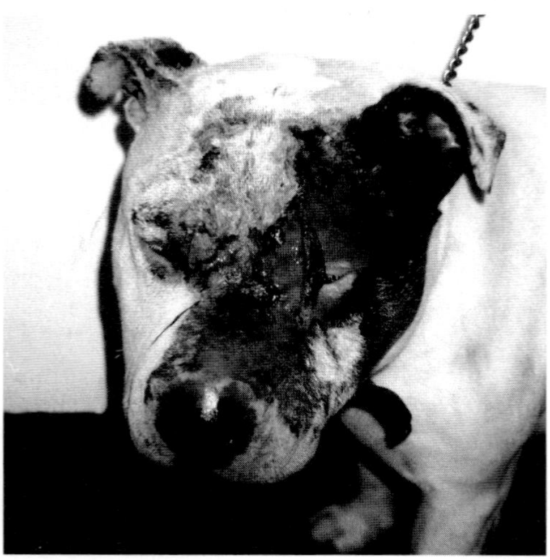

Fig. 18.4. Burns – neglect of injuries. The RSPCA were unable to prove that a Staffordshire bull terrier-type dog was deliberately set on fire. A young couple claimed the dog had climbed on to a kitchen work surface and knocked some lighter fluid on to a lit cigarette. A man and woman were charged with failing to get prompt veterinary treatment for the injury. They received a conditional discharge for 3 years, were disqualified from keeping all animals for 3 years and ordered to pay £150 costs. (Copyright RSPCA England and Wales.)

Clinical signs include the following and will depend on how recently the animal received the burns:

- singed hair;
- missing hair;
- scarring;
- redness;
- pain;
- areas of skin constriction;
- discharge;
- infection; and
- damage to other body systems, e.g. the respiratory tract.

First aid

For recent skin damage run cool tap water over the burned area (being careful not to over-cool the animal), do not touch the area with bare fingers and do not apply dressings. Broad-spectrum antibiotics, intravenous fluids and pain relief will be needed. Opioids are the drugs of choice for burns – use of corticosteroids and NSAIDs is controversial (Niles, 2009). Silver sulphadiazine cream has been used with success as a topical treatment in burns cases.

Pead and Langley-Hobbs (2007) recommend that wide margins of hair are clipped from around the burns and the animal assessed for evidence of dehydration, anaemia and hypoalbuminaemia, with cardiovascular, pulmonary and renal function evaluated and monitored for several days after the injury.

Older burns and scalds may cause significant constriction of the skin. Pope (2009) describes the creation of a caudal superficial epigastric axial pattern flap to relieve the contraction of the skin and deviation of the prepuce in the case of a Border collie that had been tied up with cable, doused with petrol and ignited.

If you suspect that caustic chemicals have caused the burn, be sure to wear suitable protective clothing (including eye protection and gloves) when you are handling the animal and rinsing the wound.

Collection of forensic evidence

Merck (2007, pp. 115–117) advises that it is imperative to take samples in all burn injuries, giving the following guidelines:

- The burn and adjacent tissue should be swabbed for accelerants or chemicals.
- Samples of the fur and skin should be taken for residue testing.
- The animal's bedding and a sample of the soil beneath the animal should be collected.
- Recommended containers are clean, uncoated paint tins.

Fighting dogs

A number of breeds have been bred and used for dog fighting, but the pit bull terrier is the most commonly involved dog (Merck, 2007).

Aggression toward other dogs, absence of aggression toward humans (to enable fighting dogs to be separated by people if necessary) and a willingness to continue to fight until death are desirable characteristics of fighting dogs (Dinnage *et al.*, 2004).

Signs that raise suspicion of dog fighting include (Sinclair *et al.*, 2006):

- bite wounds and scarring to the face (Fig. 18.5) and legs, particularly a 'ringing' or degloving injury that encircles the entire limb; and
- cropped ears and docked tail.

When dealing with suspected dog fighting, careful documentation of the dog's injuries will be reinforced by evidence of physiological stress from fighting – blood tests for dehydration, abnormal haematocrit and elevated creatinine phosphokinase levels and toxicology testing for drugs such as cocaine, amphetamines, steroids, diuretics and analgesics (Sinclair *et al.*, 2006).

Dogs used in fighting or animal baiting may present with old scars that have healed (possibly causing significant tissue constriction), torn skin and ears (if present), tooth damage and/or fresher wounds, which may be infected or infested with maggots. Bite wounds can also be accompanied by complications such as pneumothorax and subcutaneous emphysema (Barr, 2007). While some injuries will be evident on external physical examination, further diagnosis will require the use of imaging modalities such as radiography (e.g. to assess for fractures, pneumothorax and to determine the extent of subcutaneous emphysema). Magnetic resonance imaging (MRI) is also very helpful; however, MRI often requires referral to a specialist veterinary centre once the patient is stabilized (Barr, 2007).

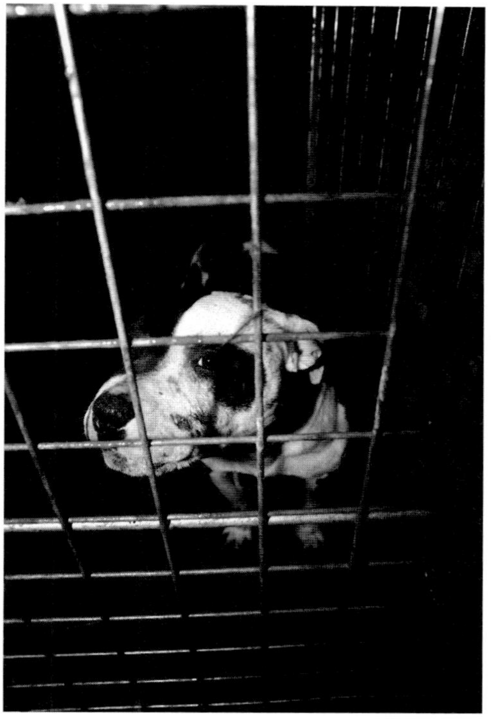

Fig. 18.5. This dog was seized by the RSPCA after a raid on a property that trained dogs to fight. Facial injuries are commonly seen in dogs used in organized fighting. (Photograph copyright RSPCA England and Wales.)

First aid

Ensure the safety of staff working with potentially aggressive animals by using suitable humane restraint such as sedation and muzzles.

First aid of fighting wounds involves stabilizing the patient, assessing for pain and providing necessary analgesia. Bite wounds should be assumed to be contaminated and will require thorough cleaning by copious (but not overly vigorous) irrigation and thorough examination to check for debris such as hair. Depending on the location and extent of the fight wounds, surgical treatment may involve placement of a drain.

Forensic techniques of investigating bite wounds are discussed in the forensic section of this book (Chapter 23).

Rehabilitation of fighting dogs

> Gentle approaches, incremental handling, and patience, patience, patience.
>
> (Somerville, 2008)

Rehabilitation of fighting dogs is possible, such as in the case of the Michael Vick-owned fighting dogs in the USA sent to Best Friends Animal Society.

These dogs received veterinary treatment and psychological rehabilitation from a committed team led by Dr Frank McMillan. Each dog received behavioural evaluation and an individualized rehabilitation protocol including patient socialization and gaining its trust, providing exercise, use of dog-appeasing pheromone (DAP), aromatherapy treatments and therapeutic massage (Somerville, 2008).

Case study: dogs seized from dog-fighting activity

RSPCA inspectors and West Midlands Police (in the UK) discovered two pit bull-type dogs and one Staffordshire bull terrier-type in a dawn raid. All of the dogs found were heavily scarred with injuries to their heads and legs. Officers discovered veterinary items used to treat injured dogs and a treadmill for training the dogs. A 29-year-old man from Birmingham was sentenced to 3 months in custody and banned from keeping animals for life. He admitted 11 charges including training dogs for fighting, causing the animals unnecessary suffering, failing to provide them with proper veterinary care and possession of items used to train dogs for fighting.

Gunshot wounds

Ballistic injuries vary depending on the calibre (diameter), mass, composition, shape and velocity of the bullets and cartridges used and the resulting degree of fragmentation within the wound (Pope, 2009). Injuries can be life threatening and, depending on the structures that have been affected and the length of time since the animal was shot, contamination and infection are risks (Pope, 2009). Initial first aid treatment in cases of gunshot involves opioid analgesia, fluid therapy and broad-spectrum antibiotics while preparing for definitive treatment.

The following case studies and photographs of gunshot wounds are provided by Dr Howard Ralph, a veterinarian who works in rescue, treatment and rehabilitation of waterbirds shot during the legal duck-shooting season.

Case study
Howard Ralph

NANKEEN NIGHT HERON, LAKE COWAL, NEW SOUTH WALES, AUSTRALIA. This bird had been shot through the wing and thereby suffered a fracture (Fig. 18.6). It was rescued from the water as it struggled to survive. After rescue, it was transported to the veterinary field hospital where antibiotics, parenteral (systemic, by injection) fluid therapy and pain relief were given. The wound was dressed and the wing strapped to

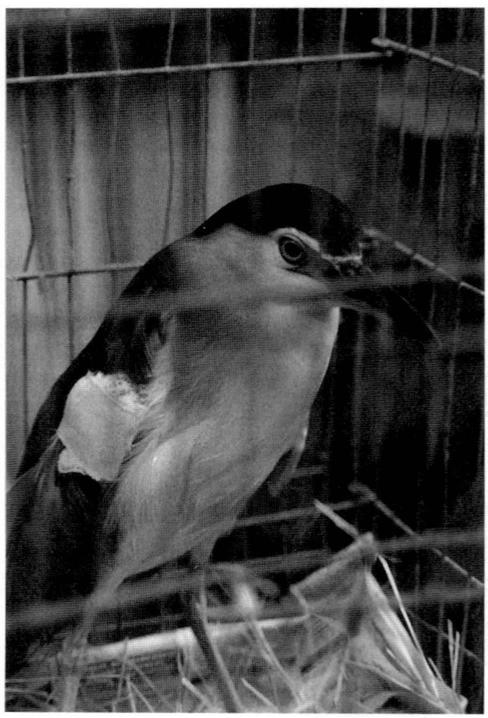

Fig. 18.6. Nankeen night heron. This bird had been shot through the wing, resulting in a fracture. Treatment included pain relief, antibiotics, fluid therapy and strapping the wing.

provide further pain relief and preclude further damage to the bone, nerves, blood vessels, skin and tendons. The heron was then settled into the intensive care section of the veterinary facility where there was warmth, quiet and limited access other than by rostered volunteers. At the appropriate time it was translocated to a safe house and later had surgery to repair the fracture, under general anaesthetic. Following a period of post-operative care that included further antibiotics and pain management, and then rehabilitation, the injury healed and the bird was released in a suitable environment, safe from shooters and able to be monitored by a compassionate neighbour.

GREY TEAL, LAKE COWAL. First aid treatment for this little bird included strapping for a shot and fractured wing, plus splinting and bandaging to a shot and fractured leg (Fig. 18.7). Shotgun wounds often result in multiple fractures and other damage to the limbs, body, spine and head. Birds with multiple bullet wounds were often alive when they fell from the sky and hit the water. Some were then killed by shooters. Some were rescued, treated and recovered. Others were too severely injured to survive and were helped to end their suffering (by euthanasia) or sought refuge in reeds (lignum) where they inevitably died eventually from starvation, predation, septicaemia, shock and other causes.

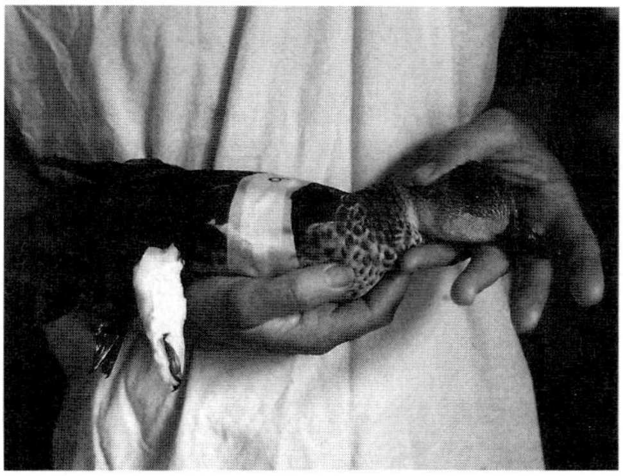

Fig. 18.7. Grey Teal. First aid treatment for this bird included strapping for a shot and fractured wing, plus splinting and bandaging to a shot and fractured leg. Shotgun wounds often result in multiple fractures and other damage to the limbs, body, spine and head.

Ingrown collar

Collars ingrown into skin

People may place ligatures, nooses, snares or overly tight collars or hobbles on animals. Any collar, halter or restraint on an animal needs to be regularly checked and loosened as the animal grows. The case in Fig. 18.8 shows a chain that had actually become embedded in the dog's neck, causing the animal suffering and clearly indicating that this had happened over a considerable length of time. Some cases of ingrown collars or halters will require surgical removal under anaesthetic, and a permanent deformity may result.

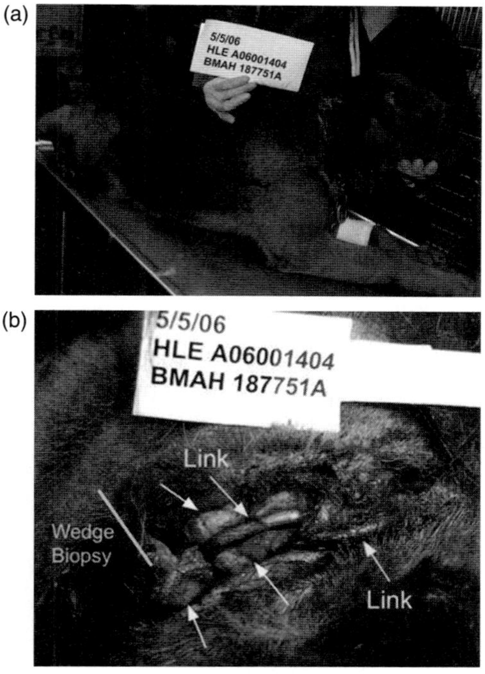

Fig. 18.8. (a) A 10-year-old German shepherd cross dog had a collar (chain) embedded in his neck, which was removed under anaesthetic. At the same time a full-thickness wedge biopsy was taken of the wound from surface to healthy tissue. The biopsy was sent for histopathology to provide an estimate of the age of the wound. (b) A close-up of the embedded chain and location of the site of the biopsy. (ASPCA/ALDF, 2011). (Photographs courtesy of ASPCA.)

Harness wounds

Working animals are prone to wounds if they are in poor condition, overworked, overloaded or have incorrectly fitting tack (Fig. 18.9).

Working equines at brick kilns in the Kathmandu valley have been overloaded with bricks and often suffer from harness wounds and lameness. Reducing the load, allowing frequent rest periods and ensuring well-fitting harnesses and healthy animals will help prevent sores (Fig. 18.10) developing. Groups such as Animal Nepal and SPANA provide veterinary care for these animals and work with the owners to educate them about animal welfare issues. McLean *et al.* (2012) undertook a welfare assessment of donkeys in Mali, West Africa and implemented an educational programme of animal welfare and donkey management in secondary schools and colleges. The authors found that while improved harnesses were greatly needed, students were enthusiastic in learning humane donkey husbandry techniques (e.g. training, donkey care and harnessing).

First aid

First aid for harness wounds involves removing the harness that is causing the injury and cleaning debris from the wound, using analgesia, antibiotic medication and fly repellent where indicated and available. Often harness wounds are seen in working animals in countries where veterinary care is infrequent or non-existent. The book *Where There is No Vet* (Forse, 1999) was written for such circumstances.

Matted hair

An animal with heavily matted hair will be in extreme discomfort. Matted hair pulls at the skin, inhibits normal mobility and renders the animal unable to groom or scratch at itself to relieve the discomfort (Patronek, 2004). Urine scalding, faecal impaction, maggot infestation, ingrown claws, infection and lameness may be seen (Patronek, 2004).

In severe cases the animal will need sedation or a full anaesthetic for clipping of the matted hair. Careful handling and speaking calmly are essential as the animal may be fearful and aggressive and unable to easily see, hear or move away from you, causing increased anxiety. Intravenous fluids during the clipping are advisable as these animals are likely to be debilitated and dehydrated. The veterinarian may opt to perform desexing, dental treatment and ear cleaning (as indicated) at the same time. Antibiotic therapy and pain relief will probably be necessary in all but the mildest of these cases. Prior blood tests help indicate if there are other health concerns (e.g. renal or hepatic disorders)

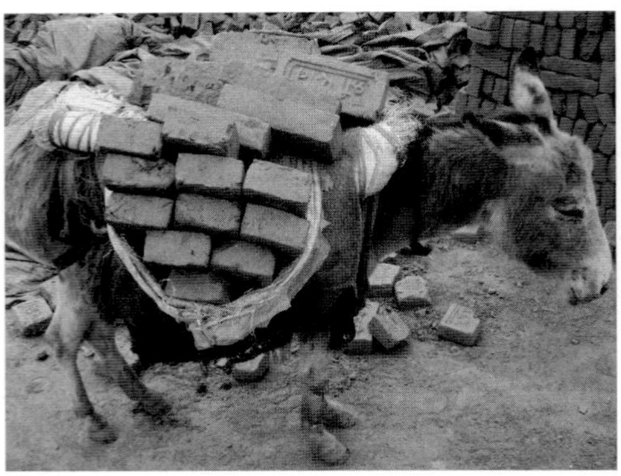

Fig. 18.9. This donkey at a brick kiln in the Kathmandu valley has been overloaded with bricks. Such animals often suffer from harness wounds and lameness. (Photograph courtesy of Lucia de Vries at Animal Nepal.)

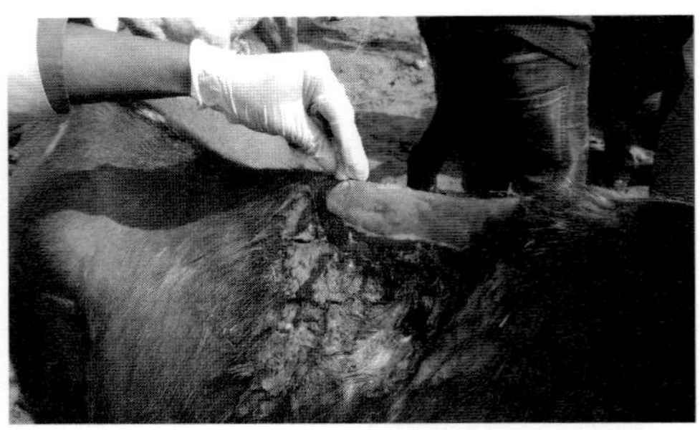

Fig. 18.10. This wound is being cleaned with iodine and will require a period of rest, daily cleaning and antibiotic cream to heal. When the animal returns to work the harness must be checked and adjusted so it is not rubbing the animal's back. Education is crucial in these cases so that the animal carers know what caused the injury and how to prevent it. (Photograph courtesy of Lucia de Vries at Animal Nepal.)

and will guide you in your decision of which drugs to use. A sample of the matted hair can be stored in a plastic zip-lock bag for use as evidence if the case becomes a court trial.

Case study: Matted hair and neglect

'Miss Bea', a 5-year-old poodle cross, was found locked in a cupboard after an anonymous tip-off to the ASPCA. Not only was her coat a solid mass of matted fur, laden with faeces, urine and filth, she also had an ear infection and overgrown nails, which had curled around and pierced her paw pads (ASPCA, n.d., Fig. 18.11). Miss Bea's muscles had atrophied and she was unable to walk or even stand without help. The extent of the neglect was so severe that the owner was immediately arrested on animal cruelty charges.

Malnutrition and starvation

Obesity or emaciation can both cause health problems.

Some animals are deliberately fed in a way that causes them to suffer. An example is the anaemia in calves farmed for veal production. In the event that a veterinarian is called to assist in a case of suspected anaemia in animals, a minimum blood test of TP and PCV (total protein and packed cell volume or haematocrit) will be needed to determine the severity of anaemia and dehydration. Treating for endo- and ectoparasites is recommended. Faecal floats can be performed to assess for parasites such as helminths and *Giardia* and a faecal egg count performed. A dental examination should be undertaken and any dental treatment administered.

Dehydration is commonly seen in cases of starvation and, whereas an animal may survive for weeks without food, water deprivation can cause death within days (Merck, 2007). An animal may be dehydrated because it has been deprived of a clean water source or has become too weak to drink (Merck, 2007). Illnesses involving diarrhoea and vomiting can also result in life-threatening dehydration, a notable example being parvovirus in dogs.

Case study: malnutrition

A 2-year-old bay thoroughbred (Fig. 18.12) had to be euthanazed after he collapsed through malnutrition. The defendant, a 68-year-old man from Leicester, failed to call for a vet and allowed him to suffer for several days. He pleaded guilty to two charges of failing to address the cause of its weight loss and diarrhoea under Section 9 of the Animal Welfare Act, and for failing to provide the gelding with adequate veterinary care and attention for its declining condition under Section 4.

Neglect/starvation/parasitism

Skin disease can be painful for the animal, contagious to other animals and zoonotic to the handler (Box 18.1). It is essential to determine the aetiology of the skin disease by performing a thorough diagnostic work-up (which can include sticky tape impressions, skin scrapings, fungal testing and biopsies). Wearing personal protective equipment (as seen in Fig. 18.13) is advisable until you have ruled out contagious/zoonotic disease. Consultation with a veterinary dermatologist is recommended in cases of which

(a) (b) (c)

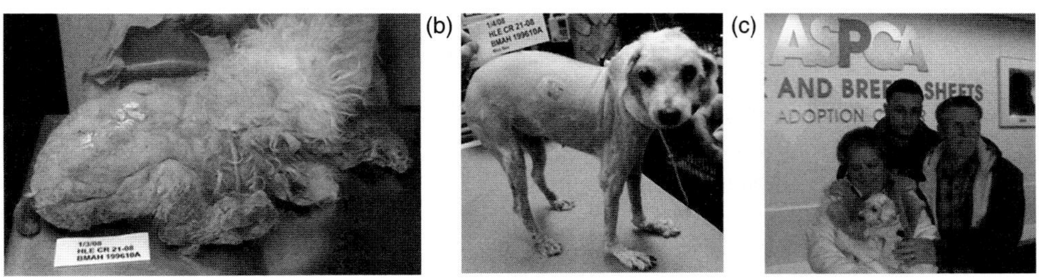

Fig. 18.11. These photographs show the disturbing level of neglect that 'Miss Bea', a poodle cross dog had suffered. (a) Her coat was a solid mass of matted fur, laden with faeces, urine and filth. (b) Miss Bea after clipping and (c) with her new family. (Photographs courtesy of ASPCA.)

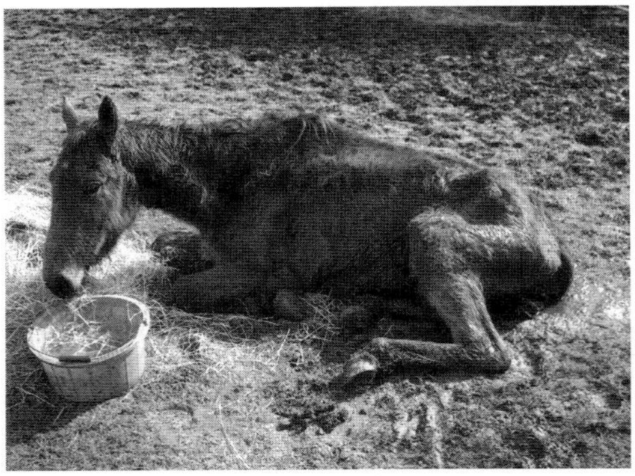

Fig. 18.12. This 2-year-old bay thoroughbred suffered without veterinary care before he had to be euthanized after collapsing through malnutrition and diarrhoea. (Copyright RSPCA England and Wales.)

you are unsure, and purchasing a good veterinary dermatology textbook to keep in the clinic or shelter is useful.

Skin disease can be diagnosed by a range of methods including thorough medical examination, looking for parasites, blood tests (for endocrinopathies), skin scrapings (for mites), biopsies, fine needle aspirates and sticky tape impressions. Allergy testing and intradermal skin tests can also be performed. In many cases, the animal seen with skin disease in an abuse/neglect scenario may have more than one presenting problem (such as demodicosis with secondary bacterial or yeast infection, an ear infection, a heavy burden of fleas, gastrointestinal parasites and malnutrition). Be aware that diagnostic tests may not be 100% accurate – ringworm will not always fluoresce under a Woods Lamp and *Demodex* mites may not be seen in skin scrapings, especially if only one scraping was performed or it was too superficial. Some cases of skin disease may be so severe it may appear initially that the animal has been burnt – one such case involved the owner bringing in his large, mixed-breed puppy with red lesions on its head, neck and forelegs. The owner accused his housemate of pouring boiling water on the animal while the owner was away. A skin scraping, however, determined that *Demodex* mites were responsible for the lesions.

Box 18.1.

Skin disease and parasitism in dogs is commonly seen in some remote Australian Indigenous communities and is a significant human and animal health issue. These dogs often live closely with the human members of the community and a strong human–animal bond between Indigenous people and dogs has been demonstrated (Constable *et al.*, 2010). Despite this, there are challenges to animal management in these communities. Overpopulation of dogs, zoonotic disease, fighting and scavenging may combine with added social problems of domestic violence, poverty, child abuse, substance abuse, low education levels and limited job opportunities (AMRRIC, 2007).

In Australia, AMRRIC (Animal Management in Rural and Remote Indigenous Communities) works with Indigenous communities and Indigenous Environmental Health Practitioners to develop sustainable and culturally appropriate animal health programmes. Recommended resources for people interested in working in Indigenous communities include those by Phelan (2007, 2010).

First aid

Debilitated animals with skin disease (as seen in Fig. 18.13) will require supportive care – intravenous fluids, medicated baths, analgesia and antibiotics may be necessary. Provision of a suitable, high-quality diet is essential. Some treatments for skin disease (e.g. certain injectable drugs and medicated washes/dips) are contraindicated for certain species and breeds, so care will be needed prior to prescribing drugs and commencing treatment.

Treatment for skin disease often requires long-term veterinary care and monitoring and a lot of dedication by the carers/owners.

Case study: neglect, starvation and parasitism

This 10-month-old female Cane Corso puppy (Fig. 18.13) had been starved and 'left outside to die' in the US winter (Reisman, 2011). She was emaciated, had a temperature of 80°F (26.6°C) and had generalized demodicosis. She was critically

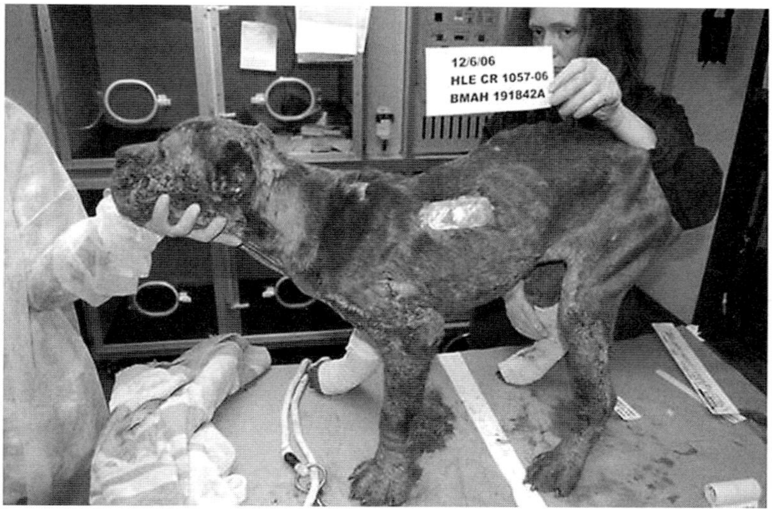

Fig. 18.13. This extremely debilitated dog was suffering from demodicosis and emaciation. Animals with skin disease will require supportive care – intravenous fluids, medicated baths, analgesia and antibiotics may be necessary. Note the protective clothing worn by the handlers in this photograph. This is a wise precaution until you have determined whether the animal's disease is zoonotic. (Photograph courtesy of ASPCA.)

ill for 5–7 days but recovered and is now living a happy life with her new owners (Reisman, 2011).

Puppy farms

Puppy farms (also known as 'factories' or 'mills') involve animal abuse on a large scale as people strive to profit by mass-producing puppies with little concern for their welfare. Any breed of dog can be involved (Fig. 18.14) but it is often the so-called 'designer dogs' such as poodle crosses that are involved. The breeding dogs, bitches and puppies in puppy factories receive inadequate care, socialization, housing and hygiene (Fig. 18.14). A range of health and welfare issues identified by the RSPCA (2010) include:

- High incidence of viral, bacterial and fungal infections, including distemper, hepatitis, parvovirus and kennel (canine) cough.
- Heavy intestinal worm burdens (tapeworm, roundworm, hookworm and whipworm) causing diarrhoea, vomiting and anaemia.
- Heartworm infection causing heart problems, respiratory problems, anaemia.
- Skin conditions such as flea infestations, sarcoptic and demodectic mange, ringworm, dermatitis, eczema, sores and abscesses from fighting, self-trauma or due to the unhygienic conditions.
- Eye conditions such as conjunctivitis, corneal ulceration and abrasions, which can lead to infection and blindness. Eye lids can be injured from fighting and foreign bodies.
- Ear infections due to lack of care and unhygienic conditions. Ear conditions can be difficult to treat after rescue as the dogs are unaccustomed to being handled by humans. Long haired, floppy eared breeds are more likely to have ear problems.
- Dental disease from poor nutrition and lack of veterinary dental care causing difficulty eating, pain, gingivitis, ulcerations and tooth loss.
- Indiscriminate breeding can lead to a number of inherited conditions such as overshot jaw and hydrocephalus.
- Reproductive problems seen include dystocia, mastitis and pyometra.
- Foot problems include interdigital dermatitis, overgrown nails and sore foot pads from the dirty environment.

First aid

Treating dogs and puppies from puppy farms depends on the presenting symptoms (see sections

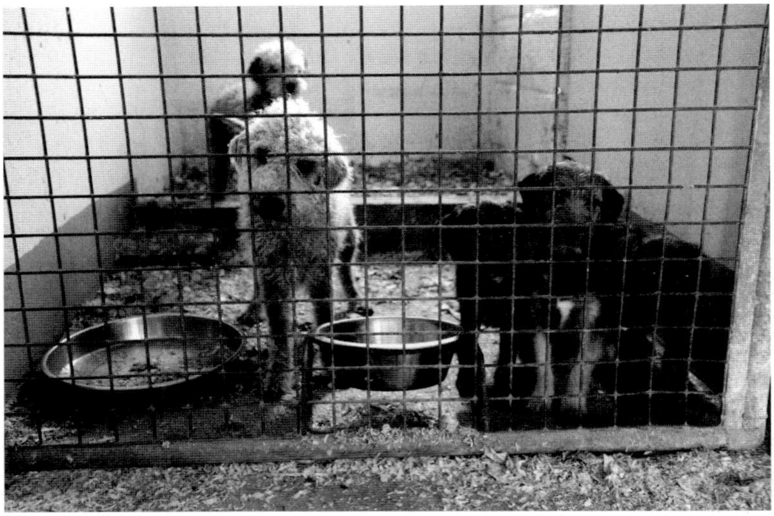

Fig. 18.14. Dogs from a puppy farm. RSPCA inspectors discovered more than 70 dogs of various breeds, some with untreated medical conditions, living in filthy and squalid kennels. Many of the dogs were living on soiled and damp bedding. (Photograph copyright RSPCA England and Wales.)

on skin disease, malnutrition and bite wounds in this chapter) and must be undertaken with an appreciation of the behavioural issues often exhibited by these poorly socialized animals (see Chapter 15 on behaviour).

Sexual abuse of animals

All case studies of sexual abuse of animals are provided by Jenny Edwards with permission of Chandler Edwards.

Jenny Edwards works as a Special Animal Crimes Investigator and has been instrumental in the arrest and conviction of animal sex offenders in Washington, Tennessee, Ohio and Florida, USA. She is a certified Private Investigator and has taught Law Enforcement officers as well as Animal Control Officers all over the USA. Jenny is a contributor to the University of Missouri Law Enforcement Training Institute, National Animal Cruelty Investigator Schools, and has authored multiple print and online publications. In 2006 Jenny worked on and appeared in the documentary film *Zoo*. Jenny may be reached at jenny.edwards@ChandlerEdwards.org. Currently, Jenny works in the Pacific Northwest region of the USA.

First aid

First aid for animal victims of sexual abuse will be to stabilize the animal and provide analgesia and/or antibiotic coverage as needed. Depending on the nature of the abuse, surgery may be required (e.g. to repair tears to the ano-genital tract). Unfortunately, some animals will be so severely injured that euthanasia is advisable.

Case study 1: suspected sexual abuse of horse

A mare was found bleeding from a large puncture wound near the vulva (Fig. 18.15). The vet suspected the mare had been raped with an object and called law enforcement. After investigation, the officer determined that the horse had likely self-injured from rubbing against a hazelnut tree on the property. (Horse hairs like the ones in the horse's tail were found on the tree trunk.)

Case study 2: sexual abuse of cat – object inserted

'Spotty' was a male cat taken to the veterinary hospital because he was unable to stand or walk. The owner suspected the cat had been raped

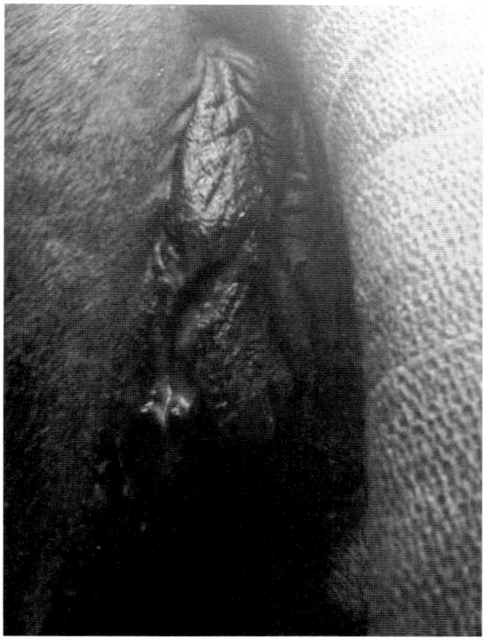

Fig. 18.15. A mare was found bleeding from a large puncture wound near the vulva. A large haematoma formed after a few days. The wound was cleaned and treated and subsequently healed normally. (Photograph courtesy of Jenny Edwards of Chandler Edwards.)

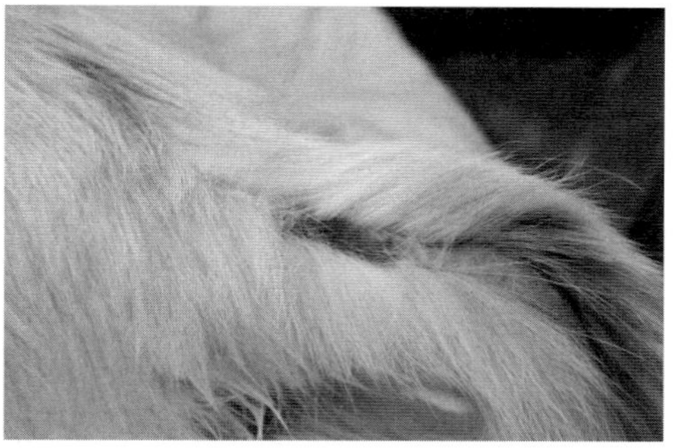

Fig. 18.16. 'Spotty', a male cat, was taken to the veterinary hospital because he was unable to stand or walk. The owner suspected the cat had been raped with an object because a month earlier she found a photo on her boyfriend's cell phone appearing to show an object being inserted into the cat's anus. There was also evidence of burn marks on the cat's tail. (Photograph courtesy of Chandler Edwards.)

with an object because a month earlier she found a photo on her boyfriend's cell phone appearing to insert something into the cat's anus. There was also evidence of burn marks on the cat's tail (Fig. 18.16). The cat was examined and determined to have internal injuries. The owner elected humane euthanasia. The case was not investigated further.

Case study 3: sexual abuse of dogs, horses and mice

Multiple animals (including one Boerbel mastiff, one Bernese mountain dog, two great Danes, two German shepherds, one Rottweiler, four warmblood stallions, 19 mice) were seized by animal control, including the stallion (Fig. 18.17) and dog (Fig. 18.18) pictured below. Videotapes and digital photographs were also seized, which depicted the owner and others having sex with the animals. The dogs were taught to mount human males, and the horses were fellated by men, so no evidence of physical injury was found in either species. The mice were found covered in a lubricating substance, and their tails were missing. All the mice were euthanized. All of the other animals were successfully rehabilitated and placed in adoptive homes. The owner was convicted of a parole violation and served 3 years in federal prison. A second person was arrested, and after serving 30 days in jail was deported to his home country.

Working with animals that have been sexually abused
Jenny Edwards

We are just beginning to study the psychological implications of animals involved in sexual abuse. From experience, I can say that they appear to suffer in much the same way as children who are sexually assaulted: anxiety, depression, reactions to stimuli that remind them of the incident (e.g. they become agitated or excited in the presence of men, or when cameras or video equipment are set up around them), and in some cases exhibit aggressive behaviour (which we believe is confusion over inappropriate training).

We have had mixed success in rehabilitating these animals. Our best success to date is with the grey warmblood stallion (Fig. 18.17). The horse received a thorough veterinary medical examination, was gelded and received dental treatment.

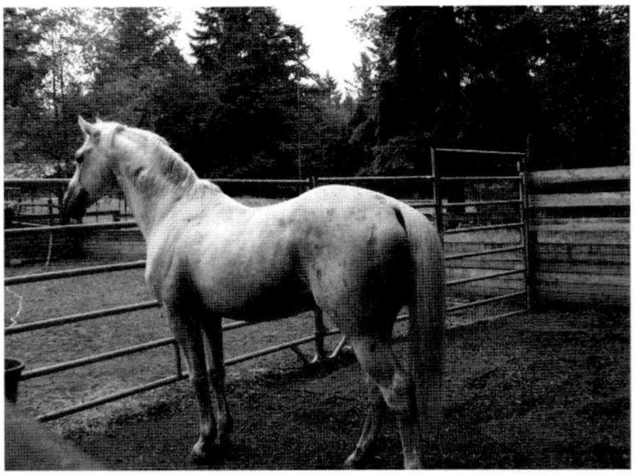

Fig. 18.17. This horse (whilst a stallion) had been sexually abused. After being seized he received veterinary care and was rehomed for rehabilitation. (Photograph courtesy of Jenny Edwards of Chandler Edwards.)

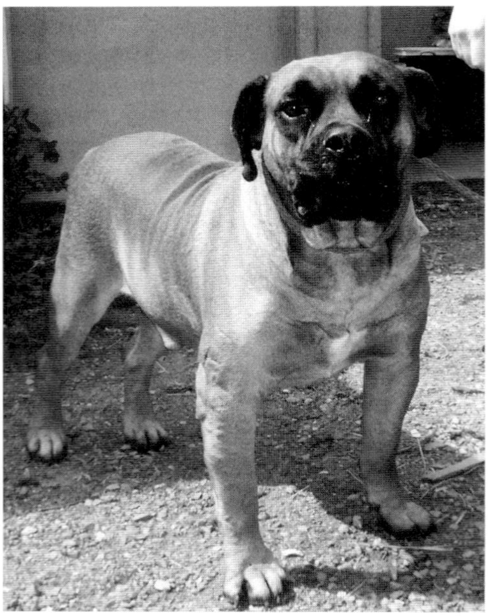

Fig. 18.18. This mastiff had been sexually abused. (Photograph courtesy of Whatcom Humane Society, Bellingham, Washington, USA; Laura Clark, executive director.)

At intake he was dangerous, untrusting and in poor shape physically. He reared, would strike and kick, and was prone to biting (at least one bite resulted in a visit to the local hospital emergency room). Whenever the horse looked at you, it was with a steely eye that said 'I can do great damage to you'. We basically left him alone for the better part of a year. He was turned out in his own paddock (in sight of other horses, but not able to connect physically), and only allowed specific volunteers to work with him. Gradually we began to work him in a round pen and then sent him to a farm that specializes in working with humans who suffer from post-traumatic stress disorder (PTSD – horses are used in the therapeutic process). There, they used a lot of the same techniques on this horse that are used with humans and today he is calm enough to be present at children's birthday parties.

Stab wound

Stab wounds can be caused by any sharp object (e.g. knives, swords, forks, sticks, screwdrivers, scissors and arrows) and although external signs of bleeding may appear minor, there may be severe internal haemorrhage and complications such as pneumothorax, haemothorax, haemopericardium and cardiac tamponade (Munro and Munro, 2008).

Forensic examination of the wound (as described by Merck, 2007, pp. 101–114) will assist in determining the type of weapon used – sharp, regular wounds suggest a sharp weapon was used, whereas a blunt instrument results in wounds with an abraded or jagged appearance.

If an animal is presented with a penetrating injury and the knife or object still embedded, care should be taken to avoid smudging fingerprints and not to remove the object in a live animal without proper preparation for treatment – withdrawal may cause more tissue damage and haemorrhage (Merck, 2007). Treatment will depend on the location of the injury once initial examination and stabilization has occurred.

Some cases of penetrative injuries have been associated with sexual abuse of animals. Some of the respondents to the veterinary survey by Munro and Thrusfield (2001c) reported animal sexual abuse cases involving stab wounds to the ano-genital area and within the vagina. Sexual abuse of animals was discussed previously in this chapter.

Case study: stabbed dog

This 6-year-old male Rottweiler cross dog was rushed to a veterinary clinic after being stabbed multiple times in the chest and head (Fig. 18.19). The incident occurred when a neighbour reportedly became annoyed by the dog's barking – the offender tried to beat the dog with a mop handle before stabbing the animal and threatening the owner, 'Do you want to be next?' (Lemmon, 2011). The dog was stabbed 13 times with a 15-cm-long blade and the offender received a jail sentence (Lemmon, 2011). Unfortunately, the dog was dead on arrival at the clinic.

Alternative/Complementary Therapies

There is increasing interest from veterinarians and owners in the use of alternative therapies for animals (Cheever, 1997). Some veterinary schools have responded to student demand by including training in complementary and alternative therapies (Kara, 2000), and a survey of international veterinary school deans found that while they supported student awareness of these therapies they strongly believed that any such inclusion in the curricula must be evidence-based (Memon and Sprunger, 2011).

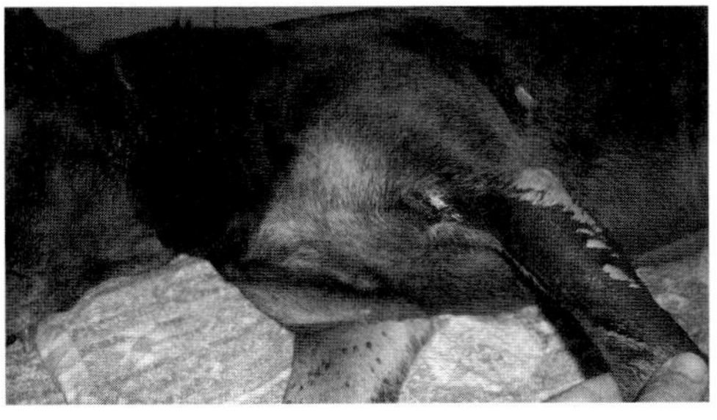

Fig. 18.19. This 6-year-old male Rottweiler cross dog was rushed to a veterinary clinic after being stabbed multiple times in the chest and head by the owner's neighbour. Unfortunately, the dog was dead on arrival at the clinic. (Photograph courtesy of Animal Welfare League Queensland Veterinary Clinic, Ipswich with the permission of the dog's owner, Mr Adam Turnbull.)

Criticism of complementary and alternative therapies among veterinarians may be because they are unfamiliar with the therapies, feel there is a lack of evidence of their efficacy and/or that any effect may be due to a placebo effect. While the placebo effect is recognized in human medicine (Finniss *et al.*, 2010), it is difficult to know if the placebo effect exists in animals and if it does, exactly what the mechanism is (McMillan, 1999). An evidence-based approach to complementary and alternative therapies is provided by Ernst *et al.* (2001). If you intend to use alternative or complementary therapies to treat animals it is advisable you seek advice from a reputable practitioner experienced in this area. Veterinary associations have special interest groups for members interested in alternative therapies and can advise about further training in this area.

Common alternative and complementary therapies used on animals include acupuncture, aromatherapy, chiropractic, flower essences, herbal medicine, homeopathy, Reiki, Shiatsu and TTouch. Whilst many people report positive results when using complementary and alternative therapies on animals, this should not replace examination, diagnosis and treatment by a qualified veterinarian. The experiences and personal opinions of one person who uses an integrative approach to animal care are described below.

Case study: Allie Phillips

Allie Phillips is an attorney who works with human and animal victims of abuse in her role as Director of the National Center for Prosecution of Animal Abuse, a programme of the National District Attorneys Association (USA). Allie is a Certified Crystal Healer and has obtained master-teaching certifications in Usui Reiki and Integrated Energy Therapy, two energy healing methods (Fig. 18.20). She uses these energy healing methods, alongside crystal healing and flower essences to help calm abused and traumatized animals. Allie volunteers with a cat shelter and says she has seen amazing results using energy healing on the animals waiting for adoption. When her own cat, Oscar, became diabetic through a disease called acromegaly, Allie used energy healing, alongside homeopathic veterinary care and insulin injections, to help Oscar cope with his illness.

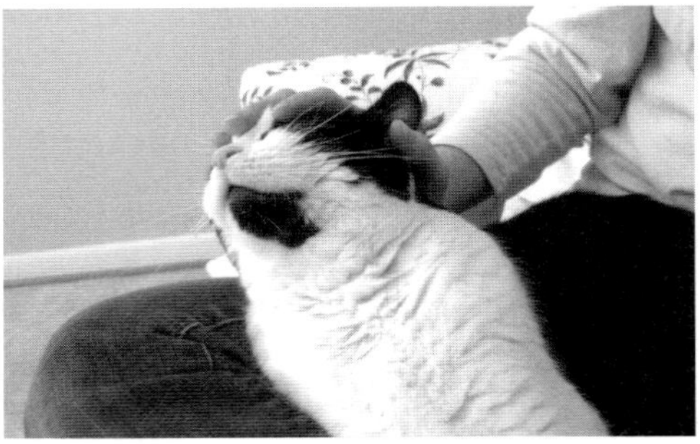

Fig. 18.20. Allie applying Reiki to her cat, Oscar. (Photograph courtesy of Allie Phillips.)

Allie explains the importance of healing animals that have suffered abuse or neglect (Phillips, 2011):

> When I read stories of how animals have been rescued from an abusive or neglectful environment, whether it was a dog, cat or cow, I am always relieved; but then my next thought goes to whether the animal is receiving any healing. When we hear of people who have been victimized, those people often undergo therapy and counselling. And while many people may think that an animal can simply 'shake off' the trauma of abuse or neglect, we cannot stop with the rescue and need to start thinking about providing healing to animals after they are in a safe place.

References

AMRRIC (2007) Animal Management in Rural and Remote Indigenous Communities – What are the Issues? Available at: http://amrric.org/2008/02/09/what-are-the-issues (accessed 31 December 2010).

ASPCA (n.d.) ASPCA Rescue Stories. Available at: http://www.aspca.org/about-us/aspca-supporter (accessed 7 January 2012).

Barr, F. (2007) Imaging techniques for the critical patient. In: King, L.G. and Boag, A. (eds) *BSAVA Manual of Canine and Feline Emergency and Critical Care*, 2nd edn. British Small Animal Veterinary Association, Quedgeley, Gloucester, UK, pp. 356–371.

Cheever, H. (1997) Alternative medicine for pets. *Good Housekeeping* 225(5), 191.

Constable, S., Dixon, R. and Dixon, R. (2010) For the love of dog: the human-dog bond in rural and remote Australian Indigenous communities. *Anthrozoos* 23(4), 337–349.

Dinnage, J., Bollen, K. and Giacoppo, S. (2004) Animal fighting. In: Miller, L. and Zawistowski, S. (eds) *Shelter Medicine for Veterinarians and Staff.* Blackwell Publishing, Ames, Iowa, pp. 511–521.

Ernst, E., Pittler, M.H., Stevinson, C. and White, A. (2001) *The Desktop Guide to Complementary and Alternative Medicine: an evidence-based approach.* Mosby, London.

Finniss, D.G., Kaptchuk, T.J., Miller, F. and Benedetti, F. (2010) Biological, clinical, and ethical advances of placebo effects. *The Lancet* 375(9715), 686–695.

Forse, B. (1999) *Where There Is No Vet.* Macmillan Press, London.

Ghaffari, M.S., Marjani, M. and Masoudifard, M. (2009) Oculocardiac reflex induced by zygomatic arch fracture in a crossbreed dog. *Journal of Veterinary Cardiology* 11(1), 67–69.

Green, P.C. and Gullone, E. (2005) Knowledge and attitudes of Australian veterinarians to animal abuse and human interpersonal violence. *Australian Veterinary Journal* 83, 619–625.

Jasani, S. (2011) *Small Animal Emergency Medicine.* Saunders Elsevier, Edinburgh, UK.

Kara, R. (2000) Alternative therapies grow in veterinary curriculums. *DVM* 31(8), pp. 1, 26.

Lemmon, K. (2011) Pet dog stabbed to death over its barking. *The Queensland Times*, October 11, pp. 1–2.

McGuinness, K., Allen, M. and Jones, B.R. (2005) Non-accidental injury in companion animals in the Republic of Ireland. *Irish Veterinary Journal* 58(7), 392–396.

McLean, A.K., Heleski, C.R., Yokoyama, M.T., Wang, W., Doumbia, A. and Dembele, B. (2012) Improving working donkey (*Equus asinus*) welfare and management in Mali, West Africa. *Journal of Veterinary Behavior* 7, 123–134.

McMillan, F.D. (1999) The placebo effect in animals. *Journal of the American Veterinary Medical Association* 215(7), 992–999.

Memon, M.A. and Sprunger, L.K. (2011) Survey of colleges and schools of veterinary medicine regarding education in complementary and alternative medicine. *Journal of the American Veterinary Medical Association* 239(5), 619–623.

Merck, M. (2007) *Veterinary Forensics – animal cruelty investigations.* Blackwell Publishing, Ames, Iowa.
Munro, H.M.C. (1999) The battered pet – signs and symptoms. In: Ascione, F.R. and Arkow, P. (eds) *Child Abuse, Domestic Violence, and Animal Abuse.* Purdue University Press, West Lafayette, Indiana.
Munro, H.M.C. and Thrusfield, M.V. (2001a) Battered pets: features that raise suspicion of non-accidental injury. *Journal of Small Animal Practice* 42, 218–226.
Munro, H.M.C. and Thrusfield, M.V. (2001b) Battered pets: non-accidental physical injuries found in dogs and cats. *Journal of Small Animal Practice* 42, 279–290.
Munro, H.M.C. and Thrusfield, M.V. (2001c). Battered pets: sexual abuse. *Journal of Small Animal Practice* 42, 333–337.
Munro, H.M.C. and Thrusfield, M.V. (2001d) Battered pets: Munchausen syndrome by proxy. *Journal of Small Animal Practice* 42, 385–389.
Munro, R. and Munro, H.M.C. (2008) Wounds and injuries. In: Munro, R. and Munro, H.M.C. (eds) *Animal Abuse and Unlawful Killing – Forensic Veterinary Pathology.* Saunders Elsevier, London, pp. 30–47.
Niles, J.D. (2009) Special considerations in wound management. In: Williams, J. and Moores, A. (eds) *BSAVA Manual of Canine and Feline Wound Management and Reconstruction*, 2nd edn. BSAVA, Quedgeley, Gloucester, UK, pp. 223–253.
Patronek, G.J. (2004) Animal cruelty, abuse, and neglect. In: Miller, L. and Zawistowski, S. (eds) *Shelter Medicine for Veterinarians and Staff.* Blackwell Publishing, Ames, Iowa, pp. 427–452.
Pead, M.J. and Langley-Hobbs, S.J. (2007) Acute management of orthopaedic and external soft tissue injuries. In: King, L.G. and Boag, A. (eds) *BSAVA Manual of Canine and Feline Emergency and Critical Care*, 2nd edn. British Small Animal Veterinary Association, Quedgeley, Gloucester, UK, pp. 251–268.
Phelan, S. (2007) Conducting dog health programs in Indigenous communities – a veterinary guide. AMRRIC and IFAW. Available at: http://www.amrric.org/sites/default/files/Conducting_dog_health_programs_june%2008.pdf (accessed 20 August 2012).
Phelan, S. (2010) *Dog Health Programs in Indigenous Communities – an environmental health practitioners guide.* AMRRIC, Darwin, Australia.
Phillips, A. (2011) Manifested harmony: don't forget to heal. Available at: http://manifestedharmony.com/?s=don%27t+forget+to+heal (accessed 20 April 2012).
Pope, J. (2009) Wound aetiology and classification. In: Williams, A. and Moores, A. (eds) *BSAVA Manual of Canine and Feline Wound Management and Reconstruction*, 2nd edn. British Small Animal Veterinary Association, Quedgeley, Gloucester, UK, pp. 15–24.
Reisman, R. (2011) The veterinarian as expert witness in animal abuse cases. Webinar. 7 December. Hosted by ALDF/NDAA/ASPCA.
RSPCA (2010) RSPCA Australia Discussion Paper – Puppy Farms. Available at: http://www.rspca.org.au/assets/files/Campaigns/RSPCAPuppyFarmDiscussionPaperJan2010.pdf (accessed 2 October 2012).
Sinclair, L., Merck, M. and Lockwood, R. (2006) *Forensic Investigation of Animal Cruelty – a guide for veterinary and law enforcement professionals.* Humane Society Press, Washington, DC.
Somerville, B. (2008) *Dogtown – a sanctuary for rescued dogs.* Sellers Publishing, Portland, Maine.

19 Humane Euthanasia

Catherine Tiplady

This chapter discusses how to assess an animal's quality of life, the decision-making process prior to euthanizing an animal, and humane euthanasia techniques to minimize the suffering of animals and staff who perform euthanasias.

To Treat or Euthanize? Assessing the Animal's Quality of Life

Where there is uncertainty whether to attempt treatment, continue treatment or euthanize, it is advisable to arrange a meeting of all members of the animal care team so everyone can discuss the patient, express their concerns and reach a consensus about the options for this animal (Lindley and Watson, 2010).

Each case will have to be assessed as an individual, keeping in mind the need for animals to have a life free of unrelenting pain and distress and the ability to move comfortably and perform natural behaviours. One suggestion to help determine an animal's quality of life is to obtain from the owner or carer a list of what they believe makes the animal happy or unhappy (Rollin, 2006). In the case of animal abuse and neglect, the foster carers or staff familiar with the individual animal will be better able to provide details to enhance an animal's quality of life.

McMillan (2003) provides guidelines that can be referred to by veterinarians and staff to maximize an animal's quality of life:

HEALTH

- Provide high-quality healthcare.
- Eliminate disease if possible. If not possible (e.g. arthritis), alleviate any discomfort.
- Mental health disorders: use of pharmacological and non-pharmacological (e.g. behavioural modification) interventions where indicated.

FOOD CONSUMPTION

- Feed a high-quality, palatable food in amounts that maintain a proper body weight.
- Offer treats in moderation.

SOCIAL RELATIONSHIPS

- Provide suitable social interaction and companionship with people and other animals.

MENTAL STIMULATION

- Provide mental stimulation suitable for the particular animal. This can include: activities, play, challenges, exploration, and other forms of mental stimulation and engagement. Specific examples include treasure hunts with food treats, interactive toys, novel objects to investigate and explore, outings, games and working for food.

STRESS

- Reduce or remove stressors.
- Enhance the animal's opportunities to adapt to the stressor by providing the means for coping (e.g. social support and predictability).

CONTROL

- Offer the animal opportunities to make choices (e.g. to go outside or inside, which food to eat, which toys to play with).
- Ensure the animal has the ability to lessen unpleasant feelings or situations (e.g. boredom, loneliness, frustration, fear, or pain), for example by having a safe place to escape or hide.

Humane Euthanasia

> It is important to us that the summation, or consummation, of their lives not involve fear, horror, pain, or suffering as the final encapsulation of their lives, particularly given that we cannot provide compensation or remedy after death.
>
> (Rollin, 2009, p. 1082)

When an animal is deemed to have a poor quality of life with no prospect of improving and is not considered a candidate for rehabilitation, treatment and rehoming then euthanasia may be considered. Involving other staff in the decision-making process is recommended as the team approach may alleviate individual feelings of grief or failure surrounding patient loss (Barton Ross and Baron-Sorensen, 2007).

Euthanasia means 'good death' and, just as no animal should suffer during life, euthanasia should not cause pain or distress to the animal.

The high staff turnover in animal shelters is believed to be related to the number, method and handling of euthanasias (Rogelberg *et al.*, 2007) – training staff in humane methods of animal handling and euthanasia (Fig. 19.1),

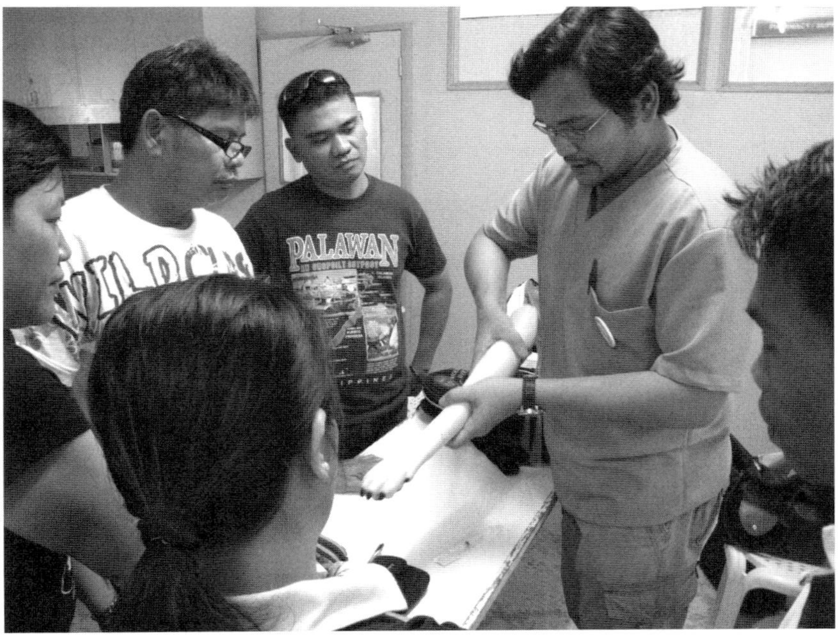

Fig. 19.1. A humane euthanasia training workshop for veterinarians in the Philippines was conducted in 2011. Rubber models of dog's legs were used to demonstrate intravenous injections into the cephalic vein. In this photo, PAWS (Philippine Animal Welfare Society) veterinarian Dr Wilford Almoro explains to the group about giving intravenous injections. Saline or water can be used in these classes to inject these rubber models. (Photograph courtesy of Natasha Lee.)

trying to increase the rehoming rate and rotating work duties so the same staff are not spending prolonged periods euthanizing will address these issues.

Euthanasia techniques

The author and publishers cannot take responsibility for the information provided on drug dosages and methods of application that are mentioned in this publication. These details must be verified by individual users by referral to the appropriate literature.

The following guidelines for choosing a method of euthanasia are among those outlined by Wolfensohn and Lloyd (1998, pp. 49–51). The guidelines were designed for laboratory animals but are equally applicable to all species.

1. Death must occur without producing pain.
2. The time required to produce loss of consciousness must be as short as possible.
3. The time required to produce death must be as short as possible.
4. The method must be reliable and non-reversible.
5. There must be minimal psychological stress on the animal.
6. There must be minimal psychological stress to the operators and observers.
7. It must be safe for personnel carrying out the procedure.
8. Any drugs used should be readily available and have minimum abuse potential.
9. The method should be economically acceptable.
10. It should be simple to carry out, with little room for error.

A 'layered' euthanasia, where the animal enters a state of relaxation prior to euthanasia, will lead to a calmer experience for the animal and staff. This can be achieved by using pre-anaesthetic drugs suitable for the individual animal. One of the objectives of pre-medication is to decrease fear and apprehension in the animal (Wolfensohn and Lloyd, 1998), something that is particularly relevant to abused and neglected animals.

Using this technique, instead of euthanizing a conscious (and possibly distressed and struggling) animal with pentobarbital injected into the vein, the animal has 'layers' of sedation, intravenous euthanasia occurring only when the animal is completely relaxed, pain free and preferably unconscious. This method is more time consuming and expensive but is well worth the extra effort. The animal is first sedated and given any necessary pain relief (e.g. by subcutaneous injection), then anaesthetized and finally euthanized intravenously. Sedation drugs used will vary depending on the species but for a dog may include sedation with an opioid and/or acepromazine administered subcutaneously or intramuscularly. Fifteen to 30 minutes later an intravenous catheter and extension set (if desired) can be placed (usually in the cephalic vein) and flushed with saline to ensure patency. Anaesthesia can be induced with a suitable intravenous anaesthetic drug. When the animal has lost consciousness, the euthanasia solution, such as pentobarbital, can be injected. Some staff may prefer simply to sedate the animal and then euthanize, or just euthanize, a conscious, tractable animal. Information about dose rates and guidance on storage and licensing of opioids and barbiturates can be obtained from veterinary drug publications.

Oral sedatives can be given in food to animals that are difficult to handle.

Small animals such as rodents and birds can be 'masked down' with anaesthetic gas (such as isoflurane) and oxygen prior to administering the barbiturate. Barbiturate can be injected into the unconscious animal via the following routes:

- intravenously (e.g. the jugular vein);
- intra-cardiac; or
- intra-hepatic or intra-peritoneal (for these methods the barbiturate should be diluted at least 50:50 with sterile NaCl or water for injection to lessen irritation from the high pH).

Euthanasias are never without stress to the operator, but a rushed and badly performed euthanasia is hard to get over and may affect your confidence in performing future euthanasias.

It is advisable to contact an expert in the species you are working with to discuss suitable methods of analgesia, anaesthesia and euthanasia.

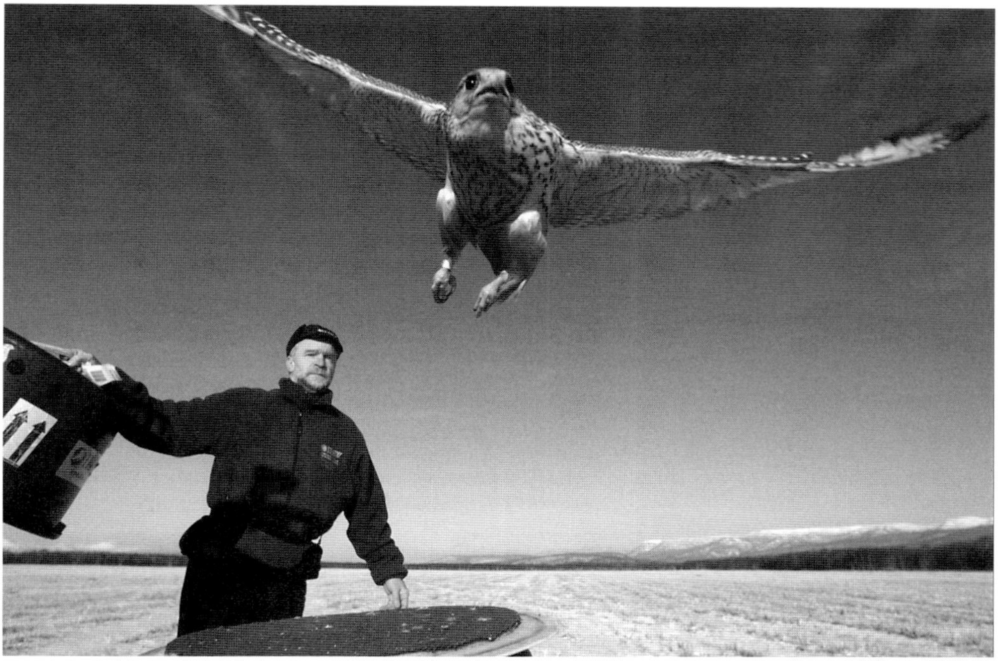

Fig. 19.2. An endangered gyrfalcon being released back into the wild in Russia after being rescued and rehabilitated from a smuggling operation in Moscow. (Photograph courtesy of IFAW.)

Remembering Animals that Died due to Abuse/Neglect

Starting a memorial wall or garden for paying tribute to animals dying due to abuse will give some comfort to those who cared for these animals. Events that serve to remember the human victims of violence could include mention of the animal victims. A short speech, poem or candle-lighting ceremony could be performed to acknowledge animal victims of abuse and provide some sense of peace to the human carers who worked to alleviate their suffering.

References

Barton Ross, C. and Baron-Sorensen, J. (2007) *Pet Loss and Human Emotion – A Guide to Recovery,* 2nd edn. Taylor and Francis Group, New York.

Lindley, S. and Watson, P. (2010) Introduction. In: Lindley, S. and Watson, P. (eds) *BSAVA Manual of Canine and Feline Rehabilitation, Supportive and Palliative Care: case studies in patient management.* British Small Animal Veterinary Association, Gloucester, UK, pp. 1–6.

McMillan, F.D. (2003) Maximising quality of life in ill animals. *Journal of the American Animal Hospital Association* 39(3), 227–235.

Rogelberg, S.G., DiGiacomo, N., Reeve, C.L., Spitzmüller, C., Clark, O.L., Teeter, L., Walker, A.G., Carter, N.T. and Starling, P.G. (2007) What shelters can do about euthanasia-related stress: an examination of recommendations from those on the front line. *Journal of Applied Animal Welfare Science* 20(4), 331–347.

Rollin, B. (2006) Euthanasia and quality of life. *Journal of the American Veterinary Medical Association* 228(7), 1014–1016.

Rollin, B. (2009) Commentary – ethics and euthanasia. *The Canadian Veterinary Journal* 50(10), 1081–1086.

Wolfensohn, S. and Lloyd, M. (1998) *Handbook of Laboratory Animal Management and Welfare,* 2nd edn. Blackwell Science, Oxford, UK.

Part V

The Science of Animal Abuse: Veterinary Forensic Investigation

Veterinary forensics plays a vital role in the investigation of animal abuse cases. In this section, several expert forensic veterinarians define veterinary forensics, explain how veterinary forensics can be used in cases of animal abuse and neglect and describe the appropriate recording, sampling, handling and storage procedures needed in a forensic investigation. Importantly, the welfare of animals as 'living evidence' is discussed and a chapter on Bitemark Analysis includes wildlife crime involving animal baiting, human interpersonal violence, dog bites of people and a suspected case of child abuse involving animals.

20 Forensics: Introduction to Veterinary Forensics

David Bailey

Forensic science is, in the simplest definition, the application of science to the resolution of legal disputes. Forensic veterinary science then is the application of veterinary science to the resolution of legal disputes that usually involve animals or their derivatives. And here, within the definition of the subject, we have the first issue that needs to be addressed. Biology and veterinary science does not fit well into this physical science-led world of forensics.

Physics is the application of the laws of motion and mathematics to nature and it helps to describe man's interaction with nature and *predict events* based on the laws of physics. We have three Newtonian laws that predict motion. These are not theories but they are laws; not the legal kind, but the laws of nature and there is no barrister who could argue with Newton.

Chemistry is the application of the science of the composition of properties and elements. There are laws of chemistry and predictable equations such as the Henderson–Hasselbalch equation and the Rate law – all neatly designed to predict what is going to happen, to predict events of the future.

Biology is a fuzzy science and the best law we have in biology is the theory of evolution – it is not a law, it is a theory just waiting there for that one-time event that has to occur or be described to allow it to become disproved. 'If man evolved from monkeys then why do we still have monkeys?' asked the barrister of Darwin. Biology is seen to others as a deceptive science. Biologists can tell what has happened and say with a degree of certainty, 'I thought that would happen', but biology lacks the predictability of physics and the certainty of the laws of chemistry, forced always to look back and say that an event did happen with expected certainty from which to make a statistical conclusion, but biology does not predict very well. It does not tell you what is going to happen as well as physics or chemistry.

Whenever a system or arrangement of complex organs made up of cells that are made up of atoms exists, then it is called a biological system and usually describes a living thing. This living thing is unpredictable and does not behave in a way that the laws of physics and chemistry expect. It is this unpredictable biological behaviour that veterinarians have to deal with, and then as forensic vets we need to marry an unpredictable biological science that is descriptive with the elements of forensic analysis that are heavily dependent upon chemical analysis and physical properties of events described by laws of physics and motion, resulting in this inevitable mismatch of the sciences. Forensics needs an answer where biology does not deliver as easily as chemistry and physics forces it to, and here is the problem. While we can tell what is *likely* to have happened and what *may* have happened, we are, as biologists, very bad at predicting what will happen *with any certainty*. Reduced to describing an event and saying 'I told you so', the court needs a better interpretation of analysis of evidence. The court expects science to tell us that something either *did* or *did not* happen, and many vets stumble into the legal arena with this as the mistaken understanding as to the guidance required for their role.

They attempt to be certain when being sure is all that is required and that being unsure is sometimes all that biology provides. Combined with the courts' expectations for good evidence and solicitors' attempts to instruct good witnesses and an adversarial system that discovers truth as a secondary consequence of winning, it makes the field of veterinary forensics a challenge that many vets are not used to and perhaps unprepared for.

'Animals are made up of atoms anyway' is the infamous quote from a court case where a vet was asked to explain that, despite having never seen a wild Bengal cat, he was able to give expert opinion on the matter as he was a vet and he knew 'all animal breeds and species'.

The reply from the barrister was appropriate for the expert:

> So you claim that veterinary science then, is applied chemistry?
> Yes, partly.
> What part?
> The chemical part.

Veterinary science is the study of biological systems, which at the atomic level individually obey the laws of chemistry and physics but together coalesce to form cells, organs and bodies – an emergent system of a living thing that is quite reluctant to yield to any laws, legal or natural.

While this is my interpretation of what veterinary forensics is, there are other views held by some to incorporate the meaning of veterinary forensics as a subsection of pathology or as a specialized interest grouping of wildlife vets. Individuals with training in welfare, ethics and law feel the use of the term 'forensics' should be applied to their particular field and guard the use of the term with some degree of jealousy, as do the holders of any specialism (recognized or not) of veterinary science who claim to be expert witnesses in their particular field of interest, qualification or expertise. Others will be surprised to discover that veterinary forensics values the use of argument, presentation and knowledge in a manner to support the prosecution *and* defence of a particular case involving animals or their derivatives. Forensics does not distinguish between a prosecution stance and a defence position – it does not align itself to pathology, ethics, law or welfare and it certainly does not allow itself to be clouded by emotional judgements or feelings of what investigators feel should have happened.

A litmus test for a forensic report is to ask yourself whether your report would have been different if you had written it for the defence or prosecution. The answer should be no.

Regardless of who instructs you and what they want you to say, you are not paid for your opinion, but the time taken to reach that opinion and that opinion needs to be the same regardless of who instructs you.

It is a similar mindset that lawyers are adept at controlling and that many non-lawyers find difficult to comprehend. It is emotionless and deals with facts, the interpretation of facts and the conclusions made from these interpretations. The law says what you can or cannot do – forensics determines if you did or did not do it.

Pathology, ethics, welfare and wildlife investigations are all a subset of forensics – forensics is certainly too broad to be placed under any heading within veterinary science, and veterinary science too is a subsection of forensics, and is therefore subservient to the rules and requirements of the forensic discipline.

Vets need to fit their mindset and training to comply with the rules and expectations of forensics, and this is a counter-intuitive process for most vets who are used to dealing with what is available rather than what is required.

I have had to deal with cases involving sexual assault of animals, the use of forged and questioned documents, firearms and ballistic investigations, DNA interpretation, bitemark analysis of a small child that was killed by a dog, toxicology and chemical analysis, blood pattern analysis and hair and feather analysis. I have provided advice and input into cases involving illegal veterinary medicine residues and import of veterinary medicines, snail bait toxicity, hoarding as well as roles in research and education in forensic reasoning and philosophy.

It is a curious mix of work and all available through the power of attachments sent via email to review case reports or as a live investigator called to a scene.

I have a busy lifestyle and it is difficult, and I enjoy it.

21 Forensics: Introduction to Veterinary Forensic Investigation

David Bailey and David Chamberlain

When called to a premises or scene to investigate a case of suspect animal cruelty, there are a few protocols that need to be established and of which the forensic vet needs to be aware.

In various worldwide legislation, as an introduction there must be pain and suffering that is likely to occur for an offence to have been committed against an animal.

This pain and suffering must also be considered 'unnecessary'.

The term 'animal' is defined as any non-human organism with a backbone.

This applies to animals that are domestic and does not apply to wild animals (they are usually ignored or covered under a separate act). In law, animals are property that is owned and there is more legislation currently dealing with the right of an individual to protect his or her property or dispose of his or her property than there is to deal with issues arising from animal abuse or property damage.

Animals are, under the law, the only piece of property that can have feelings or are sentient beings. This legal definition of animals as property can provide problems when dealing with property that is living and has needs, and especially when storing this evidence prior to a court contest.

A forensic vet then is looking for evidence of pain and suffering and this can take many different forms, such as photographs, gunshot residue, bruising, blood sample analysis, post-mortem examination (PME), hair collection for exposure to drugs, blood pattern analysis and bitemark analysis, but also in the form of documents, evidence of trophies or filming of abuse.

Owners can be difficult to deal with and crime scenes can be dangerous places for an examiner. Mental health issues are common at these scenes and while it is beyond my area of expertise to comment, I believe there is not one crime scene I have been asked to attend where I did not suspect mental health issues were involved.

Vets must adapt the PREGS protocol for dealing with a crime scene. This mnemonic stands for:

- **P**rotect
- **R**ecord
- **E**xamine
- **G**ather
- **S**tore

Each aspect of a (PREGS) scene examination is open to challenge and scrutiny by an opposing barrister and needs to be followed meticulously.

If an animal is found at a crime scene and is living but near death, then efforts need to be made to resuscitate it. It is not acceptable to enter a crime scene where there is a dying animal and allow it to die in order to preserve evidence. Even if it means that the owner may escape a conviction, your first obligation is to promote the life of the animal and then gather evidence later. During the recent bushfires in Australia large areas of bush land were declared crime scenes, and this meant that no one could enter the area to provide care for the affected animals. If there has been human death or a human crime at a scene involving animals that are dead or dying, then it may not be permitted to enter the crime scene in order to provide relief of pain and suffering to those animals as there is a risk that you may contaminate the scene.

This is one of the few examples where an animal's pain suffering may be deemed necessary. Legislation designed to protect animals does not guarantee them an existence free from pain and suffering, but an existence free from unnecessary pain and suffering. A vet may be criticized for allowing pain and suffering to occur, but can justify this if, for example this pain and suffering is deemed necessary to catch a murderer. The animal is left alone, injured and unattended at a crime scene, as the priority is gathering of evidence and avoidance of contamination, not the freedom of that animal from pain and suffering.

Dead animals can be taken away for further examination. They should be photographed *in situ* and then placed in a bag, sealed, labelled and taken away and frozen. The type of bag depends on the evidence required: wet items need to be in plastic bags and frozen; dry items need to be in paper bags and stored on a shelf.

Living animals can be seized if it is likely that they are going to be in a position where pain and suffering is likely to occur or if it has already happened. They must be photographed and identified (see Chapter 22 on 'Animals as living evidence') and then removed and transported to appropriate housing and looked after as living evidence. This invariably means that the animal that is healthy and nurtured by the time the case goes to court is not the same animal that was seized, and so the evidence has changed.

Radiographic interpretation can be useful to determine if previous injuries exist – but on its own it is not a very discriminating tool. On its own, any one single piece of evidence is unhelpful in a cruelty case. You need multiple pieces of evidence, and the crucial aspect of multiple evidence is that it must be independent. So, ten radiographs can help to demonstrate that a dog has received prior injuries. But ten radiographs *and* signs of healing wounds *and* reflected UV light showing an old injury are three independent types of evidence all pointing to a similar conclusion.

While there is too much detail to provide within an introduction to this topic, a further detailed approach to the retrieval of post-mortem samples for toxicology is provided below.

Post-mortem Toxicology and Toxicokinetics

Introduction

For definitions of terms, see Glossary. Toxicologists may be requested to perform investigations in situations where toxicants are thought to have contributed to the death of a human or animal. The death may have occurred as a consequence of acts that may have been:

- deliberate, poisoning/arson;
- accidental, therapeutic mistakes (over-medication); or
- natural, therapeutic mistakes (under-medication).

(Toxicologists are also often involved with anti-doping procedures.)

When considering post-mortem examinations (PME), it is also important to pay regard to gross pathological changes (e.g. injection sites, unabsorbed toxicant within the stomach, pulmonary oedema).

From PME samples the toxicologist has to determine:

- What toxicants were involved?
- What dose did the individual take?
- When was the dose taken?
- Did the toxicant contribute to the individual's death?

Post-mortem (PM) toxicokinetics are different from ante-mortem toxicokinetics. After death, absorption, metabolism/biotransformation and excretion of toxicants occur at a much lower rate than before death. However, the significance of PM toxicokinetics has recently been recognized particularly in respect to the PM distribution of drugs (Bailey and Shaw, 1980; Stevens, 1984; Preskorn, 1998; Cook *et al.*,

2000; Drummer and Gerostamoulos, 2002; Flanagan and Connally, 2005).

After death, many toxicants present redistribute around the body differently to the situation prior to death. After death a number of PM changes are responsible for this altered distribution of toxicants:

- Once the circulation stops, toxicants tend to gravitate to the most dependent parts of the body.
- pH changes in the blood and tissue influence solubility and the ability of toxicants to cross cell membranes. The pH of body fluids falls PM, releasing many toxicants from their binding sites (Forrest, 1993).
- Toxicants that were intracellular may become extracellular and vice versa.
- Toxicants that were in interstitial fluids may enter the plasma and vice versa.
- There may be continued absorption form organs such as the skin, bladder, lungs or stomach.
- Some metabolism/biotransformation of toxicants may continue as a consequence of autolysis/putrefaction or the action of microorganisms (bacteria) from the parent body detritivores (Stevens, 1984; Regional Laboratory for Toxicology, 2007).

After death there is an inevitable change in cellular biochemistry. Autolysis, the destruction of a cell through the action of its own enzymes, begins and consequently toxicants may be released from intracellular sites or biotransformed by the enzymes of autolysis. Toxicants may continue to be passively absorbed from or eliminated into organs.

Ante-mortem toxicants within plasma are relatively uniformly distributed throughout this fluid compartment. However, PM distribution of toxicants within plasma can demonstrate up to a tenfold difference in concentration, which is dependent upon the sampling site, method of sampling and volume of blood collected (Regional Laboratory for Toxicology, 2007). In animals, sampling from the femoral vein is recommended. However, the toxicant concentrations from PM samples may not reflect those at the time of death.

It is also possible to observe differences in the concentration of certain drugs obtained from different tissue sampling sites for liver and lung.

While it is the role of the pathologist and toxicologist to prepare, analyse and interpret PME samples, it may be the role of the forensic scientist to collect, identify, preserve and introduce the PME samples to the 'chain of custody' (Richardson, 2000).

PM sample collection for toxicology

Collection of samples for toxicological analysis from a body as soon as possible after death will prevent further artefactual changes as a result of:

- medication or toxicant redistribution;
- creation of artefactual toxicants through the action of microorganisms or autolysis and putrefaction of the body; or
- the loss of toxicants through biotransformation action of microorganisms or autolysis and putrefaction of the body.

If sample collection or PME cannot be performed promptly then the body should be frozen.

The standard procedure for toxological examination in most laboratories requires blood and urine samples with other additional samples when appropriate (Regional Laboratory for Toxicology, 2007). However, more detailed sampling procedures are suggested in specific orders to minimize the risks of sample contamination (Forrest, 1993; Richardson, 2000). These include, in the following order:

1. Blood.
2. Urine.
3. Gastric contents.
4. Vitreous humour.
5. Liver and bile.
6. Brain.

General considerations

The normal crime scene and evidence collection practices must be adhered to. Before removing a body from a crime scene for freezing or conducting the PME, written communication from the competent authority indicating their authorization must be obtained together with any specific requests of direction.

As with all evidence collection, the first priority has to be health and safety considerations. Before handling a body or embarking on a PME and specimen collection, it is important that the person conducting the examination has all of the necessary personal protective equipment (PPE). Protection against zoonotic microorganisms or opportunistic pathogens is important and, if necessary, a preliminary blood smear stained with polychromatic methylene blue for anthrax may be prudent.

Some intoxicants may prove a hazard for the individuals conducting the examination, so PPE and procedures to avoid contamination must be utilized.

Before commencing the PME the position of the dead animal at the scene should be recorded, possibly utilizing photography or video along with any demographic information available. Information regarding previous medical history and medication could greatly assist any toxicological analysis. Advanced decomposition of a body or protracted immersion in water can concentrate certain toxicants such as cyanide (Richardson, 2000).

Care must be taken not to introduce any potential toxicants as part of the sampling process. Do not use surgical spirit to swab areas before sampling, or lubricants, especially those containing lignocaine, if urethral catheters are used.

Ideally the person conducting the PME and collecting the specimens is witnessed, videoed and assisted by a second person. Samples collected must be identified, including left or right, placed in suitable containers with tamperproof seals and introduced into the chain of custody for evidence. Ideally duplicate samples are produced if there is sufficient material.

Specimen containers

If PME and sample collection cannot occur promptly and the body or part of the body is going to be frozen until it can proceed then the remains should be placed in a body bag, sealed and identified, introduced to the chain of custody and taken to a place where they can be frozen promptly.

For the collection of PME specimens, glass containers are preferable because they are inert. Where rubber or plastic is present on lids of jars or bungs or tubes they should be covered with aluminium foil before the lid is replaced. In most situations no preservatives should be present in the tube or jar or added to the tube or jar once the specimen is collected.

The presence of microorganisms and nutrients in fluids of dead bodies can result in fermentation and the production of ethanol. This process can result in PM artefact results for ethanol concentrations of up to 1500 mg/l in blood where there may be many bacteria and fermentable nutrients. Other body fluids such as urine and vitreous humour are less prone to fermentation because there are fewer bacteria or fermentable nutrients.

Tubes containing 2% w/v sodium fluoride (Karch, 2008) are required as a preservative to inhibit bacterial production of analytes such as alcohol, gamma-hydroxybutyric acid (GHB) and cyanide, and to prevent bacterial degradation of labile drugs (Analytical Services International Ltd, n.d.). These can be used to collect both blood and urine, usually in 5 ml volumes.

Nylon specimen bags can be used for tissue samples of brain, adipose tissue, kidney and lung (Analytical Services International Ltd, n.d.; Keren, 2004; Regional Laboratory for Toxicology, 2007; Rao, 2012).

Blood

Blood samples are essential for the toxicological analysis of some common poisons such as salicylate, paracetamol, iron and ethylene glycol. Although the volume of the blood sample depends on the size of the animal and the amount of blood available, from 3 to 10 ml from each femoral vein is a guide (Table 21.1). Blood samples from the following should be *avoided*:

- Blood from large central, thoracic and abdominal vessels should be avoided because toxicant concentrations can be falsely elevated by factors of up to tenfold.
- Cardiac blood (according to some authorities, ethanol can diffuse from the stomach to the heart; Richardson, 2000).

Table 21.1. Summary of PM toxological samples, collection techniques and storage.

Specimen (including collection order)	Sample site/technique	Sample volume	Container(s)	Storage
Blood	Aspiration of the femoral veins × 2	Small animals, two samples of 3–10 ml each from left and right	Glass tubes with aluminium foil over the rubber bung. Fill with minimal air gap 5 ml as above with 2% sodium fluoride	Transport to lab at 4°C immediately or freeze at –20°C. Keep out of light
Urine	Open cystocentesis of the bladder	All urine present	Glass jars with aluminium foil over the lid. Fill with minimal air gap 5 ml with 2% sodium fluoride as for blood	Transport to lab at 4°C immediately or freeze but *not* below –16°C. Keep out of light
Gastric contents	Ligate the stomach sphincters, remove the stomach and examine contents in receptacle	60 ml plus any undigested evidence of medication or toxicant for gross identification	Glass jars with aluminium foil over the lid. Fill with minimal air gap	Transport to lab at 4°C immediately or freeze at –20°C. Keep out of light
Vitreous humour	Aspirate the posterior chamber of eye with a 16 G needle and 5 ml syringe; insert needle at 60° to the axis of the eye, direct to centre	2–3 ml from each eye, left and right	Glass tubes with aluminium foil over the rubber bung. Fill with minimal air gap 2 ml as above with 2% sodium fluoride	Transport to lab at 4°C immediately or freeze at –20°C. Keep out of light
Liver	Dissect and remove the right lobe	60 g	Glass jars with aluminium foil over the lid, or nylon bags	Transport to lab at 4°C immediately or freeze at –20°C. Keep out of light
Bile	Aspirate gall bladder	Small animals, 3–15 ml	Glass tubes with aluminium foil over the rubber bung. Fill with minimal air gap	Transport to lab at 4°C immediately or freeze at –20°C. Keep out of light.
Lungs		10–60 g	Glass jars with aluminium foil over the lid, or nylon bags.	Transport to lab at 4°C immediately or freeze at –20°C. Keep out of light
Brain	Post-mortem total craniotomy	10–60 g	Glass jars with aluminium foil over the lid, or nylon bags	Transport to lab at 4°C immediately or freeze at –20°C. Keep out of light
Hair	Pluck or cut	20 shafts to 10 g	Folded into paper then placed in a plastic bag and sealed. If cut, identify proximal end (not needed if plucked)	Robust and unaffected by normal environmental temperatures

- Haemorrhaged blood present in body cavities.
- Areas where there is ante-mortem venous stasis.
- Areas of haemolysis.
- Vessels that have been used to administer fluids or medication.

Ideally, blood samples should be collected from the peripheral vessels such as the femoral veins, but it is unlikely that samples of 40 ml could be obtained from the majority of small animals. Indeed, attempting to draw large volumes of blood from the femoral veins of small animals could result in blood being drawn from central sites, which is undesirable. In reality it is probably wise to draw only 5 ml of blood from each femoral vein in small animals (Regional Laboratory for Toxicology, 2007). It would be prudent to label samples from both left and right femoral veins separately and indicate the side of the animal's recumbency in death.

In most cases plain glass blood tubes (red top) used clinically for serum collection are the best containers for blood.

Analysis of volatile compounds requires sample collection into all-glass containers to prevent the volatile compound leeching into plastic tubes or rubber bungs and seals. In practice, this is achieved by using glass serum tubes, removing the rubber bung, wrapping the base with aluminium foil and replacing the bung into the tube.

Where it is thought the presence of ethanol or cyanide could have contributed to the death, it is necessary to decant 10% of the total sample into separate tubes and add sodium fluoride to the blood samples (Forrest, 1993).

It has been demonstrated that the sodium fluoride concentration in the fluoride/oxalate blood sample tubes (grey top) used clinically for determination of blood glucose levels is insufficient to inhibit the changes in ethanol concentrations that occur in PM specimens after sampling. A sodium fluoride concentration of 1.5% in the blood is required to prevent PM changes in ethanol concentration in PM samples (Richardson, 2000). If cyanide poisoning is suspected it is necessary to store blood in 2% sodium fluoride to prevent PM production of cyanide by bacterial action (Regional Laboratory for Toxicology, 2007).

Lithium in blood collection tubes (purple) interferes with high-performance liquid chromatography (HPLC) (Richardson, 2000) and should be avoided.

Urine

Analysis of toxicants in urine is easier than in blood because at PME it is a much cleaner specimen and is often free of putrefaction products and there is no protein binding as there is in blood, which hinders extraction and can interfere with analytical methods. Urine is useful for qualitative analysis and confirmation of blood results. As the bladder is a confined compartment, largely free from bacteria, in human toxicology it is of particular value in quantifying alcohol, where the validity of the blood result is in question.

Drugs and their metabolites are usually present in urine in much higher concentrations than in blood and are detectable for much longer periods following ingestion. Depending on the half-life of the toxicant and the sensitivity of the assay, it may be possible to detect the toxicants in urine for a few days or even a week after ingestion. However, this also means that the presence of the toxicant in the urine does not necessarily suggest that it was in the blood and exerting a toxicological effect at the time of death (Analytical Services International Ltd, n.d.).

Urine is usually collected by cystocentesis at the time of PME, and all available urine should be collected in one container and the sample then divided in two and placed into two clean, sterile 60 ml containers. Some laboratories will wash containers with 1 ml of methanol prior to filling (Richardson, 2000). Boric acid containers should not be used and, if the presence of ethanol is important, a 5 ml aliquot of urine should be collected in a tube containing sufficient sodium fluoride to provide a 2% concentration.

Gastric contents

In cases of oral overdose with a medication or ingestion of a toxicant, large amounts of unabsorbed medication or toxicant may remain in the stomach. Consequently concentrations will be substantially higher in gastric contents than in any other body fluid. It may be possible to identify medication present in the stomach from its gross appearance using a 'tablet identification reference' (TICTAC, n.d.).

Ideally, 60 ml of gastric contents should be submitted. However, some pathologists recommend ligation of the cardiac and pyloric sphincters and removal and submission of the whole stomach. It may be beneficial to collect the entire stomach contents in a suitably sized container so that they can be grossly examined.

Vitreous humour

The vitreous is in the relatively contained compartment of the posterior chamber of the eye, which is behind the lens. The vitreous is not as prone to PM changes as the blood. It is relatively resistant to putrefaction because its structure protects it from bacterial infiltration and there are few nutrients present to support PM fermentation. Its structure also protects it against trauma, so vitreous can often be extracted from intact eyes even if an individual has been extensively burnt.

While vitreous is largely free of protein and other complex substances so analysis is relatively straightforward, toxicant concentrations are difficult to interpret due to lack of reference data.

It is essential that the specimen is collected correctly, because excessive suction during sampling can cause significant changes in the concentration of several analytes. A 16-gauge needle attached to a 5 ml syringe is suitable. The eyelid should be firmly retracted and the sclera punctured at a latitude of about 60°, taking the pupil as the North Pole, with the needle being directed towards the centre of the eyeball. Gentle aspiration usually yields 2–3 ml of vitreous humour (in humans). All vitreous humour should be collected from both eyes and an aliquot should be preserved in a tube containing 2% sodium fluoride.

A 2 ml sample of vitreous humour in 2% sodium fluoride for glucose, lactate, acetone, insulin and C-peptide with a blood sample for the analysis of HbA1c (glycosolated haemoglobin) can provide an indication of ante-mortem glycaemic control. This can provide valuable information where insulin overdose is suspected as a cause of death (Analytical Services International Ltd, n.d.).

Liver and bile

Liver samples are particularly valuable when it has proved difficult or impossible to obtain adequate blood samples. If the liver is absent, muscle could be collected as an alternative (Analytical Services International Ltd, n.d.). Ideally, take a 60 g representative specimen of liver from the right lobe to avoid bile contamination and redistribution artefacts from the stomach (Analytical Services International Ltd, n.d.) and place in a plain glass jar. Do not add formalin because it is a reactive agent.

Collect 60 ml of bile by aspiration of the gall bladder at PME then place the sample in a separate glass container. Bile can be very useful when trying to detect toxicants or their metabolites. Such substances may be present in bile long after levels in blood are undetectable (Forrest, 1993).

Lungs

For the diagnosis of death by inhalation of toxic gases and vapours, some pathologists submit entire lungs. Detection of common gases and solvents can readily be performed on blood collected in plain glass blood tubes. Lung tissue samples should be placed in glass containers or nylon bags (Rao, 2012) with no preservatives and immediately chilled to 4°C or frozen (Regional Laboratory for Toxicology, 2007).

Brain

Ideally, 60 g of brain should be collected, especially if centrally active toxicants or drugs are suspected. Brain is also helpful when there is a suspicion of gas or volatile agents contributing to the animal's death. Brain samples should be placed in glass containers or nylon bags with no preservatives and immediately frozen (Regional Laboratory for Toxicology, 2007).

Other samples can also be collected, such as:

- Kidney tissue samples collected in a similar way to liver samples (Forrest, 1993).
- Adipose tissue, like liver, kidney, lung and brain, can be useful for the identification of volatile substances (solvents) (Analytical Services International Ltd, n.d.).
- Hair is resistant to contamination during handling and degradation. It provides a historic record of toxicants. It can be collected and stored in paper and sealed in a plastic bag. The proximal end should be identified if the hair is cut (Regional Laboratory for Toxicology, 2007) – this is not necessary if it is plucked (Forrest, 1993). Plucking the hair is more useful than shaved hair for DNA analysis.
- Feathers, similar to hair. The plumulaceous region of feathers is the ideal region for bird identification; this is the downy part of the feather and is not to be confused with down or contour feathers. For analysis you need the calamus or the shaft, and there are subsampling variations that occur depending on what you are looking for and the area subsampled.
- Saliva can be used to detect toxicants, but concentrations are lower and their presence is often fleeting.
- Nail and bone may be useful in the investigation of chronic heavy metal poisoning, e.g. arsenic and lead (Regional Laboratory for Toxicology, 2007).
- Milk: toxicants diffuse into milk but are also attracted by calcium and lipids within milk.
- Meconium, from new-borns, can be a potential source of information.
- Cerebrospinal fluid (CSF), via cisterna puncture (Forrest, 1993).
- Subdural and epidural clots may provide useful information but are very difficult to sample.
- Bone marrow may be useful in putrefied samples (Forrest, 1993).
- Semen.
- Larvae of detritivores accumulate toxicants as they feed on decomposing bodies. However, entomotoxicology is very much an emerging science and interpretation of results could be complicated (Analytical Services International Ltd, n.d.).
- Vomit and faeces, if present at a scene could provide information regarding recently ingested toxicants or the metabolites of toxicants previously ingested, respectively.

Storage of samples for toxicological analysis

Specimens should be chilled to 4°C before being promptly transported to a laboratory (Regional Laboratory for Toxicology, 2007). If transport is delayed, samples should either be frozen and stored until they can be transported or transported frozen. Freezing at temperatures below −16°C can result in the loss of some toxicants from frozen urine (Richardson, 2000).

Some toxicants can be decomposed if exposed to light (Richardson, 2000), so specimens should be transported in light-proof containers.

Conclusion

Once an animal dies the process of redistribution of toxicants starts. It is impossible to reverse this process, but prompt collection provides the best opportunity for samples with minimal possible PM artefactual changes.

Before beginning a PME of an animal to collect samples for toxological analysis, it is important to ensure that an adequate number of suitable containers are available. Glass tubes and jars that are clean, preferably sterile and without preservative, need to be to hand. Aluminium foil is needed to protect the specimens from any rubber bungs or plastic lids. A source of sodium fluoride needs to be available to add to blood, urine and vitreous humour as a preservative at a 2% w/v concentration.

Once samples are collected the majority can be frozen at −20°C and kept away from light. It may be prudent to freeze urine between −10°C and −15°C.

If a PME and sample collection cannot proceed promptly, then the animal's body should be placed in a body bag and frozen until a PME can be organized.

Glossary

Toxicant definitions

Name	Description
Xenobiotic	A foreign substance taken into the body, which may produce beneficial effects (nutrients) or be toxic
Toxicant	A substance that causes an adverse biological effect
Toxin	A specific protein produced by a living organism (e.g. tetanus toxin)
Organic toxin	A substance that was originally derived from a living organism (large carbon-based molecules)
Inorganic toxin	A chemical or mixture of chemicals, which may not have constant composition, not derived from living organisms (molecules consisting of a few atoms)
Systemic toxin	Affects the entire body or multiple organs
Organ/tissue toxin	Affects only specific organs or tissue types, the remainder of the body being unaffected
Analyte	A substance or chemical constituent that is of interest in an analytical procedure

Dose definitions

Name	Description
Exposure dose	The amount of xenobiotic encountered in the environment
Absorbed dose	The amount of the exposed dose that enters the body
Administered dose	The quantity administered, usually orally or by injection
Total dose	The sum of all the individual doses
Fractionating a total dose	May reduce toxicity because the body has an opportunity to repair the effect of each sub-toxic dose if sufficient time passes before receiving the next dose
Dose response	Correlates exposures and the spectrum of induced effects usually depicted as a bell-shaped standard distribution curve for a population of individuals. Dose responses are commonly presented as mean ± 1 SD (standard deviation), which incorporates 68% of the individuals. The variance may also be presented as two standard deviations, which incorporates 95% of the responses
Dose–response curve	The dose–response curve normally takes a sigmoid form. It conforms to a smooth curve as close as possible to the individual data points. For most effects, small doses are not toxic. The point at which toxicity first appears is known as the threshold dose level. A threshold for toxic effects occurs at the point where the body's ability to detoxify a xenobiotic or repair toxic injury has been exceeded
LD_{50}	A common dose estimate for acute toxicity, which is a statistically derived dose at which 50% of the individuals will be expected to die
Effective doses (EDs)	Are used to indicate the effectiveness of a substance. Normally, effective dose refers to a beneficial effect (*relief of pain*). It might also represent a harmful effect (*paralysis*). Thus the specific endpoint must be indicated
Toxic doses (TDs)	Are utilized to indicate doses that cause adverse toxic effects

Therapeutic safety definitions

Name	Description
Therapeutic index (TI)	Is used to compare the therapeutically effective dose to the toxic dose. The TI is a statement of relative safety of a drug. It is the ratio of the dose producing toxicity to that needed to produce the desired therapeutic response. The common method used to derive the TI is to use the 50% dose-response points. For example, if the LD_{50} is 200 mg and the ED_{50} is 20 mg, the TI would be 10 (200/20)
Margin of safety (MOS)	The MOS is usually calculated as the ratio of the dose that is just within the lethal range (LD_{01}) to the dose that is 99% effective (ED_{99}). The MOS = LD_{01}/ED_{99}. A physician must use caution in prescribing a drug in which the MOS is less than 1
No observed adverse effect level (NOAEL)	The highest dose at which there was no observable toxic effect; this is the threshold dose for a toxic effect. Since NOAEL is to set exposure limits, it is very important
Low observed adverse effect level (LOAEL)	The lowest dose at which there was an observable toxic effect

References

Analytical Services International Ltd (n.d.) Guidelines for Obtaining Specimens for Post mortem Toxicological Analysis. St George's – University of London. Available at: http://www.forensic-toxicology.org/Sample_Collection_Guidelines_2011.pdf (accessed 4 June 2012).

Bailey, D.N. and Shaw, R.F. (1980) Interpretation of blood and tissue concentrations in fatal self-ingested overdose involving amitriptyline: an update (1978–1979). *Journal of Analytical Toxicology* 4(5), 232–236.

Cook, D.S., Braithwaite, R.A. and Hale, K.A. (2000) Estimating ante mortem drug concentrations from post-mortem blood samples: the influence of post-mortem redistribution. *Journal of Clinical Pathology* 53, 282–285.

Drummer, O.H. and Gerostamoulos, J. (2002) Postmortem drug analysis: analytical and toxicological aspects. *Therapeutic Drug Monitoring* 24(2), 199–209 (Abstract).

Flanagan, R.J. and Connally, G. (2005) Interpretation of analytical toxicology results in life and at post-mortem. *Toxicological Reviews* 24(1), 51–62 (Abstract).

Forrest, A.W.R. (1993) Obtaining samples at post-mortem examination for toxicological and biochemical analysis. *Journal of Clinical Pathology* 46, 292–296.

Karch, S.B. (2008) (ed.) *Postmortem Toxicology of Abused Drugs.* CRC Press, Boca Raton, Florida.

Keren, B. (2004) How to obtain specimens at post mortem for analytical toxicology. Available at: http://cyanidepoisoning.blogspot.com/2004/10/how-to-obtain-specimens-at-post-mortem.html (accessed 4 June 2012).

Preskorn, S.H. (1998) What happened to Tommy? *Journal of Practical Psychiatry and Behavioral Health* 4(6), 363–367.

Rao, D. (2012) General toxicology. Available at: http://forensicpathologyonline.com/index.php?option=com_content&view=article&id=91&Itemid=100 (accessed 4 June 2012).

Regional Laboratory for Toxicology (2007) Guide to Obtaining Specimens at Post-mortem for Analytical Toxicology. Available at: http://www.toxlab.co.uk/postmort.htm (accessed 4 June 2012).

Richardson, T. (2000) Pitfalls in forensic toxicology. *Annals of Clinical Biochemistry* 37, 20–44.

Stevens, H.M. (1984) The stability of some drugs and poisons in putrefying human liver tissue. *Journal of the Forensic Science Society* 24(6), 577–589 (Abstract).

TICTAC (n.d.) TICTAC for Law and Order – Drug Identification Database. Available at: http://www.tictac.org.uk/Law/ (accessed 4 June 2012).

22 Forensics: the Animal as Living Evidence

David Bailey and Pippa Swan

Although animals are regarded in law as property there are limitations to ownership. An animal's owner may use it, sell it or destroy it as they choose but may *not* cause or allow it to suffer. If a law enforcement officer suspects that an animal is suffering, or has done so, they may take steps to seize the animal and begin legal proceedings. A veterinarian is likely to become involved at this point and examine the animal in order to determine if it is suffering, or is likely to suffer, if its circumstances do not change. Where in the opinion of the veterinarian the suffering can practicably be relieved, a decision may be made to seize the animal and treat it or move it to a place of safety for treatment. Any dependent offspring will also need to be assessed and seized along with their mother.

Animals might similarly be seized if it appears that they have been used in any type of animal fighting. A dog that appears to be of a banned breed or type, or certain types of dangerous wild animals, might also be legally seized.

The forensic handling of live animals presents particular problems. Forensic evidence in court would normally consist of reports and photographs (sometimes exhibits) based on physical items, from large to microscopic or even molecular. These physical items will normally be handled in specific ways in order to preserve them in the state in which they were found at the time of seizure, to minimize contamination and store them in a way that allows them to be re-examined where necessary or possible. This will usually involve placing the item or substance in a sealed bag or container, which can be uniquely identified and sealed in such a way as to make any tampering evident, and attaching a form identifying those people who are in charge of it over time, thus ensuring 'continuity of evidence'. When carried out correctly, this should make the results and any conclusions of forensic examinations and tests valid and capable of withstanding challenge in court. Unlike evidence such as illegal drugs, blood-soaked clothing or DNA samples, which can be bagged, sealed and stored, animals must be treated first and foremost as sentient beings. They cannot be packaged to insulate them from their surroundings or handlers, and their ongoing 'storage' presents problems of continuity and potentially considerable costs.

Animals involved in legal proceedings will often be in a poor, or very poor, state of welfare. The veterinarian's first and overriding priority is to attend to the animal and take whatever steps are necessary to relieve any pain or distress. This might involve euthanasia, the administration of drugs or immediate removal of the animal from its situation. The issue therefore of preserving evidence in its original state as required by forensic protocols must take secondary place in these situations. Much information, and the ability to record it, about the state of the animal or the offence that might have been committed may well be lost after the animal's poor welfare has been treated. Notes or photographs can be made as soon as practicable explaining or illustrating the situation and the reasons for any actions taken. Should the case end up in court it is unlikely that criticism will be made of any actions designed to relieve pain and distress, despite the inherent problems this might create for the usual testing of evidence.

The identification of individual animals in general often presents problems and this is particularly so in a forensic context. Microchips are commonly used in companion animals, and often in exotic animals or birds, but these are inserted beneath the skin and can only be read with a microchip scanner. Large farm animals may be individually marked with ear tags that bear a unique number, but these may be difficult to read if they become damaged or dirty, can become lost and can only be properly seen when very close to the animal. Smaller animals such as pigs may bear tattoos but poultry are unlikely to be individually marked at all.

Initially, temporary collars or tags can be placed around an animal's neck to hold information about the evidence number, the time and date of seizure and its location. But animals may interfere with them or they may become soiled, so their use as a long-term identification method is limited. Larger numbers can be used while taking photographs to help identify the animal for the purposes of photographic evidence, but these would need to be held manually. A spray marker could also be used for some animals. Information about the evidence number given to each animal, the time, date and place of seizure should be recorded in an evidence log. This can also be linked to sketches and photographs of the site or premises where the animal(s) were initially found.

Any method of identification in common usage is likely to be considered acceptable on welfare and legal grounds and may include ear tags, microchips, leg rings and marker sprays. The numbers contained in a microchip are unique but there is no way to show externally that an animal contains one, and not all the people who are in charge of the animal after seizure will necessarily have access to a scanner. It would be possible for a veterinarian to make a statement that the animal in question had been microchipped (if not already) and scanned by them and subsequently rescanned, thus confirming that the animal was positively identified to their satisfaction.

Ensuring unequivocal identification for the purposes of continuity over a period of time presents challenges, particularly when dealing with large numbers of animals and when they need to be moved. Identifying numbers or marks can be used to provide a connection to records held about each animal relating to its management, veterinary treatment and any movements, and will provide whatever level of continuity is possible in each case. Movement of an animal to a different place or a change in care should be additionally recorded in the evidence log. Animals are naturally subject to change, especially when they are recovering from a period of poor welfare, and in the strictest sense a 'living' piece of evidence is not the same piece of evidence seized several weeks or months earlier, although those very changes may prove to be significant in court. Many seized animals will be held at veterinary surgeries initially and then at charitable rescue centres, which will often have procedures in place for dealing with them. This may be a problem if no such rescue centres are available.

There may be situations where animals do not need to be kept for the purposes of a prosecution beyond the initial period of gathering forensic evidence. However, there are additional considerations when dealing with animals beyond their role as evidence or property. Where animals have been taken from owners or situations that compromised their welfare, it would seem self-evident that they should not be placed back there without significant changes being made. In reality the necessary changes may not happen, since undertakings to improve will in all likelihood have failed in the period preceding seizure. The aim of many welfare prosecutions is to prevent the defendant from owning or keeping animals in the future. With this possibility it would be desirable to hold any animals until a ruling is made, but this can generate huge costs given the needs of animals for food, shelter and human care. It may be possible in some circumstances for animals to be rehomed or destroyed once forensic evidence has been collected, and this might be desirable both in terms of welfare and reducing burdensome costs.

23 Forensics: Bitemark Analysis

David Bailey and Stephen Drew

Analysis of bitemarks is a developing and specialized field of forensic veterinary science. Bitemark analysts often are required to give professional and expert testimony in court on bitemarks from an animal that may have bitten another animal or person, and in cases where humans may have bitten animals.

Animal-to-animal bites may involve investigation of a crime involving wildlife, such as badger baiting by dogs. The bitemarks viewed and examined on the dogs need to be identified as being more likely to be from a badger than from any other animal, or even if the injuries were caused by objects such as barbed wire or undergrowth.

People who are bitten by animals are often injured by the event, and efforts to treat the injured person may not always have a forensic focus, thus leaving uncollected a large amount of valuable evidence that could have been retrieved at the time. On non-pigmented human skin, exposure to certain light wavelengths by forensic imaging techniques can allow visualization of a bitemark pattern long after visual wound healing has occurred (see: http://www.company7.com/library/nikon/Reflected_UV_Imaging_for_Forensics_V2.pdf).

In some instances, this can allow a stronger case to be presented in a report or courtroom if a claim is subsequently made against a responsible party. Dogs that are presented with a bite received from a human may not always be identified correctly as a bite or a human bite, and the correct examination techniques, analysis and interpretation of these events requires considerable skill.

I have examined bitemarks where dogs have been involved in fights with other dogs (see Fig. 23.1) and dogs that have been bitten by badgers – a protected species in the UK (Fig. 23.2).

Figure 23.3 shows an example where a human pathologist would require the assistance of a veterinary forensic bitemark analyst to assist when a dog is suspected of biting a human.

Man and dog have long enjoyed a close relationship, with the dog adopting various roles from working animal and protector to family companion. Inevitably this close association may sometimes result in conflict. Over 1 million dog bites occur every year in the USA alone (De Munnynck and Van de Voorde, 2002). Severe injury, disfigurement and occasionally fatalities occur, attracting significant media and public attention as they often involve young children and the family pet. An individual who owns, or is in control of a dog, is legally liable should that dog cause harm to another person. This provides an opportunity for the Forensic Veterinarian, acting as an expert witness, to aid the courts by employing bitemark analysis in the resolution of such legal disputes. However, in the absence of a victim with visible injuries, an assailant (the dog) and an owner with adequate insurance, there may not be reasonable grounds to pursue a case.

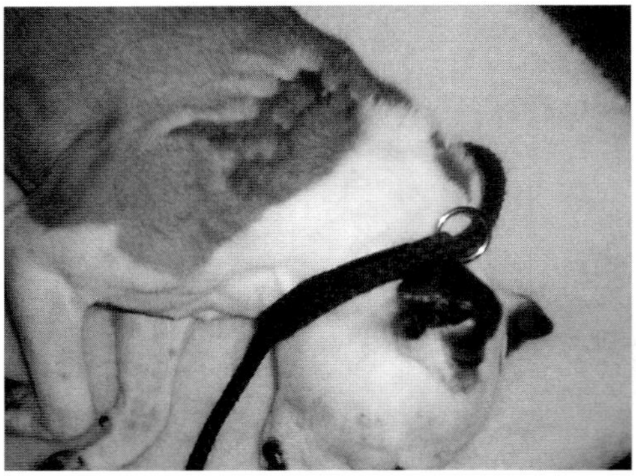

Fig. 23.1. A dog that had been seized and had been in a fight. The owner claimed the wound on its back was due to him accidentally dropping a cup of very hot tea on the dog's back. It was the opinion of the author (David Bailey) that this bite was more likely to have been inflicted by another dog in a fight. The owner pleaded guilty prior to contest. (Copyright David Bailey.)

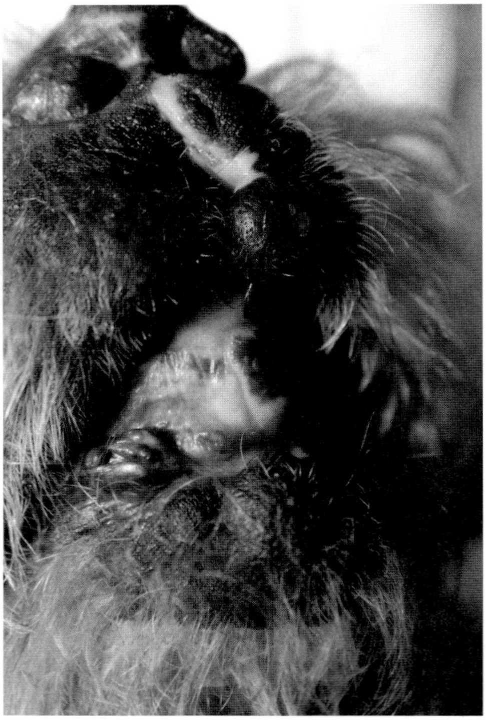

Fig. 23.2. Image of a dog's muzzle that had been de-gloved after being bitten by a badger. The dog in this photo has had most of its bottom lip removed. Badgers have very blunt canine teeth and their bites tend to crush and tear rather than puncture. The microbiology from wounds is also of important evidential value. A bite with anaerobes is likely to be a puncture wound from a sharp canine, whereas a blunt canine tooth injury could return a culture of aerobes. Bitemark analysis as a sole determinant of a badger bite, and therefore of evidence of interfering with a badger could not be determined from this analysis alone and a conviction was not successful against the owner. (Photograph copyright David Bailey.)

An accurate description of the distribution and nature of the injuries is essential. Weiss *et al.* (1998) found that only 30% of dog bite wounds to adults were on the head and neck, whereas 73% of injuries to children were on the face, head and neck. Brogan *et al.* (1995) and De Munnynck and Van de Voorde (2002) also identified this pattern of injuries to children. A veterinarian is *not* entitled to directly examine the injuries to a human or pass expert opinion on such injuries. This is outside of their area of expertise and should be left to suitably qualified medical personnel. A veterinarian can only examine the *images* obtained of any bitemarks on a human. A bitemark may be defined as 'a pattern produced by human or animal dentitions and associated structures in any substance capable of being marked by these means' (Clark, 1992). The importance of bitemarks on a victim's skin, and on inanimate objects connected with a crime scene such as food items, bottle tops and pencils, has long been recognized in human forensic investigations. In 1979 at the trial of the infamous serial killer Theodore 'Ted' Bundy, the correlation between an outline of his front teeth and a bitemark on the left buttock of one of his victims was a pivotal piece of evidence in his conviction and subsequent execution. A forensic odontologist is 'an expert whose knowledge of dental anatomy is made use of within a legal context' (Jackson and Jackson, 2011). Both the British Association for Forensic Odontology (BAFO) and the American Board of Forensic Odontology (ABFO) produce guidance for personnel involved in the photography of such wounds. ABFO recommends that 'when bitemarks are photographed as evidence, attempts are made to carefully control perspective variables in an effort to obtain an accurate representation of the bitemark for later comparative analysis' (ABFO, n.d.).

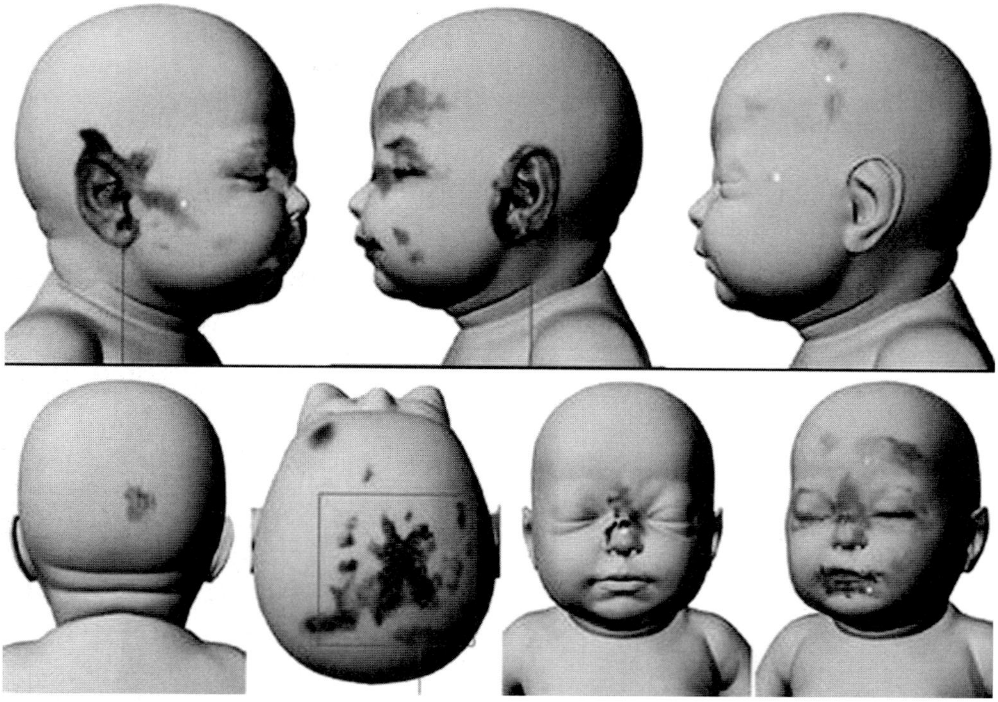

Fig. 23.3. Representations of injuries received by a baby in the UK who had died as a result of injuries received from its carers. Some of the wounds were suspected to have been dog bites. The suspect dog was not able to be examined as the owner had had him destroyed. The lack of neck injuries to the victim was indicative, in this expert's opinion, of the dog having been held by a lead and allowed to attack the face and head and not allowed to kill the baby quickly. Bruises and healing wounds on the victim suggest that the abuse had been long term. (Copyright David Bailey.)

Photography of bite marks and similar types of two- and three-dimensional physical evidence should have the following features (Bowers and Johansen, 2004):

- Presence of a scale (Fig. 23.4) oriented on the same plane as the bitemark.
- The orientation of the camera back and the scale is parallel.
- The scale is on the same plane as the bitemark, thus eliminating parallax distortion. The scale is used to reproduce a life-size image of the object. Its displacement below or above the object will make this later process inaccurate.

Both distant (for orientation) and close-up photographs should be obtained and provided for examination. As long as these are focused,

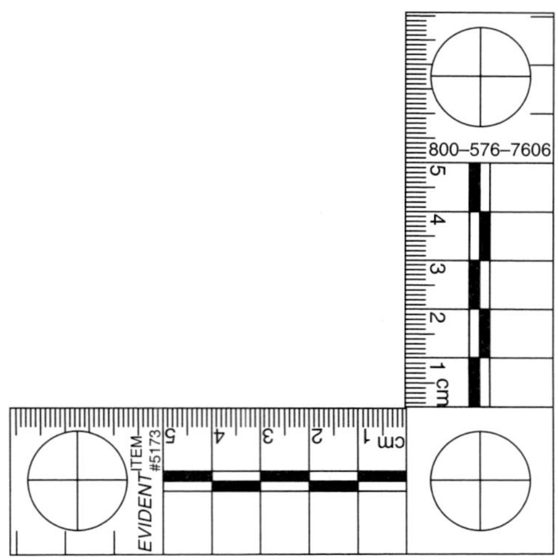

Fig. 23.4. Forensic scale (Copyright S. Drew).

clearly labelled, 1:1 scaled images of the bitemark then they can be used for further analysis.

Human or Canine?

If there is no witness to the injury then it may be necessary to ascertain whether it is a dog (canine) bite. Children may bite themselves or each other and may also be bitten by adults in cases of abuse. The distribution of injuries is again important in this respect. For example, a child is not able to bite themselves on the face or neck and the larger adult human bitemarks found on abused children are more likely to be in a less overt location. Bitemarks to the buttocks and breasts are not uncommon in human sexual assault cases. The anterior portion of the dental arch is much narrower in dogs than in humans and the canine teeth much larger, with a curved and more conical outline (Clark, 1992) (Fig. 23.5).

Lessig *et al.* (2006) describe the characteristic human bite as 'superficial abrasion and/or sub-surface haemorrhage looking like an arch'.

The canine teeth of a dog anchor the victim, while other teeth bite and tear tissues.

De Munnynck and Van de Voorde (2002) suggested that the features to be considered 'pathognomic' for dog bites were:

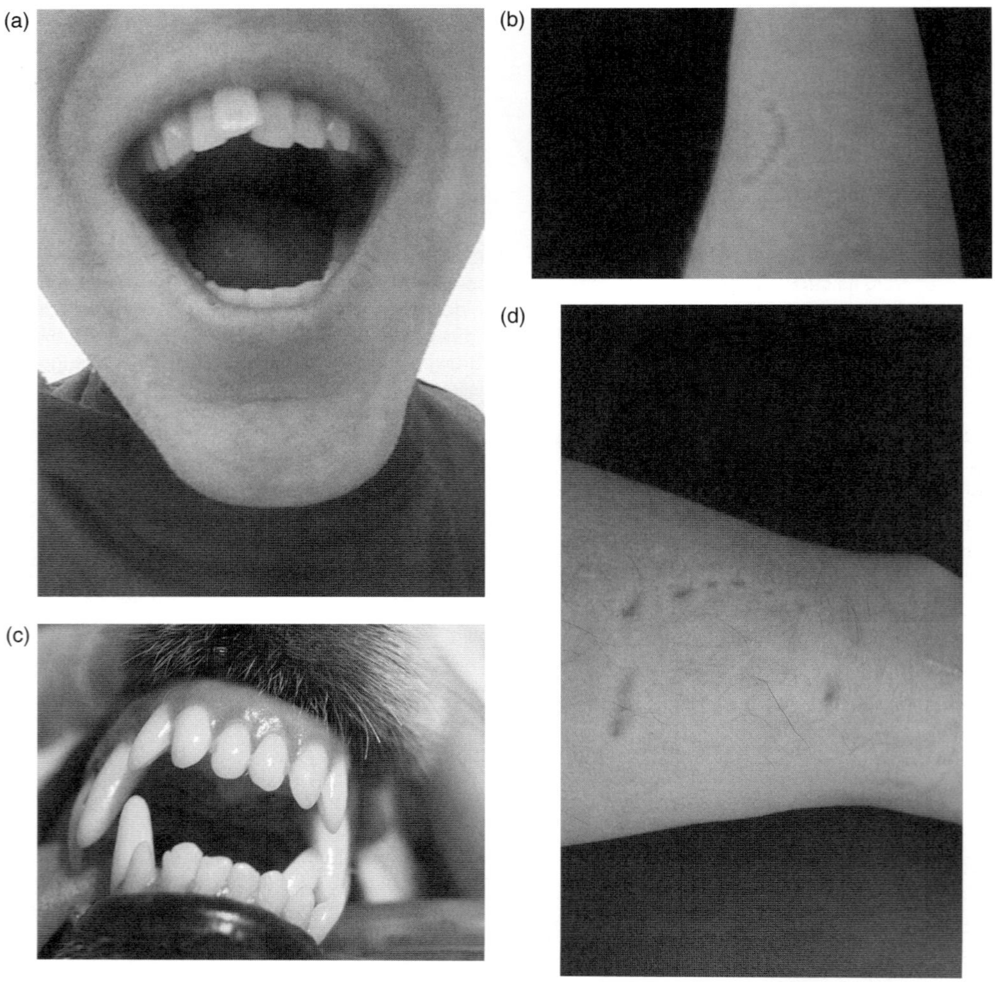

Fig. 23.5. (a) Human dentition and (b) resultant bitemark compared with (c and d) dog. (Copyright S. Drew)

- puncture wound(s)(caused by canine tooth);
- wounds with ragged irregular edges – stretch lacerations (caused by other teeth in the process of biting, shaking and tearing and sometimes including avulsed tissue with irregular borders resembling a dental arch outline); and
- claw marks (multiple, parallel, linear scratches or drying scuff abrasions).

In both humans and dogs the level of violence accompanying the bite, the size/breed of the assailant, the area of the body bitten, the position of the body part at the time of being bitten and the constitution of the skin (e.g. elderly versus young) can all cause distortions and variations to the bitemark, making analysis and interpretation challenging. It may be possible to draw a conclusion that the injury is likely or unlikely to be a dog bite, although it may also be inconclusive. If this is the case, or if the suspected dog is not available for comparative examination, then there would be very little rationale to proceed.

Detailed Examination of the Bitemark

It must be remembered that the image of the bitemark used for analysis shows the bruising, puncture wounds and lacerations made by the teeth. It is *not* an accurate representation of individual teeth. Unique features such as those created by missing teeth, abnormally aligned teeth or damaged teeth form useful reference points. Measurements may also be taken between certain prominent marks, the commonest measurement taken being the inter-canine width (Fig. 23.6) as detailed by Murmann *et al.* (2006) and Tedeschi-Oliveira *et al.* (2011).

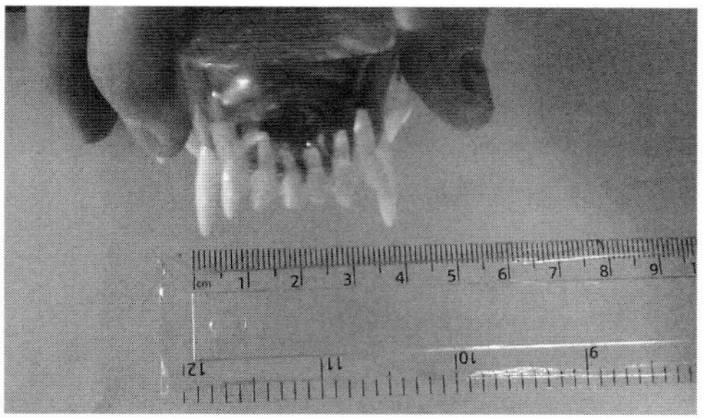

Fig. 23.6. Inter-canine width. (Copyright S. Drew)

Examination of the Dog

The dog is a living piece of evidence (see Chapter 22). It is also an animal with a history of aggression. All appropriate precautions (such as a muzzle and the use of chemical restraint) must be taken to protect personnel involved in the examination while preserving the animal's welfare and following appropriate recording, sampling, handling and storage procedures to preserve the integrity and evidential value of any forensic evidence obtained. A full medical history should be ascertained prior to a thorough physical examination. Has there been any prior history of aggression? Have there been any previous injuries to the dog that may have contributed to its propensity to bite? (Biting may be a defensive response if the dog itself has been a victim of abuse.)

The examination should be performed as soon as possible after the incident. There may be blood and other visible, or trace, evidence from the victim present on the dog. This is more likely in severe and sustained attacks. A sterile swab should be taken from the dog's mouth and appropriately labelled and packaged for DNA analysis by a laboratory capable of analysing both human and canine short tandem repeats (STRs). According to Locard's Principle of Exchange, 'every contact leaves a trace'. The ability to demonstrate the two-way transfer of DNA between the dog and the victim, i.e. the dog's DNA in the wounds of the victim and the victim's DNA in the mouth of the dog, is of greater evidential value than bitemark analysis alone, which is purely comparative. It is of course reliant on a swab of the victim's wounds being taken prior to medical treatment being implemented. Eichmann *et al.* (2004), Tsuji *et al.* (2008) and Clarke and Vandenberg (2010) all document the use of DNA analysis in the forensic investigation of dog bites on humans. When examining the mouth it would be recommended to use a dental chart such as that in Fig. 23.7, along with photographs, to aid the identification and recording of distinguishing features

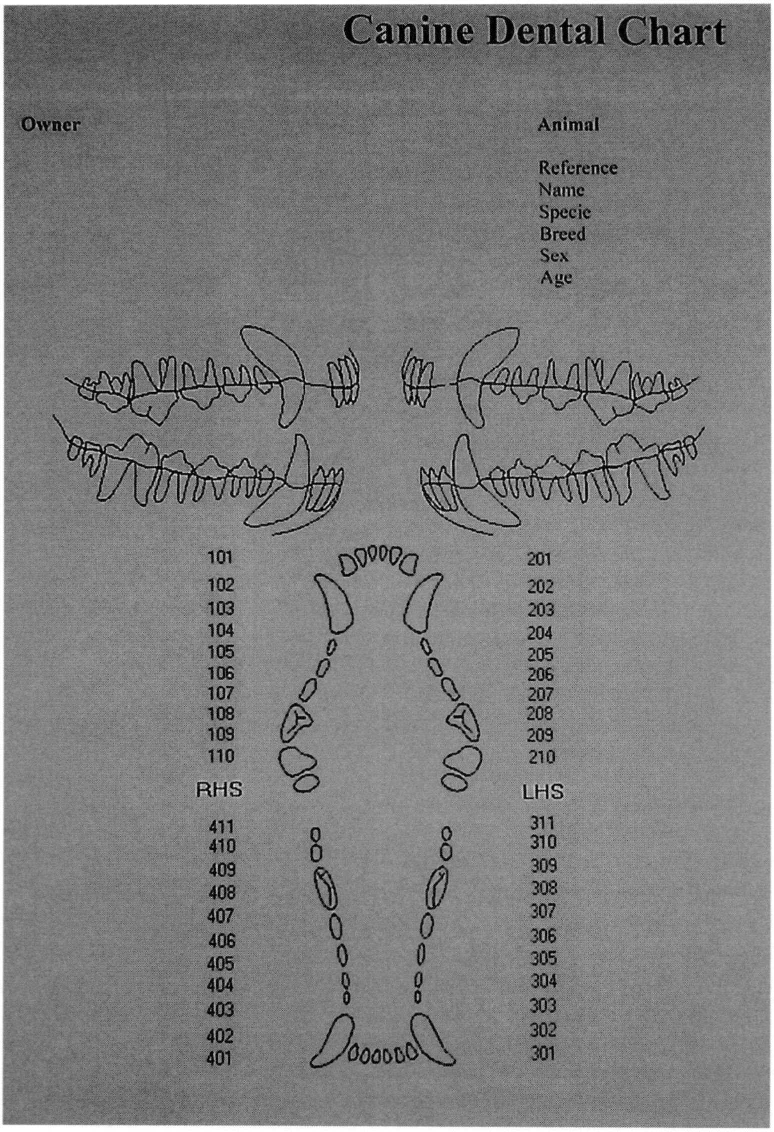

Fig. 23.7. Canine dental chart. (Copyright S. Drew.)

such as missing, broken or misaligned teeth. Impressions taken of the upper and lower dental arcades using plasticine or wax can be photographed, following the same principles already discussed, and computer programs such as Microsoft Paint® or Adobe Photoshop® used to generate images that can be accurately measured and overlaid on to the images of the bitemark from the victim in order to compare them.

Interpretation and Conclusion

The process of bitemark comparison involves the superimposition of a suspect's dentition on the image of the bitemark, the aim being to identify sufficient correspondence between the size and shape of the two patterns to draw a valid, substantiated conclusion. The potential for distortion and inaccuracy during evidence collection and interpretation can render bitemark comparison evidence highly controversial. Bernitz *et al.* (2012) 'warn against over interpretation of poor quality bite marks and a final conclusion of absolute certainty'. Pomara *et al.* (2011) cite evidence from a case where the son of the victim of a fatal dog pack attack was convicted for manslaughter and 'bitemark analysis provided conclusive evidence in identifying the offending animals'. It may be argued that the only truly valid conclusion is one of exclusion, i.e. that an individual was very highly unlikely to have created the bitemark in question. The conclusion that a particular individual was very highly likely to have caused the bitemark may be difficult to achieve and would almost certainly rely on additional forensic evidence such as DNA analysis, as well as the skill and experience of the forensic veterinarian.

References

ABFO (n.d.) Bitemark standards and guidelines. American Board of Forensic Odontology. Available at: http://www.forensic.to/webhome/bitemarks/#ABFO (accessed 8 June 2012).

Bernitz, H., Bernitz, Z., Steenkamp, G., Blumenthal, R. and Stols, G. (2012) The individualisation of a dog bite mark: a case study highlighting the bite mark analysis, with emphasis on differences between dog and human bite marks. *International Journal of Legal Medicine* 126(3), 441–446.

Bowers, C.M. and Johansen, R. (2004) Issues in Human and Animal Bite mark (Bitemark) Analysis. Available at: http://www.forensic.to/webhome/bitemarks/#ABFO Bitemark Terminology Guidelines (accessed 8 June 2012).

Brogan, T.V., Bratton, S.L., Dowd, M.D. and Hegenbarth, M.A. (1995) Severe dog bites in children. *Paediatrics* 96(5 Pt1), 947–950.

Clark, D.H. (ed.) (1992) *Practical Forensic Odontology*. Butterworth Heinemann, Oxford, UK.

Clarke, M. and Vandenberg, N. (2010) Dog attack: the application of canine DNA profiling in forensic casework. *Forensic Science, Medicine, and Pathology* 6, 151–157.

De Munnynck, K. and Van de Voorde, W. (2002) Forensic approach of fatal dog attacks: a case report and literature review. *International Journal of Legal Medicine* 116(5), 295–300.

Eichmann, C., Berger, B., Reinhold, M., Lutz, M. and Parson, W. (2004) Canine-specific STR typing of saliva traces on dog bite wounds. *International Journal of Legal Medicine* 118(6), 337–342.

Jackson, A.R.W. and Jackson, J.M. (2011) Bite Marks. In: *Forensic Science*, 3rd edn. Pearson Education, Harlow, Essex, UK, p. 126.

Lessig, R., Wenzel, V. and Weber, M. (2006) Bite mark analysis in forensic routine case work. *Experimental and Clinical Sciences International Online Journal* 5, 93–102.

Murmann, D.C., Brumit, P.C., Schrader, B.A. and Senn, D.R. (2006) A comparison of animal jaws and bite mark patterns. *Journal of Forensic Science* 51(4), 846–860.

Pomara, C., D'Errico, S., Jarussi, V., Turillazzi, E. and Fineschi, V. (2011) Cave canem: bite mark analysis in a fatal dog pack attack. *American Journal of Forensic Medicine and Pathology* 32(1), 50–54.

Tedeschi-Oliveira, S.V., Trigueiro, M., Oliveira, R.N. and Melani, R.F.H. (2011) Intercanine distance in the analysis of human and domestic dog dental arches. *Journal of Forensic Odontostomatology* 29(1), 30–36.

Tsuji, A., Ishiko, A., Kimura, H., Nurimoto, M., Kudo, K. and Ikeda, N. (2008) Unusual death of a baby: a dog attack and confirmation using human and canine STRs. *International Journal of Legal Medicine* 122, 59–62.

Weiss, H.B., Friedman, D.I. and Coben, J.H. (1998) Incidence of dog bite injuries treated in emergency departments. *Journal of the American Medical Association* 279, 51–53.

Part VI

Interviews with People who Work with Animal Abuse

This section includes interviews with eight people who are involved with animal abuse in various fields around the world, including veterinarians (in practice and a scientific officer in a welfare organization), people working in animal advocacy, law, journalism and campaigning. Providing these interviews highlights the range of people working with a common goal of increasing awareness of animal abuse and alleviating animal suffering.

Interview 1: The Veterinarian

Interview with Andrew Knight PhD, CertAW, MRCVS, FOCAE

Andrew completed his veterinary degree in Western Australia in 2001 and spent nearly a decade practising veterinary medicine, most of it in the UK. He was awarded a Certificate in Animal Welfare Science from the Cambridge E-Learning Institute in 2005 and in 2009 was awarded a Fellowship of the Oxford Centre for Animal Ethics. In 2010 Andrew received a PhD from Australia's Griffith University for a thesis critically analysing the human clinical, toxicological and educational utility of animal experimental models. This expanded to become a book, *The Costs and Benefits of Animal Experiments*, published by Palgrave-Macmillan. In 2011 Andrew became a European Veterinary Specialist in Welfare Science, Ethics and Law, and in 2013 he became an Associate Professor for Animal Welfare and Ethics at Ross University School of Veterinary Medicine, St Kitts, in the Caribbean.

How do you define animal abuse?

Animal abuse has traditionally been understood to include physical acts such as acts of obvious cruelty, or the severe withholding of food. For a long time such acts have been outlawed within the UK and in other countries with animal protection legislation. In 2006, however, the UK's Animal Welfare Act also imposed a duty of care on animal owners, which aims to ensure their animals do not needlessly suffer through neglect. The Act seeks to ensure that animals have a reasonable quality of life. Owners are now arguably required to seek veterinary attention for their animals where warranted, for example.

I agree with this wider definition of animal abuse. It is no longer enough to simply prevent suffering; we must take active steps where these are warranted to ensure our animals are able to enjoy a reasonable quality of life. This includes opportunities for positive experiences, as well. If we keep animals in captivity and prevent them from living lives free of human interference, and we also deny them a reasonable quality of life, I think that constitutes abuse. It is certainly an abuse of our power over them.

It is sometimes argued that animal killing, providing it is conducted humanely, without stress or physical suffering, is ethical, and does not constitute abuse. I disagree. Animals have a broad range of interests they seek to fulfil during their lives. The interest in achieving a state of positive physical and psychological well-being is but one example. Death prevents the achievement of virtually all of the interests important to any animal, and therefore constitutes one of the most profound abuses that may be inflicted.

A rare exception occurs when there is an overwhelming interest in avoiding severe and intractable suffering caused by illness or injury. In this case physical and psychological well-being may be elevated from a profoundly negative to a 'null' state, through death. When humanely performed such killing constitutes genuine *euthanasia*, that is, a 'good death' – one clearly in the animal's best interests.

When did you first become interested in working to prevent animal abuse?

When in my 20s, I started volunteering with human charities, including those working to advance human rights. I briefly volunteered for the Red Cross, the International Campaign to Ban Land Mines and Amnesty International. Whilst working with Amnesty, Kuwait was invaded by Iraq. I read a detailed report about the horrific human rights violations inflicted on the Kuwaitis, and I learnt that such atrocities are inflicted on people around the world by oppressive regimes.

Then I learned that animals suffer similar abuses in intensive farms and laboratories. Similar, at least, in the suffering caused. However, the numbers of animals affected seemed to be millions of times greater. Differences in animal cognitive capacities might possibly have decreased some forms of suffering, but their suffering was hardly millions of times less. Upon realizing this I switched my primary focus to animal issues, because my primary goal is to maximize my impact in decreasing suffering. However, I still support campaigns for human rights and environmental protection.

Who or what inspired you to work in this area?

I think many children are intrinsically compassionate towards animals. When I was 8, my parents gave me a book on baby animals. I looked at the baby deer and other animals and declared to my parents that I was going vegetarian!

Later, I grew up. Now I'm older my interest in animal issues and animal ethics is very strongly based in reason and evidence, rather than emotion, although emotions can be positive too, of course.

What do you find most challenging about your work?

The ideal of being a veterinarian is fantastic – we should be able to make a major difference for animals and their owners. Unfortunately, the reality is often very different. Severe financial limitations of owners, lack of more than a cursory interest in the welfare of their animals, and veterinary practices interested in cutting costs in terms of drugs and equipment in order to maximize profits, combine to markedly limit what we're able to do to assist our patients. This is extremely frustrating and, combined with long hours and unrealistic or unappreciative clients, markedly contributes to the high levels of stress commonly experienced by veterinarians.

What do you find most rewarding about your work?

Those occasions when we really can make a major, positive impact on the welfare of the animals we treat.

How do you cope with the emotional stress of working with abused animals?

Unfortunately, it's inevitable that we become desensitized to a degree to all of the animal suffering we see. When this allows us to function more professionally and therefore effectively, this is a good thing. It's important, however, not to allow this to go too far, which can result in decreasing ethical and animal welfare standards.

When abuse is serious, we're also able to report it to authorities such as the RSPCA.

I think it's very important to try to maintain some balance though, so I also try to take time off after hours, with longer breaks during the year, for travel or other fun activities. This is an area I'd definitely like to work on more!

What advice would you have to others keen to follow your path in working to help stop animal abuse?

It helps to pick perhaps one or two issues that are potentially winnable, and that will provide the greatest positive impacts for animals in return for the time, money and effort you invest. Then you should research your issue, and argue your case, reasonably and rationally.

Additionally, I strongly advise those who are in a position to do so, to consider gaining formal qualifications, thereby becoming a science-based advocate for animals. Good examples are medicine, veterinary medicine, dietetics or environmental science. Law is also brilliant. Such skills increase your knowledge of animal issues, ability to argue scientifically and effectively, and your public credibility. They can also provide the financial means to support both you and your campaigns.

The movement also needs support skills such as IT, graphic design, photography and videography, management, marketing and fundraising.

What do you feel are the biggest animal abuse problems in the world today?

Intensive farming typically involves involuntary confinement, which can be severe, social disruption, a variety of surgical mutilations, often conducted without painkillers or anaesthesia, all followed by a very premature death. Many millions of animals are farmed in these ways. I think intensive farming is perhaps the greatest source of suffering on Earth today, particularly in the case of caged hens and pigs.

How do you feel the UK compares with other countries with how they work to protect animals from abuse?

The UK has a reputation as a 'nation of animal lovers', but the reality for animals is very different. Millions of animals still suffer in intensive farms, laboratories and private homes through neglect.

Within the veterinary profession, it's been said that the UK leads the world in standards of 'compassionate care'. As stated, however, the clinical standards within veterinary practice often fall well below what they should be. The UK may lead simply because we rarely conduct the cosmetic surgeries and convenience 'euthanasias' more common in other countries. Unfortunately, this is not much to be proud of. The UK can, and should, do much better than it does. The same is true of most countries.

Interview 2: The Animal Campaigner

Interview with Jan Creamer

Jan Creamer is the Chief Executive of Animal Defenders International (ADI), an animal advocacy group, which has offices in London, Bogota and Los Angeles.

How did you first get interested in animal advocacy work?

I joined the campaign against animal experiments in 1976, when I was given a leaflet in the street. There had been an exposé in a national newspaper about forcing beagle dogs to inhale cigarette smoke and I had been appalled – a short while afterwards, I met volunteers from the National Anti-Vivisection Society (NAVS) of the UK, and joined to help. I am also Chief Executive of the NAVS (we founded ADI in 1990). I started as a volunteer, and became the society's magazine editor in 1982, becoming Chief Executive in 1986.

What are your background qualifications and training?

Actually my background is very different – graphic design and some copy writing – however, becoming informed about animal rights and the suffering of animals at the hands of humankind was life-changing, not only my planned career path and interests, but lifestyle, too. I came to the conclusion that my chosen career simply did not feel as important as the issues before me.

What does your work involve?

Public speaking, writing, lobbying, strategy, media, investigations, animal rescues, relocating animals and educational campaigns to push forward human understanding about the other species that share our planet and change our thinking, as a species. We are unusual in that we are a holistic organization covering all dimensions of a campaign; we can take an issue from initial research and investigation through to public awareness and then legislation – we enjoy the challenge of seeing things through.

I have photographed horrific suffering in laboratories, circuses, slaughterhouses and other places and feel that it is important, where possible, for a Chief Executive to maintain that connection with the issues we are trying to address and the drive that comes with that understanding.

Our recent work in Bolivia highlights many aspects of our work. There had been no undercover investigations of animal circuses in South America, so we embedded a team in the industry for almost 2 years. They worked in many circuses and even followed them from one country to another. We filmed a nightmare world: elephants, lions and tigers being punched, kicked and beaten, dogs being beaten with metal bars, an elderly chimpanzee being beaten with a chain. We compiled all the evidence into a detailed empirical and scientific report, with videos from each country. We do that work in-house in our offices in London – we are lucky in that our Campaigns Director, Tim Phillips, is a professional video maker. We then launched our report and videos in Bolivia, Brazil, Colombia, Ecuador, Peru and later Chile. We followed up with massive awareness campaigns, engaging the public, persuading local authorities to ban animal circuses, which led to proposals for new laws in Bolivia, Brazil, Peru, Colombia and Chile. The first to be passed was Bolivia (followed in 2011 by Peru).

The Bolivian authorities then asked for help with enforcement of the new law. After all, this is the next question for all governments – what do we do with the animals? One circus handed its animals over immediately, another defied the ban and lobbied others to defy. We tracked down every circus and raided them with government wildlife officials, rescuing every animal. We set up a temporary field station in Santa Cruz where we had to nurse 25 lions back to health ready for relocation. In total we flew 29 lions to the USA – 25 in one airlift, the biggest of its kind ever. In the USA we've provided them with enclosures of up to 25 acres of natural savanna-type habit with underground dens. We also ensured that the lions were kept in natural family groups, with up to eight in a pride. So in addition to what is the most effective governmental enforcement operation of its kind ever, we've also been involved in raising the bar on how captive wild animals should be housed.

It was very satisfying to have the opportunity to see things through from start to finish.

Who or what inspired you to get involved in this area?

Although the writings of Singer, Beddow Bayly, Ryder, Melville and Johnson helped to consolidate my thoughts, the spur for me, originally, was the 'smoking beagles' story and the exposure of the government-led cloak of secrecy on animal experiments. Once I started studying the subject in more detail, I resolved to take action; but nothing drives me more than the suffering that I have seen, the grim reality is that millions upon millions of animals suffer daily and it does not have to be that way. I photographed a monkey called Elisa in a laboratory in London. She'd had bolts and metal plates screwed into her head, and her large hands were reaching out, as if imploring for mercy. The images I took have been used all over the world to engage people and give them an understanding of life and death for laboratory animals. Nothing can drive you more than to look into these animals' eyes. Ultimately this is not a purely academic or philosophical exercise, it is about identifying suffering and finding a way to end it.

What do you find most challenging about your work?

Getting the truth to people and changing minds; the enormous amount of work that needs to be done and our lack of resources – we are changing the world and our team is small. However, it is important not to let the size of the task overwhelm or deter us – our opposition is mostly rich and powerful industries and sometimes individuals with a vested interest in using animals – this makes it all the more important for us to keep moving forwards, success is now inevitable. It is obviously very distressing when we are confronted with animal suffering, but probably the hardest thing to cope with is having to keep going when you are continually being frustrated. We have to constantly deal with misinformation and even downright lies – we will film a circus beating an animal and they will simply deny it is them or claim it is actors employed by ADI; sometimes their extreme statements are quite ludicrous. Politically, we have to contend with enormous frustrations. For example, wild animals in circuses in the UK, where there has been overwhelming support for a ban for a decade – every time you get close there seems to be another reason for a delay. We expose shocking violence in a British circus and during the public and media furore action is promised, then the outcry dies down and there is delay after delay followed by – nothing. Then a year or two years later, we release film of another elephant chained down and being beaten, and again we are promised action. The biggest challenge? You just have to keep going.

How do you cope with the emotional stress of the work?

We experience extreme highs and extreme lows; the ebb and flow of political and social change swirls around us constantly. There are moments when we see animals we have rescued walk free after we have taken them from hell, or when we secure a major piece of legislation such as ending cosmetics testing on animals in Europe, or getting animal circuses banned in a country; you have to hold on to those moments. And when you are confronted by terrible suffering, that must be a driver, too. One has to hold on to the goal – the determination to succeed. Winning saves lives.

What advice would you have to others keen to follow your path in working to help stop animal abuse?

My best advice would be to always remember that this is a life that makes a difference. Hang on to that. This is the most challenging work in the world, intellectually, emotionally and even sometimes, physically. We have to provide expert evidence on a whole range of subjects. Pushing at the boundaries of society's preconceptions and self-interest will always be tough, but the rewards are incredible. Not financial, but deeply satisfying and rewarding when a sea change in human perceptions takes place – it could be in the way our species views another, or a legal change to protect animals, or a change of attitude or habits. And always to remember that the social change that is taking place now, means that success is inevitable. How hard we work is what makes the difference between sooner or later.

It is certainly not for the faint-hearted and requires determination and resilience – but these do actually grow from the challenges on the way.

Interview 3: The Animal Welfare Lawyer

Interview with Jed Goodfellow

Jed's work in animal protection started when he became a volunteer animal attendant at an RSPCA shelter. Later, he worked as a cruelty inspector for 5 years with the RSPCA, before qualifying as a lawyer. Currently, he works for RSPCA Australia in animal welfare policy and is undertaking a PhD in animal welfare regulation within the agricultural sectors.

When you were working as a cruelty inspector, did you ever find it hard, the things you would see and be confronted with?

Yes, all the time, especially the first 6 months or so, not being exposed to that cruelty in the past, you'd often see pictures on TV or the Internet but to see it in person is quite confronting. To deal with the people who commit the crimes was very confronting as well. In many cases they could be quite defensive or aggressive. But after a number of months of being exposed to it your emotions adapt and learn to deal with it. I guess you never get completely desensitized to it but there is I think a process of desensitization at work. As long as you are conscious of the fact that you're perhaps being slightly desensitized to what you're seeing and you still act in the same way as when you first started, i.e. you recognize how shocking the neglect or abuse is and you act accordingly, then I don't think there is any detriment to becoming slightly desensitized. Actually, I think it enables you to be more professional about your duties, to be able to concentrate on doing your job, gathering evidence and enforcing the legislation.

Was there one thing that inspired you to start volunteering, becoming an inspector and going into law?

I was getting interested in animal welfare from around the age of 16 but couldn't conceptualize why I was interested. I saw certain advertisements from organizations like the World Society for the Protection of Animals with their bear bile and dancing bear campaigns and that really struck a chord with me. I didn't know why at that stage but now I rationalize it as being an issue of injustice. That's the sole reason why I'm interested in animal protection – I see it as an issue of social justice.

How do you cope or how did you cope with emotionally distressing things you have encountered in your work?

Now I work in policy I don't really have the same confrontations out in the field. The confrontations I have now are different in nature, we deal with people from agribusiness industries who are seeking to oppose the animal welfare law reforms that we are seeking to introduce basically on economic grounds. That's confronting also because it's animal abuse in a very conscious way, because they are essentially prioritizing commercial considerations above animal welfare considerations. When I was an inspector, I dealt with it purely by knowing that the law was there, even though in some respects it was deficient, it was still there to enable me to either prevent further harm from occurring to that particular animal or if the harm had already occurred, it provided a mechanism for seeking justice for that particular animal or animals. So knowing there was that legislative framework in place to provide options for dealing with certain situations gave me the ability to deal with the confronting things I was seeing. Very rarely were there situations where you couldn't do anything. The legislation's designed to enable inspectors to be able to deal with all sorts of scenarios, whether they are very minor animal welfare incidences or very serious. Emotionally, in terms of psychological issues, I really didn't have any issues ... Occasionally you would go home and think about a certain case at night and that would be distressing, but I developed an ability to be able to switch off essentially, when I finished my shifts. I think when inspectors get too involved in their cases and continually think about the suffering they are witnessing out of work hours that can be really detrimental to their health. So, I guess it's just developing those mental abilities to be able to separate your personal life from your professional life.

Did you find your family and friends didn't want to hear about your day at work?

I never bring it up proactively. I guess part of my switching off at the end of the day is that I don't think about it and don't bring it up in conversation. Unless it was a particularly interesting case or something unusual happened. But I do get that reaction quite often. Actually, it's funny because a lot of people will ask you (after you tell them you were a cruelty inspector) 'What is your worst animal cruelty case you've ever seen?' and then when you go to tell them they say 'I don't want to hear any more details!' so it certainly shocks other people who haven't been exposed to those sort of things.

Did the inspectors ever talk to each other about things to get things off their chest?

Yes, in an informal way. When I was an inspector there wasn't any formal process of debriefing or psychological counselling offered. I think there may be now. When I was an inspector it was just dealt with informally. I think most inspectors were able to cope quite well with what they were seeing, after a number of months of getting used to it. Just a general chat in the office after work, after the shift, was all that happened in my experience.

What do you think is the biggest animal abuse problem in the world today?

Certainly the development of intensive farming methods in developing countries, the development of factory farming in India and China, especially with the growing meat consumption levels in those countries, particularly in China. And also, the inadequate animal protection legislation that they have in those countries, again especially China. Factory farming is a big enough issue in developed countries but I think there is a pathway forward for essentially phasing out intensive farming in developed countries but at the moment I don't think there is a clear pathway to doing the same in developing countries. I think that will certainly be the biggest animal welfare issue for many, many years to come unfortunately, simply because of the numbers involved, the duration of the suffering and therefore the quantity of their suffering.

Interview 4: The District Attorney

Interview with Diane Balkin

Diane graduated from law school in Colorado, USA in 1977 and since 1979 has worked at the Office of the Denver District Attorney. Diane is now Chief Deputy District Attorney (trial attorney). Her work includes handling all investigations and prosecutions of state-level crimes against animals; liaison to all agencies and the media for crimes against animals and she is also Director of the Juvenile Court Division and the Family Violence Unit. In July 2011 Diane joined the Animal Legal Defence Fund as a Contract Attorney. She provides resources to prosecutors, animal control officers, law enforcement, judges and veterinarians nationwide in cases involving animal cruelty, neglect, hoarding and fighting.

When did you first become interested in working to prevent animal abuse?

I have always been an animal lover and have dedicated my professional career to be an advocate for all types of victims. In 2000 I volunteered to investigate allegations against a local disc jockey who solicited listeners to bring an animal into the radio station for a contest. He arranged to have a chicken thrown from a balcony to see if it could fly. The ground was frozen and the chicken survived the first round. He then had the chicken taken up to a balcony on a floor that was higher. The chicken survived with minor injuries. After a full investigation I decided to file animal cruelty charges against him. He was convicted by a jury.

I then began studying the link between cruelty to animals and violence towards humans. I also handled local investigations and prosecutions of serious animal cruelty and abuse cases.

I was appointed by the Governor of Colorado to serve as a public member on the Colorado State Board of Veterinary Medicine. I served for 8 years and created close relationships with the veterinary community.

I have also been very active in legislative issues to try to strengthen our cruelty laws and to further protect animals and humans.

Who or what inspired you to get involved in this area?

I have always been inspired by the 'underdog' – the victim that cannot speak for itself or themselves.

What have you found most challenging about your work?

Changing the attitudes of individuals who minimize the seriousness of crimes involving animals. It is also challenging to find any type of financing to assist in cruelty investigations and prosecution.

How do you cope with any emotional stress of the work?

By concentrating on the victories and knowing you have not only saved one animal but may be saving other animals and humans.

What advice would you have to others keen to follow your path of becoming a district attorney?

I have been so fortunate to have had a career path that has been challenging, fulfilling and never boring. Also, the advancements that I have seen and experienced in (veterinary) forensics have been very exciting.

What do you feel are the biggest animal abuse problems in the world today?

Changing long-held attitudes. Some of my greatest challenges have been in the law enforcement community. They resist change and often minimize the seriousness of these crimes.

What could be done about this and how can people help prevent animal abuse?

Education!

A key to all types of crime prevention is education, intervention and collaboration. It takes a community to make a change.

How do you feel the USA compares with other countries with how you protect animals from abuse?

We have made measurable progress in the short time that I have been involved with these types of cases. It has been based on baby steps but there has been progress none the less.

Even within the USA enforcement and attitudes vary greatly. Also one has to take into consideration local religions and cultures.

What is your definition of 'animal abuse'?

I tend to feel that animal abuse and cruelty includes most any form of neglect or mistreatment of any creature. Of course, the seriousness can vary greatly and would also vary depending on the perpetrator's intent at the time. It can encompass anything from act to omission, from teasing to torture and from accidental to premeditated.

Interview 5: The Animal Advocate

Interview with Carol J. Adams

Carol J. Adams is an animal advocate and the author of many books, including *The Sexual Politics of Meat: A Feminist-Vegetarian Critical Theory*.

What inspired you to want to help prevent abuse to animals?

I grew up with horses and ponies and one day my pony was shot ... When I was eating a hamburger, I thought 'This is from a dead cow, I would not eat Jimmy, I would not eat this pony which is lying dead, aren't I a hypocrite? Is it only animals I don't know that I'll eat?' This raised so many questions for me, I was already a feminist but I knew I had to become a vegetarian.

Once you start opening yourself up to animals and realizing what kind of connections existed, my gosh, how much is going on? It just keeps growing, so I became a vegetarian but then it became obvious that vegetarian doesn't cover the issue of dairy and eggs and I became vegan and that if I cared about animals that were being consumed then wouldn't I be concerned about animals that were being experimented upon, animals in zoos, animals in circuses, so I guess the way my mind works is to make connections and I just kept finding that the way we treat animals is unacceptable and we have to protect them. That's why I became aware of animal issues.

You've mentioned about people having 'traumatic knowledge' (regarding knowledge of animal abuse). How do you cope with your 'traumatic knowledge' and how do you recommend others (such as vets) can cope with their 'traumatic knowledge'?

Well, I think some days are better than others. I think people are afraid to care about or learn about what's happening to animals because they are afraid their grief will kill them or paralyse them. I think one thing we need to do is show people that grief doesn't kill us, we live with a grief every day about what's going on but it doesn't paralyse us, it doesn't destroy our spirit, it actually allows us to be more connected to the world. The people who are afraid close themselves off. Their feeling that's dominating their life is fear of feeling connected, which is sort of paradoxical in many ways. So, one of the things I did was to start writing prayers. We started taking care of homeless bunnies here in Dallas and when this one bunny died, I had nursed her since she was little, I could hold her in my hand, she was so small when she came into our lives and it took a lot of care to nurture her and when she died I was so heartbroken. After that, I started writing a prayer a day to work with my own feelings and grief and that was very helpful. So I think one way you deal with traumatic knowledge is this is what we have to experience, because animals give us so much. Animals are a part of our lives and they give us so much, all they ask for us to do is to engage with their lives and we do that even though it is a very wrenching experience. So I think of traumatic knowledge, it's a knowledge that not to act is worse than acting, even though acting is painful.

What advice would you have for others who want to help the animals and stop animal abuse?

There are personal, political, organizational and theoretical things that have to be done and we need to identify our strengths. In identifying our strengths we should never fragment ourselves. Being a vegan is a part of it, being a vegan isn't enough, but being a vegan is a way of saying, 'OK, I'm not going to participate in what I can control', there's a lot more that can be done. Organizationally, we try and support groups that are doing the kind of change work we believe in. It can be small things like taking towels to animal shelters, checking with animal shelters about what they need. Then there's systemic change and we have to decide which groups are working for the kind of systemic change we want and how can we help them. Then there's theoretical change, always calling the media for failing to understand an issue. All of those things we could be doing, it's like taking awareness to the next level, creating a whole aura of what awareness means as I go through my life.

What do you feel are the biggest animal abuse problems in the world today?

With any individual animal, the biggest abuse issue is what's happening to them, to any individual animal. So, for circus elephants the biggest abuse issue is what's happening to them. I think abuse is something that is experienced at a very individual level and we always have to be aware of all the ramifications of labelling or conceptualizing something but all that said, I think animal abuse through animal agriculture is huge.

How would you define animal abuse yourself?

Actions or treatment that impede an animal's ability to move or to live in a way that is integral to who they are. Harm or injury to animals that are in one way or another dependent on you, harm or injury to animals that can't escape, harm or injury to animals who, because of social situations, allow you to act against them with impunity and specifically harm or injury to an animal because our society places them in tenuous situations where they are unable to protect themselves and nobody else is protecting them either.

Do you think the shared experience of abuse (between battered women and their abused companion animals) means that some women are more compassionate toward animals and more closely bonded to them?

I think there is a very good potential for that and I think it is not always realized. In one of my articles I talk about a woman whose husband was choking her and suddenly she realized 'He says he loves me and yet he wants to kill me' and he had his hands around her neck and she thought 'and I say I love animals and yet I'm eating them'. So that was a moment of profound illumination for her. So, she got up, she was able to escape him, he did not kill her and she went and started a vegan-vegetarian society. I think the recognition of the way animals are harmed in battering really provides a way for us to think about how dominance works. The kind of dominance and control that is used against an individual woman or disenfranchised person in abusive behaviour. That kind of controlling behaviour isn't specific only to batterers, I think it is politically enacted as well. It's a sign that they really recognize how connected we are, it's a perverse sign and it's a cruel sign and again that's another example of traumatic knowledge, working around domestic violence. Judith Herman, who wrote this great book called *Trauma and Recovery*, said there's no bystanders to violence, you are either standing with the victim or you are standing with the perpetrator. There's no bystanders. A bystander, by definition is standing with the perpetrator. So, back to traumatic knowledge, at least we know who we're standing with. We know that we have to take a stand against the perpetrator and that should be empowering.

You know, we might need to cry every day or every week.

Twenty years ago we started a programme to teach domestic violence shelters to help animal activists in our community create a foster care for animals so that battered women leaving, we would foster their animals and they could get out of the shelter because there wasn't anything in the States at that point and that was Feminists for Animal Rights. But another woman and I went to this huge conference in Texas and we led this workshop around harm to animals, there were maybe eight or nine women who worked in domestic violence shelters and we were all crying by the end because of the stories of what had happened to the animals and here these women had seen awful, awful things, but there's something about the complete vulnerability of the animals who, you know ... one story was about this woman who was running out of the house to try to survive and just then the little dachshund ran out and the batterer stepped on it. We all cried. We were all crying by the end. And I felt like we provided an opportunity that had never been provided before. It's not as though those experiences had not happened. It's that we had never created a space to discuss those experiences happening and that's traumatic knowledge. To avoid traumatic knowledge is to avoid acknowledging that it already exists out there. How do we help? So that goes back to naming and challenging.

The whole point is that to get batterers to stop being abusive ... the insight by Mike Jackson that this is the area that batterers didn't want to acknowledge, that they harmed animals, because it showed how controlling they were. How could they defend: 'so I walked inside, I got the gun, I walked outside, I called the dog and I shot the dog'? All the steps show how deliberate the battering is, the control is. So, it exposes the lie that battering is about impulse control or battering is about anger. All the lies about battery. When you look at what happens in one of these battering situations it really makes clear the controlling behaviour and this is why batterers would not want to have that too closely examined.

Interview 6: The RSPCA Scientific Officer

Interview with Jade Norris[1]

Dr Jade Norris is a veterinarian who graduated with a Bachelor of Veterinary Science, First Class Honours from the University of Sydney. After graduating, Jade worked as a small animal veterinarian in clinical practice for 5 years. Currently, Jade is a scientific officer with RSPCA Australia.

What does your work involve?

I do the science research that underpins RSPCA policies, positions and campaigns.

My job also involves providing advice to the public and other stakeholders, media work, reviewing policy documents and representing the RSPCA on various committees.

When did you first become interested in working to prevent animal abuse?

I was 18 and in my first year of university when I was first exposed to intensive farming practices. It was a great shock to see the poor conditions the animals were kept in. That was the catalyst for wanting to work on big picture animal welfare issues.

Who or what inspired you to get involved in this area?

Animals are the main inspiration and the many people who genuinely care about the welfare of animals.

What have you found most challenging about your work?

There are many challenges but the rewards far outweigh any of the challenges.

[1] Jade preferred to answer some of the questions using the word 'welfare' rather than 'abuse'.

How do you cope with any emotional stress of the work?

I focus on the positives. Animal welfare science is a growing field and there are a lot of steps forward taking place to improve the welfare of animals, which is heartening.

What advice would you have to others keen to follow your path of becoming a scientific officer for a welfare group?

The more people interested in working to improve the welfare of animals, the better.

If you're genuinely interested and passionate about animal welfare then you'll likely find work in the field if you persevere. If you follow your interests in work you will be naturally rewarded.

Keep an eye out for job opportunities and research what sort of qualifications and career pathways are usually associated with this type of work.

How can others help to improve the welfare of animals?

Many things can be done to improve the welfare of animals and to prevent the suffering of animals.

The main areas include:

- Community awareness and education – becoming informed is a great catalyst for positive change and improvements in animal welfare.
- Legislation to ensure animals are protected.
- Engaging with key stakeholders (e.g. industry and government) to bring about positive change and improvements in animal welfare.

Interview 7: The Waterbird Campaigner

Interview with Laurie Levy

The Coalition Against Duck Shooting (CADS) was started by Laurie in 1985. The first year they went out to the wetlands in Victoria (Australia) was at the opening of the 1986 duck-shooting season and there were only 15 rescuers going out against 100,000 duck shooters.

What is your background – did you work with animals prior to starting the Coalition Against Duck Shooting?

I'm a television camera person. I was at Channel 9 for most of my working life, I just decided to go out and work on issues I believed in.

In the 1970s, I campaigned with Project Jonah to protect whales in Australian waters, which was done by the federal government in 1980. Then we started rescuing stranded whales in 1981. This led to the establishment of the Whale Rescue Centre and to state and national whale rescue plans. And I worked on the Greenpeace campaign in 1986 to ban high sea driftnets in Australian waters, which was put into federal law later that year.

The media has been our major weapon.

What we've been able to do over the last 25 years is reduce the number of duck shooters in Victoria through public opinion from 100,000 in 1986 down to around 20,000 today. This represents only about 0.4% of the state's population. Also, a Roy Morgan Poll commissioned in 2007 showed that at least three out of four Victorians want duck shooting to be banned.

We've also seen duck shooting banned in three states, Western Australia in 1990, New South Wales in 1995 and Queensland in 2005.

What inspired you to get involved to help the waterbirds?

I just thought it was an injustice. When we first went out (to the wetlands) all the media came out and birds were falling out of the sky everywhere ... duck shooting was all about brutality, it was about violence, shooting birds out of the sky and killing and maiming native waterbirds. What we did that was different was taking out a mobile veterinary clinic so for the first time ever, wounded birds were picked up by our rescuers and taken to the mobile veterinary clinic where they were treated on the spot, on the wetlands by bird vets. And that's how it all started ... so suddenly there was a new component, a very simple component added to duck shooting and that was duck rescue and *caring* for our beautiful native waterbirds. Looking after the wounded. I've always seen our role as being similar to the Red Cross, we go into a war zone to help the innocent victims.

I've heard that one of the rescuers got shot and injured in the face, does that happen very often?

That is the first time in 25 years. That was at the opening of the duck shooting season in 2011. It was at 9.20am, virtually 2 hours after the opening of the season that a rescuer was shot in the face. Thankfully the pellets missed her eyes. The rescuer had about 15 pellets lodged in her face, and was taken to hospital. She has recovered now but the trauma is probably still there because it would take a long time to get over. This year all rescuers will be forced to wear safety goggles or face masks to protect their eyes, although you can't buy safety glasses or goggles that will stand up to a shotgun blast. However, they will protect rescuers if pellets are bouncing off the water or if they're at the end of the range of the shotgun.

(Catherine: After the interview we managed to obtain military ballistic safety goggles for rescuers, the same goggles that Australia's ground forces use overseas.)

How many vets and nurses work in the mobile vet hospitals?

Two or three vets and four or five vet nurses – they do a fantastic job because often what happens is the birds receive immediate first aid treatment, then they come back to Melbourne where they can be X-rayed and operated on and they go to wildlife carers for 2 or 3 months or however long as needed before they can be released in the wild again.

What do you find keeps you going in this work? It must be really stressful watching all this suffering all the time.

A lot of our rescuers find it traumatic because it's not easy for sensitive people to see beautiful native waterbirds blown out of the sky. And that level of brutality inflicted on them for no reason other than duck shooters like shooting live targets. Often, you'll see a bird flying over by itself and you'll have guns going off and once they hit it, all the shooters will cheer at the same time. So, this bird that's obviously suffering enormous pain and shock falls out of the sky and the shooters will be laughing. It's that type of incident that keeps our rescuers going. We thought about not going out this year after a rescuer was shot in the face last year, but without our rescue teams out there, there'd be nobody out there helping the birds. So, we have to be out there, we don't have a choice. And we can't walk away from their plight.

Is it mainly men who go shooting?

It is mainly. It's always very much been a male, macho activity and in fact when we first went out to the wetlands, 50–70% of our rescue team would be women and shooters had trouble accepting women out on the wetlands. They thought the wetlands were male territory only. They were also sexist in reverse because they couldn't understand males being out there in the rescue team, caring about and feeling emotions towards those birds. They didn't understand that. So, on one hand they couldn't understand women having the courage to be out there and they couldn't understand males being out there because they kept saying males did the killing and they shouldn't feel any empathy for the birds and they shouldn't be concerned or upset about the brutality that they inflict on the birds. So, it was a double-edged sword.

What advice would you have to others who are keen to help these wild birds?

If they want to join CADS they can go to the website www.duck.org.au and there's a volunteer page where they can sign up and join the rescue team. They can also write to (the relevant politician) and tell him or her they want the recreational shooting of native waterbirds banned and that this sort of brutality and violence is unacceptable in this day and age and it has to come to an end.

Interview 8: The Television Journalist

Interview with Sarah Ferguson

Sarah Ferguson is a journalist with the Australian Broadcasting Corporation who was part of the Gold Walkley award-winning Four Corners team who exposed cruelty to cattle in the Australian live cattle export trade. Broadcast of the animal cruelty in May 2011 resulted in the suspension of the live cattle export trade from Australia to Indonesia.

When I saw the broadcast of your story (of the cruelty to cattle slaughtered in Indonesia), I thought that must have been so harrowing to be there, I'd love to hear what your experiences were ...

Well, in a strange way, actually not so harrowing in the end. We do see a lot of harrowing things. I just wouldn't choose the word harrowing, I've seen harrowing things, we saw some terrible things. Let me just explain, when we first saw footage of what was going on in Indonesia I couldn't look at the screen, I am squeamish and some of the images were so distressing I had to look away or fidget with my pen or take my eye of the screen at the key moment. When we got to Indonesia, I thought, this will be interesting, but it's just sort of work takes over and you just have to get on with it so you do.

Do you think seeing some footage beforehand helped get you used to what you might be seeing?

Not really. I think in some ways, it's a weird thing but the act of being in a place where you have to do a job is so overpowering in terms of concentration that there just isn't time for anything else, you just have to do it. So, in some ways watching footage is worse than actually watching the real thing, oddly. There were moments when I got frustrated, our producer and I turned to each other at one point watching an animal crashing down on a concrete slope and particularly because the design of the (restraint) boxes in those abattoirs which the Australian (meat) industry has put in were so bad it was so frustrating to watch that happening because this wasn't just a matter of ingrained ignorance, this was something that a sophisticated country had spent money installing. Each time we saw an animal crash down and smash its head that was one of the things I found most difficult because it was just such a poor piece of work and so avoidable, to have that unnecessary suffering added into the picture.

Did you ever feel you wanted to run forward and shout at the abattoir staff or stop them?

Not shout ... I've thought that in other stories but not that case. I think in this case what we were seeing was so much a part of the process, i.e. that it was so much part of what they were used to doing, that they'd accepted it was the right thing to do, that the process seemed to be set, it's not like seeing something in the street that happens spontaneously, this is something that had been trained (albeit badly), but none the less, this was a *modus operandi* that was well established. So in fact it didn't have that effect on me that I wanted to lean over and stop it.

Do you think animal cruelty scenes will ever be too shocking to be displayed to the public at home?

There are lots of people who couldn't watch our story and in a sense there was a limit to what we could show. We showed an awful lot and it was much too much for lots of the audience, but we had 20 hours of material. We certainly couldn't show all of that in one go, even if you had a programme that was that long. There were certain scenes that were so grotesque that went on and on and on where there is a point when you're watching something where as a viewer you just say 'Stop it! You don't need to keep showing me that, I get it' and they get annoyed. There was a particular scene that Lyn White from Animals Australia had filmed of a very, very poor animal that had fallen over and broken its leg and the worker was trying to get it to move and make it stand up so they kicked it, they beat it, they forced water up its nose, they put their fingers in its eyes, gouged deep into its eye sockets, broke its tail, just 20 minutes of torture. In the original version of that we showed more of it and we all decided on viewing that we had to do what we would call 'cut away', so that we would go back to Lyn White talking about it in interview and we just shifted the amount of time we spent on Lyn away from the animal in the second version, in the fine cut, because it was just too relentless. So, yes, there is a limit, there's a point where people get cross, they've got it and they don't want to see it anymore.

Do your personal feelings towards animals make it easier or harder to work on this sort of story?

I don't think they change it. I hope I have an evolved person's view that any cruelty or unkindness to animals is unacceptable. I think anything short of that is a sickness in a human being. I eat meat but cruelty without purpose or through carelessness is not acceptable in any way. I would regard that as a universal view of any civilized country.

What do you see as the media's role in educating people about animal cruelty issues?

It's just essential. One of the most important consequences of this programme was that it really did change the paradigm, it made animal welfare occupy a more prominent role in the national debate than it ever has. I think it's changed it forever, just pushed it into the mainstream in a place that it wasn't before and it means that other stories on the same subject get more attention than they did before.

Appendix 1: The Glasgow Composite Pain Scale

The Short Form Composite Measure Pain Score (CMPS-SF) can be applied quickly and reliably in a clinical setting and has been designed as a clinical decision-making tool, which was developed for dogs in acute pain. It includes 30 descriptor options within six behavioural categories, including mobility. Within each category, the descriptors are ranked numerically according to their associated pain severity and the person carrying out the assessment chooses the descriptor within each category that best fits the dog's behaviour/condition. It is important to carry out the assessment procedure as described on the questionnaire, following the protocol closely. The pain score is the sum of the rank scores. The maximum score for the six categories is 24, or 20 if mobility is impossible to assess. The total CMPS-SF score has been shown to be a useful indicator of analgesic requirement and the recommended analgesic intervention level is 6/24 or 5/20.

SHORT FORM OF THE GLASGOW COMPOSITE PAIN SCALE

Dog's name ______________________________

Hospital Number __________ **Date** / / **Time**

Surgery Yes/No (delete as appropriate)

Procedure or Condition______________________________

____

In the sections below please circle the appropriate score in each list and sum these to give the total score.

A. Look at dog in Kennel

Is the dog?

(i)		(ii)	
Quiet	0	Ignoring any wound or painful area	0
Crying or whimpering	1	Looking at wound or painful area	1
Groaning	2	Licking wound or painful area	2
Screaming	3	Rubbing wound or painful area	3
		Chewing wound or painful area	4

In the case of spinal, pelvic or multiple limb fractures, or where assistance is required to aid locomotion do not carry out section **B** and proceed to **C**
Please tick if this is the case ☐ then proceed to C.

B. Put lead on dog and lead out of the kennel.

When the dog rises/walks is it?

(iii)	
Normal	0
Lame	1
Slow or reluctant	2
Stiff	3
It refuses to move	4

C. If it has a wound or painful area including abdomen, apply gentle pressure 2 inches round the site.

Does it?

(iv)	
Do nothing	0
Look round	1
Flinch	2
Growl or guard area	3
Snap	4
Cry	5

D. Overall

Is the dog?

(v)	
Happy and content or happy and bouncy	0
Quiet	1
Indifferent or non-responsive to surroundings	2
Nervous or anxious or fearful	3
Depressed or non-responsive to stimulation	4

Is the dog?

(vi)	
Comfortable	0
Unsettled	1
Restless	2
Hunched or tense	3
Rigid	4

Total Score (i+ii+iii+iv+v+vi) = ______

Appendix 2: ASPCA Medical Evaluation/Examination Form

Label	The Bergh Memorial Animal Hospital of the ASPCA 424 E 92nd Street, New York, N.Y. 10128 (212) 876-7700 Law Enforcement Agent ___________________ Doctor _______________ Date / /

Forensic Veterinary Medical Evaluation

Medical History: Date/Time of ATH:

Date/Time of injury:

Weigh Animal 3X

Exam	T	P	R	1.	2.	3.

Behavior: Assess strength, activity and interaction with people and animals I **Strength:** Normal Decreased Weak Very Weak

F FS M MN **Age (est.)** Age consistent with Hx? Y N If no , explain (e.g., dentition, nucl. sclerosis, gen. appearance etc.)

Sensorium	N Abn	L. nodes	N Abn	Nose	N Abn	Heart	N Abn	MuscSkel	N Abn
Hydration	N Abn	Eyes	N Abn	Mouth	N Abn NE	Lungs	N Abn	Neurol.	N Abn
Integ.	N Abn	Ears	N Abn	Throat	N Abn	Abdomen	N Abn	Urogen.	N Abn

**** If animal is underweight, circle 2 Body Condition Scores**** ***Purina Body Condition Scale***

Emaciated (1) Very Underweight (2) Thin (3) Underweight/Lean (4) Ideal (5) Overweight

Comfort Discomfort Distress Pain

If this is a cat, is the cat declawed? front paws ***yes no****, hind paws* ***yes no***

Assessment

Plan

Basic Wellness Screen (Dog) Super Feline Profile (Cat) Fecal O&P/G PCV/TS Babesia PCR (NC State) for Pit Bulls

Urine collection method _____________ Microchip scan Neg Pos _____________(#)

Rabies / / DHPP / / Bordetella Injectable SQ / / FVRCP / /

Vaccine Labels

ASPCA

Appendix 3: Chandler Edwards' Non-accidental Injury and Death Form – questions for vets to ask clients when suspecting animal abuse[1]

This protocol was adapted by Catherine Tiplady from materials produced by Chandler Edwards, included here with permission of Jenny Edwards.

Sample questions during intake examination when animal cruelty may be suspected

Observe Owner Behaviour during Questions

- Angry
- Suspicious
- Apathetic
- Uneasy
- Embarrassed
- Other (describe)..

Medical Questions

- When was the last time your pet saw the vet?
- What was the reason for that visit? (describe)...
- Whom did you see?
- Has your animal previously had
  - Head injury?
  - Eye/ear problems?
  - Loss of consciousness?

[1] Information gained from this interview should be attached unedited to your preliminary report. These statements are not admissible in court unless they are repeated to an animal control or law enforcement officer. The exception is if the person implicates himself in making a statement, e.g. 'I hit the dog with my fist'.

  - Convulsions/seizures?
  - Other? (describe)..

Observe Animal Behaviour

Does the animal exhibit:

- Dullness?
- Depression?
- Anxiety?
- Showing appeasing behaviours to the owner, e.g. clinginess, hand licking?
- Fear towards the owner?
  - Cowering
  - Urination or defecation
  - Vocalization
- Does the behaviour change if the owner leaves the room?
- Does it recur with person of same gender, body type, height?
- Do objects/actions induce anxiety or specific response?
  - Camera
  - Eyeglasses
  - Caps
  - Anything resembling a 'weapon'
  - Anxiety/reaction to your hands when you go to examine the animal
  - Reacting to certain body parts being handled (e.g. fearful of collar/neck being handled)
  - Acceptance of inserting a rectal thermometer and compliance during rectal/genital area examination may indicate the animal has been desensitized to having that area touched, possibly due to being trained to accept sexual abuse from humans

If NAID is Suspected, ASK:

- Who has access to the animal?
- Where did the injury occur?
- When did the event occur?
- How did it happen?
- Why did it happen?
- When the animal was found, was there any blood, body fluids, faeces or urine present?
- Is the animal normally confined?
- How is the animal confined?
- Does the animal have access to the outside?
- Is the animal supervised when it is outside?

Possible Owner/Witness Explanations

The animal fell. ASK:

- Where was the animal when it fell?
- How high/far was the fall?
- Did anyone else see the animal fall?
- What did the animal do after it fell? (e.g. roll, run away or hide, vocalize, lick the injury)

The animal was hit by a car. ASK:

- How fast was the vehicle going?
- Where was the animal when it was hit?

- Where did the car hit the animal (e.g. head)?
- Was the animal knocked to the side? Tumble under the car?
- Did the animal try to bite or scratch you (or anyone) when you approached?

If Behaviour (of Person or Animal) is Questionable, ASK:

- What does your pet do that gets him in trouble?
- What do you do when that happens?
- What does your pet do that you like?
- Do you have any concerns that you haven't mentioned?
- Do you have any other pets?
  Name Dog/Cat/Other Age

If Domestic Violence is Suspected, ASK:

- Has anyone you know injured or threatened your pet?
- Has anyone in your home ever killed a pet?
- Do you have a safe place for your pet if you seek shelter?
- Are you aware that pets may be included in personal protection orders (or whichever domestic violence order is relevant in your jurisdiction)?
- Are you aware of pet fostering services, which will care for pets while the owner seeks safe accommodation and/or refuges that house people and pets together?
- What are some of the things that are currently stressful for you?
- Offer contact details (if safe to do so) of support services for people and pets encountering domestic violence.
- Avoid making negative comments about the person's partner as this is likely to alienate them.

If Sexual Abuse is Suspected:

- Remain neutral and objective.
- Abuser may feel s/he is keeping a secret or is misunderstood.
- Interview each person in private and away from the suspected abuser.
- **Ask:** Do you mind if I ask a few questions? (to establish that the person being interviewed has 'status').
- **Do not ask leading questions,** such as 'Do you think your husband sexually abused your dog?'
- Let them tell the story and write down EVERYTHING.
- Avoid questions with a Yes or No answer. Ask 'How do you discipline the dog?' rather than 'Do you discipline the dog?'

Appendix 4: Professional Quality Of Life Scale

This ProQOL scale is included with permission of the author Beth Hudnall Stamm (2009).

PROFESSIONAL QUALITY OF LIFE SCALE: COMPASSION SATISFACTION AND COMPASSION FATIGUE (PROQOL) VERSION 5

When you work to help animals and people you have direct contact with their lives. As you may have found, your compassion for those you help can affect you in positive and negative ways.

Below are some questions about your experiences, both positive and negative, as a veterinarian/animal carer. Consider each of the following questions about you and your current work situation. Select the number that honestly reflects how frequently you experienced these things in the *last 30 days*.

1=Never 2=Rarely 3=Sometimes 4=Often 5=Very Often

_____ 1. I am happy.
_____ 2. I am preoccupied with more than one animal/person I help.
_____ 3. I get satisfaction from being able to help animals/people.
_____ 4. I feel connected to others.
_____ 5. I jump or am startled by unexpected sounds.
_____ 6. I feel invigorated after working with those animals/people I help.
_____ 7. I find it difficult to separate my personal life from my life as a veterinarian/animal carer.
_____ 8. I am not as productive at work because I am losing sleep over traumatic experiences of an animal/person I help.
_____ 9. I think that I might have been affected by the traumatic stress of those animals/people I help.
_____ 10. I feel trapped by my job as a veterinarian/animal carer.
_____ 11. Because of my work, I have felt "on edge" about various things.
_____ 12. I like my work as a veterinarian/animal carer.
_____ 13. I feel depressed because of the traumatic experiences of the animals/people I help.
_____ 14. I feel as though I am experiencing the trauma of an animal/person I have helped.
_____ 15. I have beliefs that sustain me.
_____ 16. I am pleased with how I am able to keep up with veterinary/animal care techniques and protocols.

_____ 17. I am the person I always wanted to be.
_____ 18. My work makes me feel satisfied.
_____ 19. I feel worn out because of my work as a veterinarian/animal carer.
_____ 20. I have happy thoughts and feelings about those animals and people I help and how I could help them.
_____ 21. I feel overwhelmed because my case work load seems endless.
_____ 22. I believe I can make a difference through my work.
_____ 23. I avoid certain activities or situations because they remind me of frightening experiences of the animals and people I help.
_____ 24. I am proud of what I can do to help animals and people.
_____ 25. As a result of my work, I have intrusive, frightening thoughts.
_____ 26. I feel "bogged down" by the system.
_____ 27. I have thoughts that I am a "success" as a veterinarian/animal carer.
_____ 28. I can't recall important parts of my work with abused animals/people.
_____ 29. I am a very caring person.
_____ 30. I am happy that I chose to do this work.

Stamm, B.H. (2009) The ProQOL (Professional quality of life scale: Compassion satisfaction and compassion fatigue). Pocatello, Idaho. Available at: http://www.proqol.org (accessed 6 May 2011).

YOUR SCORES ON THE PROQOL: PROFESSIONAL QUALITY OF LIFE SCREENING

Based on your responses, place your personal scores below. If you have any concerns, you should discuss them with a physical or mental health care professional.

Compassion Satisfaction

Compassion satisfaction is about the pleasure you derive from being able to do your work well. For example, you may feel like it is a pleasure to help animals and people through your work. You may feel positively about your colleagues or your ability to contribute to the work setting or even the greater good of society. Higher scores on this scale represent a greater satisfaction related to your ability to be an effective caregiver in your job.

The average score is 50 (SD 10; alpha scale reliability .88). About 25% of people score higher than 57 and about 25% of people score below 43. If you are in the higher range, you probably derive a good deal of professional satisfaction from your position. If your scores are below 40, you may either find problems with your job, or there may be some other reason—for example, you might derive your satisfaction from activities other than your job.

Burnout

Most people have an intuitive idea of what burnout is. From the research perspective, burnout is one of the elements of Compassion Fatigue (CF). It is associated with feelings of hopelessness and difficulties in dealing with work or in doing your job effectively. These negative feelings usually have a gradual onset. They can reflect the feeling that your efforts make no difference, or they can be associated with a very high workload or a non-supportive work environment. Higher scores on this scale mean that you are at higher risk for burnout.

The average score on the burnout scale is 50 (SD 10; alpha scale reliability .75). About 25% of people score above 57 and about 25% of people score below 43. If your score is below 18, this probably reflects positive feelings about your ability to be effective in your work. If you score above 57 you may wish to think about what at work makes you feel like you are not effective in your position. Your score may reflect your mood; perhaps you were having a "bad day" or are in need of some time off. If the high score persists or if it is reflective of other worries, it may be a cause for concern.

Secondary Traumatic Stress

The second component of Compassion Fatigue (CF) is secondary traumatic stress (STS). It is about your work related, secondary exposure to extremely or traumatically stressful events. Developing problems due to exposure to others' trauma is somewhat rare but does happen to many people who care for those who have experienced extremely or traumatically stressful events. For example, you may repeatedly hear stories about the traumatic things that happen to animals and other people, commonly called Vicarious Traumatization. If your work puts you directly in the path of danger, for example, field work in a war or area of civil violence, this is not secondary exposure; your exposure is primary. However, if you are exposed to others' traumatic events as a result of your work, for example, as a therapist or an emergency worker, this is secondary exposure. The symptoms of STS are usually rapid in onset and associated with a particular event. They may include being afraid, having difficulty sleeping, having images of the upsetting event pop into your mind, or avoiding things that remind you of the event.

The average score on this scale is 50 (SD 10; alpha scale reliability .81). About 25% of people score below 43 and about 25% of people score above 57. If your score is above 57, you may want to take some time to think about what at work may be frightening to you or if there is some other reason for the elevated score. While higher scores do not mean that you do have a problem, they are an indication that you may want to examine how you feel about your work and your work environment. You may wish to discuss this with your supervisor, a colleague, or a health care professional.

WHAT IS MY SCORE AND WHAT DOES IT MEAN?

In this section, you will score your test and then you can compare your score to the interpretation below. To find your score on each section, total the questions listed on the left in each section and then find your score in the table on the right of the section.

Compassion Satisfaction Scale

Copy your rating on each of these questions on to this table and add them up. When you have added the[m] up you can find your score on the table to the right.

3. ____
6. ____
12. ____
16. ____
18. ____
20. ____
22. ____
24. ____
27. ____
30. ____

Total: ____

The Sum of my Compassion Satisfaction questions	So My Score Equals	My Level of Compassion
22 or less	43 or less	Low
Between 23 and 41	Around 50	Average
42 or more	57 or more	High

Burnout Scale

On the burnout scale you will need to take an extra step. Starred items are "reverse scored." If you scored the item 1, write a 5 beside it. The reason we ask you to reverse the scores is because scientifically the measure works better when these questions are asked in a positive way though they can tell us more about their negative form. For example, question 1. "I am happy" tells us more about the effects of helping when you are *not* happy so you reverse the score.

You Wrote	Change to
1	5
2	4
3	3
4	2
5	1

*1. _____ = _____
*4. _____ = _____
8. _____
10. _____
*15. _____ = _____
*17. _____ = _____
19. _____
21. _____
26. _____
*29. _____ = _____
Total: _____

The sum of my Burnout Questions	So My Score Equals	My Level of Burnout
22 or less	43 or less	Low
Between 23 and 41	Around 50	Average
42 or more	57 or more	High

Secondary Trauma Scale

Just like you did on Compassion Satisfaction, copy your rating on each of these questions on to this table and add them up. When you have added the[m] up you can find your score on the table to the right.

2. _____
5. _____
7. _____
9. _____
11. _____
13. _____
14. _____
23. _____
25. _____
28. _____
Total: _____

The sum of my Secondary Traumatic Stress questions	So My Score Equals	My Level of Secondary Traumatic Stress
22 or less	43 or less	Low
Between 23 and 41	Around 50	Average
42 or more	57 or more	High

Index